PRAISE FOR *BIRGITTA GALLO'S EXPECTING FITNESS*

". . . [Birgitta] provides a fresh, new insight into pregnancy fitness, which has been generally lacking from a conventional medical and over paternalistic approach to pregnancy care. This book will teach women how to avoid the consequences of poor fitness in pregnancy such as dietary deficiencies, postural and pelvic muscle weakness, and associated bladder, bowel, and sexual dysfunction."

—*John F. Kerin, M.D.*
Professor of Obstetrics and Gynecology, UCLA School of Medicine, and past director of the Reproductive Medicine Program, Cedar Sinai Medical Center, Los Angeles

"Exploding changes in technology and in the practice of medicine are exciting. Birgitta Gallo's book is truly a dictionary. Congratulations to Birgitta on becoming a communicator and a motivator!"

—*Jack R. Robertson, M.D.*
University of Nevada School of Medicine

"I've had a lot of other professional trainers in Hollywood, but Birgitta's technique is very different. Birgitta has such gentle ways of training, yet you really feel like you get a great work out."

—*Mary Stavin*
Miss World 1978 and Bond girl in *Octopussy* and *A License to Kill*

"Birgitta—she's here! She is perfect. Thank you so much for your help! Love, Kathy."

—*Kathy Najimy*
New mother and actress on *Veronica's Closet* and in *Sister Act*

Birgitta Gallo's Expecting Fitness

birgitta gallo's

expecting fitness

birgitta gallo

with Sheryl Ross, M.D.

Renaissance Books
Los Angeles

To access the latest prenatal fitness information or to order prenatal fitness wear and exercise accessories, visit Birgitta's Web site at:

www.expecting-fitness.com

Grateful acknowledgment is made to the following organizations and individual for permission to adapt and/or reprint information from their publications: American College of Obstetricians and Gynecologists, the March of Dimes Birth Defects Foundation, and Raul Artal, M.D., author of *Exercise in Pregnancy* (Baltimore: Williams & Wilkins, 1991).

Library of Congress Catalog Card Number: 99-067292
ISBN: 1-58063-064-2

10 9 8 7 6 5 4 3 2

Design by Lisa-Theresa Lenthall
Exercises photographed by Anthony Nex
Models: Kayleigh Conrad, Kelly Cooper, Yesenia Guzman
Illustrations by Mary Bryson

Published by Renaissance Books
Distributed by St. Martin's Press
Manufactured in the United States of America

This book is dedicated to every woman contemplating pregnancy or already pregnant who has any questions or hesitations about exercise at this special time in her life.

And, to the person who helped this book get into the right hands, but unfortunately did not get to see it through the end—my friend, Arnold Ashkenazy.

contents

Foreword by Jane Seymour

The first time I met Birgitta, it was at the request of my doctor, Sheryl Ross, M.D. I was three and a half months pregnant with twins, and Sheryl told me that I needed to exercise to counteract the effects that this pregnancy would have on my body. My show, *Dr. Quinn, Medicine Woman*, was on hiatus, so it was a good time to start an exercise program. This pregnancy at this stage in my life was very different from my previous pregnancies, which I also exercised through. Back then I was pregnant with only one child and I did floor exercises at Jane Fonda's Workout Center. Now, with twins, I was a "high risk" pregnancy, and I wasn't sure what I would be able to do.

Birgitta assessed me and conferred with Dr. Ross about everything we were to do. We started out with some light toning exercises that she gradually made more difficult. In the beginning we would alternate indoor workouts with pool workouts. We did a lot of squats, outer thigh exercises, abdominals, upper body movements on the Pilates machine, breathing exercises, and those eternal Kegels. She would throw in Kegels everywhere, at the bottom of a squat, in the middle of a stomach contraction, and even during stretching. Working in the pool was a lot of fun. Birgitta had all kinds of pool toys that we used for resistance. Sometimes my time was so constrained that Birgitta had to come to the set to work me out. It must have been quite a sight—me exercising in a big crinoline dress, hat and all.

She always encouraged me to work to my capacity, but also to listen to my body and slow down and rest when I needed to. She kept it fun and varied and modified the workout according to my advancing condition. Toward the end I was put on bed-rest just to be on the safe side. I was supposed to remain in bed for most of the day, but about the only time that I did was during our workouts. Birgitta somehow managed to modify and redesign my whole workout to be done in bed. Being pregnant with twins became a gruesome experience, but she kept my spirits and strengths up. It was always about staying strong and healthy, never about vanity—and I'm proud to say, I never waddled once.

Exercising during a pregnancy is like a metaphor for life. It can be difficult, at times when you feel like giving up, when you're aching and tired and overwhelmed. But you keep going. Finally, when those boys were born, the purpose was clear. I did it for them as much as for me, but postpartum it was all for me. Three days later, Birgitta came to the hospital handing me a sheet of three "little" exercises to do until I saw her in two weeks. I got no break at all. I was back in shape in no time. With a Golden Globe nomination, it was a good thing. Hollywood can be very cruel, especially at awards—we have to look fabulous.

We continued working out, gradually making me stronger, and by the time my boys were six months old, I felt and was back to normal.

As you read on, you'll be impressed with Birgitta's dedicated and thorough research and incredible knowledge on pre- and postnatal fitness. This book is full of useful information that you won't find anywhere else.

Thank you Birgitta.

—Jane Seymour

Preface

We are living in very exciting times. Gone are the days of submissively accepting the idea that pregnancy is a disease that requires total confinement and inactivity, and the fear that the pregnant body can't be trusted. The outmoded Western belief that a pregnant woman should be sedentary is cultural and not based on physiological need. New studies show that exercise and pregnancy actually complement each other to be "feto-protective." There is actually more that a pregnant woman *can* do than *can't* do, but if you haven't exercised before you will need to begin slowly.

I designed this book to be as comprehensive as possible, covering everything you need to know to enjoy a healthy pregnancy, including exercise and nutritional guidelines, information on the changes the pregnant body goes through, answers to many pregnancy-related questions, and much more. Although some of this information has been published, a lot has never before been made available to the public. It is all based on the latest research from medical journals (primarily the groundbreaking work of Drs. Raul Artal and James F. Clapp III) and institutions including the American College of Obstetricians and Gynecologists and the American College of Sports Medicine, as well as my years of personal experience working with pregnant moms. You may find some sections to be a bit technical, but it's not necessary for you to study and learn every detail. Even if you just skim through some of the medical chapters, you will still gain an understanding of the whys, hows, dos, and don'ts of pre- and postnatal fitness.

Birgitta Gallo's Expecting Fitness is the first book to offer recommendations on how to modify specific sports and fitness activities during pregnancy. It covers practically every sport and fitness activity, with instructions on how to adapt each one. There are some activities that should be avoided altogether during pregnancy, but you'll be surprised how much you *can* do, with some modifications. In addition to teaching you to adapt your current activities, I'll also lead you through exercises to tone, stretch, and strengthen every part of your body.

You should consult your OB/GYN prior to beginning any fitness program or participating in any sport or activity. You know your body best, however, and if you feel your doctor's guidelines are too restrictive, you should consider getting a second opinion. Unfortunately, there are some doctors out there who don't keep up with the latest scientific data on exercise and pregnancy, and some who cling to outmoded fitness recommendations. Make sure you choose a doctor you feel comfortable with. For advice on how to find the right doctor, I recommend the book *Doctor Shopping: How to Choose the Right Doctor for You and Your Family* by Hal Apiar.

The benefits of exercise during pregnancy are tremendous. These benefits include increased energy levels, reduced pregnancy discomfort, fewer delivery complications, decreased labor time, and speedier recovery time. Exercise will give you better control of your pregnant body, because a strong and fit body can better support the growth and changes in a pregnant woman. Exercising when pregnant also helps your circulation, relieves tension, and helps with balance and coordination. You will gain less weight and regain your pre-pregnancy shape sooner. Most importantly, recent research has proven my personal theory to be correct—your baby will derive substantial health benefits.

Realizing that your pregnant body is beautiful, strong, and healthy will do wonders for your self-esteem, confidence, and emotional well-being. With an educated and positive outlook on the changes of pregnancy, you will move and enjoy your body much more. With a better understanding of your pregnant body, knowing how to minimize discomfort and prevent complications, your mind will be more at ease throughout your pregnancy and as you anticipate motherhood.

Being able to motivate and inspire women to confidently go through their pregnancies strong, fit, and healthy, and to educate them about their pregnant bodies is extremely fulfilling and exciting. Part of my goal in writing this book was to answer your questions about prenatal fitness, so that you can confidently exercise your right to a healthy pregnancy by staying as fit and strong as you can. Just by picking up this book you are demonstrating an interest in giving your baby the best possible start in life. Being pregnant is definitely not the time to stop moving—stay active and enjoy the nine months of quiet before the storm.

Also look for Jane Seymour's upcoming book on having twins, to be released in the spring of 2001.

E-mail me with any questions at ftness@aol.com or look for my newsletter at www.expecting-fitness.com.

—Birgitta Gallo

Acknowledgments

I would like to thank all of those people who have in one way or another influenced, inspired, promoted, and helped me with this book. Starting at the beginning, my appreciation goes to:

Renee Greiff—my first "official" prenatal client, who got me hooked on and obsessed with keeping pregnant moms fit and healthy.

Rick Rayle—the attorney and friend who, believing so strongly in my special niche of work, is responsible for convincing me that I had to write this book.

John F. Kerin, M.D.—one of the world's leading fertility experts, and a living, walking gynecological encyclopedia, who let me pick his medical brain for hours at a time, with a million questions and theories, whenever he visited Los Angeles.

Paul Crane, M.D.—a top Beverly Hills OB/GYN and my client, who patiently listened to all of my questions during our workouts and gave me the medical literature that was otherwise not available to me.

Sheryl Ross, M.D.—an exercising mother of three and one of Los Angeles's best OB/GYNs, who spent hours and hours with me and on her own, making sure that everything I wrote was medically accurate, who has approved my prenatal fitness programs, and who refers and entrusts her "high-risk" pregnant patients to me—one of them being:

Jane Seymour—a great lady, who, being the professional that she is, worked out no matter what and never complained, and who also included me in her family's activities and put me in the spotlight.

Jim Miller—a dear friend who straightened me out when things went crazy and made sure I had proper legal representation by:

Ron Litz—my terrific attorney and friend, who helped me immeasurably with all things legal.

Arnold Aschkenazy—a dear old friend who is responsible for this book getting into the right hands.

Renaissance Books and my editor, Brenda Scott Royce—who so wholeheartedly believed in me and my book and has been such a pleasure to work with.

My sister Annette—for always being there, through thick and thin, believing in me and encouraging any and all of my endeavors with all of her heart—a true sister.

All my friends—Sandra, Dama, Gloria, Pam, Laurie, Lauren, Anne, Ron, Marvin, Mimi—who have, through the years, been so supportive and always promoted me and my book to anyone who cared to listen, even when it looked like a lost cause. Thank you.

All my clients—pregnant and not-so-pregnant, who inspired this book, believed in me and my productive, but sometimes controversial, methods and theories of training and nutrition, and who have patiently been waiting for the arrival of my book-baby.

Michael Canale—my hairdresser, who acts like my manager, sending me famous clients, and who invented hair color just for pregnant women—right up my alley.

Nike—my diligent, loving little dog, who sat in my lap and kept me sane while I was writing this book.

Introduction

JACK R. ROBERTSON, M.D. is one of our country's top urologists, a professor emeritus at the University of Nevada School of Medicine, and a friend and colleague of Dr. Arnold Kegel (inventor of the Kegel exercise) and Dr. John Frankenberg (Jane Seymour's late father and a top gynecologist in England).

Birgitta Gallo's Expecting Fitness, is truly a dictionary. My advice to the pregnant reader is that you first must call your doctor to ask if he or she recommends exercise during your pregnancy. If not, you should call another doctor for a second opinion. There are, of course, a few contraindications to exercise during pregnancy, but the relationship between the doctor and the patient is very important—so start out with the right doctor for you.

Exploding changes in technology and the practice of medicine are exciting. The standard textbook of obstetrics at the time of my graduation from medical school (1950) contained only one paragraph on exercise.

One of the great things about humans is that they can change their attitudes. A positive attitude releases chemicals in the brain that promote a feeling of well-being. Negative thoughts lead to a lack of energy and depression. The best medications we have are a positive attitude, exercise, and humor.

If you are already blessed with children, they should be involved in the whole pregnancy process, including the exercise. Now that we have sturdy strollers, the whole family can become involved in walking. It is my opinion that with very few exceptions, everyone should exercise for life, not just during pregnancy. However this is the best time to exercise, and a very important time to get the family group involved.

The most important muscles in a woman's body, other than her heart muscles, are the ones that make up the pelvic floor. They are called the *levator ani* (translation: elevate the anus). These muscles are out of sight and tend to be neglected.

Doctor Arnold Kegel, who first described the exercises of the pelvic floor muscles that now bear his name, is a friend of mine. We worked together at the University of Southern California (USC)–Los Angeles County hospital in the 1970s. Kegel was a communicator and a motivator. He was like the coach getting a team ready for Saturday's game. He checked his patients weekly for their progress. In today's medicine this is unlikely to happen, given the time constraints and reluctance to refer to specialists, although the health maintenance organizations (HMOs) should take heed because down the line many medical costs can be saved.

Simple instructions as to how to do the pelvic exercises, such as "stopping your urine," are of little or no benefit. I talked to a patient this week who, having been "taught" Kegels after the birth of her now seven-year-old daughter, was still starting her exercises with "stopping her urine." This is not only bad for the bladder, but points out the inadequacies of incomplete instruction in the proper method of performing the pelvic floor muscle exercises. The author's advice about checking with a sexual partner is wise. The importance of bringing the force of the muscles to squeeze into the vagina can be verified. If there is no sexual partner, the woman can place a finger in her vagina and feel the finger being gripped.

It is to be hoped that this book will support the concept of exercise for life, not just during pregnancy, but this is a good start. The chapter on relaxation is well written. I wish to stress its importance. It should be left open for constant referral. Congratulations to Birgitta on becoming a communicator and a motivator!

—*Jack R. Robertson, M.D.*

RAUL ARTAL, M.D. *is professor and chairman of the department of obstetrics and gynecology at SUNY Health Science Center in Syracuse, and fellow at both the American College of Obstetricians and Gynecologists and the American College of Sports Medicine.*

It is well recognized that 40 percent of all medical conditions in our urbanized society are behavior related, that is, they arise because of sedentary lifestyle and poor nutritional habits that result in obesity, cardiovascular disease, diabetes, and hypertension.

Pregnancy provides a unique opportunity for behavioral modification. The increased awareness for well-being in pregnancy provides a strong impetus for lifestyle changes. Pregnancy-acquired lifestyle changes ultimately impact on the well-being of the entire family. It is laudable that prominent individuals in the entertainment industry such as Jane Seymour have taken upon themselves to promote a healthy lifestyle for the public at large. These initiatives have a significant influence on behavior modification.

Today's women are better informed and usually assume the key role in issues that relate to family health. Most of the women in today's society combine a career with pregnancy and motherhood and wish to remain physically active. We as health-care providers should promote these trends.

Contrary to the beliefs and practices of previous generations, we should change the perception that pregnancy is a state of confinement. It is not! Women can and should continue to derive health benefits from an active lifestyle during their pregnancy.

The immediate benefits of exercise and fitness in pregnancy include the ability to better cope with the rapid anatomical changes of pregnancy: to maintain better posture, ambulate more easily, experience less back pain, and maintain a better overall psychological outlook. Fit women also appear to cope better with labor and delivery.

Throughout history, attitudes toward pregnancy and fitness have changed dramatically, although misconceptions and misinformation persist to this day. To the Victorian lady, pregnancy was a state of confinement and it was considered unseemly for pregnant women to engage in active recreational or social activities. It was even inappropriate to be seen outside her family setting.

The same attitude toward pregnant women persisted in the beginning of the century in the United States. In 1913, a handbook for pregnant women advised:

> Walking is the best kind of exercise. Most women who are pregnant find that a two to three mile walk daily is all they enjoy, and very few are inclined to indulge in six miles, which is generally accepted as the upper limit. Very few outdoor sports can be unconditionally recommended to the prospective mother. Because athletic exercise is either too violent or else jolts the body a great deal, it is especially dangerous in the early months of pregnancy. All kinds of violent exertion should be avoided—a rule which at once excludes sweeping, scrubbing, laundry work, lifting anything that is heavy, and going up and down stairs hurriedly or frequently. The use of a sewing machine is also emphatically forbidden.

These attitudes have gradually and slowly changed. By 1949, the U.S. Children's Bureau recommended:

> A moderate amount of exercise is good for anyone, and this is particularly true for pregnant women. Unless you have been ill or unless there is some complication, you can continue your housework, gardening, daily walks . . . and even swim occasionally.

Grantly Dich-Read, a South African obstetrician practicing in London, emphasized knowledge, relaxation, and some specific prenatal exercises to reduce the need for pain medication in labor. A Russian physician named Velvovsky developed a psychoprophylaxis regimen for "painless" childbirth, which was introduced to the West in the 1950s by Dr. Fernand Lamaze and brought to the United States by one of his patients, Marjorie Karmel.

Most childbirth preparation classes thereafter focused on relaxation techniques intended to ease the perception of pain and minimize the administration of pain medication. Some called this technique *natural labor*, a term that was utilized earlier in the century to describe home deliveries. At that time, hospital deliveries were associated with a high incidence of maternal mortality, primarily due to infections. The hospital environment was considered dangerous, unnatural, and a last resort.

Realities and perceptions have changed. Modern hospitals and facilities are certainly the safest locations for labor and deliveries; prospective mothers are educated, inquisitive, in control of their bodies, eager to stay fit and derive health benefits from a healthy lifestyle. In the past ten years, significant research has demonstrated that exercise during pregnancy is not only safe, it is also desirable.

Safe guidelines for exercise in pregnancy have been developed and published by the American College of Obstetricians and Gynecologists. Pregnant women are well-advised to participate in programs that incorporate these guidelines; however, it's always wise to also consult your obstetrician.

Birgitta Gallo has authored with Dr. Sheryl Ross this very practical book on fitness and pregnancy. This book is an excellent, balanced source of information that should find its way to each pregnant woman who desires to remain active in pregnancy!

—Raul Artal, M.D.

Birgitta Gallo's Expecting Fitness

Chapter One

the pregnancy/exercise connection

IN THIS CHAPTER

- *The benefits of exercise during pregnancy*
- *Dispelling the myths about pregnancy and exercise*
- *How exercise affects your pregnancy—and pregnancy affects your ability to exercise*

Pregnancy is a nine-month physical and emotional roller-coaster adventure to motherhood. There is so much information on pregnancy, but do we really understand it? Myths and unsubstantiated theories are perpetually thrown at us. New books come out all the time without updating their information or researching all of the new medical studies on the subject, many of which have been published in just the last five years. Many books dispense facts about pregnancy but leave out the all-important *why*.

This chapter begins by detailing the benefits of prenatal exercise and dispelling the myths that had earlier generations of women afraid to leave their rocking chairs during pregnancy. Next, it describes the basics of the pregnancy/exercise connection, helping you to understand *why* exercise is not just okay but important during a pregnancy, benefiting both mother and child, and how and why pregnancy will affect the way you can exercise.

why you need to exercise

Let's begin with the reasons why you should exercise during all stages of your pregnancy. Most of these will be discussed in greater detail elsewhere in this book, but I wanted to start off by listing the many benefits—to you and your baby—of a good pre- and postnatal fitness program:

PRENATAL BENEFITS

- improves your fertility
- reduces the unpleasant effects of the biomechanical changes in your body
- eliminates or reduces pregnancy-related discomforts
- prevents and treats pregnancy-induced diabetes
- improves calcium absorption, preventing hypertension, preeclampsia, and future osteoporosis
- relieves tension, stress, and possible depression
- increases your general strength, improving your ability to carry your larger belly
- reduces the strain on your upper back
- reduces the strain and pressure on your lower back and sciatic nerve
- prevents "round shoulders" and improper posture
- increases energy, particularly in the last trimester
- improves your immunity
- less excess weight gain
- a better looking pregnant body
- increases your self-esteem and improves your self-image
- gives you a sense of achievement
- gives you a more positive outlook on your pregnancy and motherhood
- strengthens, tones, and gives you better control of your pelvic floor muscles during labor
- improves your endurance, fitness level, and muscle control, for a faster, easier, and less painful labor
- prevents or reduces the risk of labor complications
- reduces your chance of needing a C-section
- reduces the chance of birth defects
- increases the chance of delivering a child with higher Apgar scores (tests taken at one and five minutes after birth—low scores usually indicate a problem with the baby's health)

POSTPARTUM BENEFITS

- minimizes stretch marks
- minimizes postpartum blues or depression
- minimizes present and future incontinence (urinary leaking) and organ prolapse problems
- allows faster recovery from pregnancy and labor
- helps you get back into shape easier, faster, and more safely
- reduces back strain from carrying and nursing your newborn
- increases energy and allows you to keep up with your baby
- gives you time for yourself
- improves your child's health
- keeps your child calmer
- minimizes your child's chances of having a weight problem
- improves your child's neurological, mental, and physical development

myths

Now, let's get some of those pesky myths out of the way. There have been so many misconceptions about what pregnant women should or should not be allowed to do. There have been even bigger misconceptions about the entire concept of "prenatal exercise," perpetuated by both the fitness industry and the medical community, mainly due to the lack of knowledge on how exercise can and should be modified during pregnancy. Many of these myths grew out of fear or ignorance, and they have been disproved by modern medical research.

Following is a list of things regular exercise during pregnancy *was thought* to cause:

- miscarriage
- hormonal imbalance
- overstressing of the joints, increasing risk of injury
- redirecting blood flow away from the fetus to the muscles, reducing oxygen and nutrient supply for the fetus
- overheating the fetus in the womb
- uterine bleeding
- displacement or rupture of the placenta (the placenta moving to cover the opening of the cervix, preventing the baby from coming out during labor)

Children born of fit pregnancies are leaner, healthier, and more intelligent.

- entangled umbilical cord (the cord wrapping around the baby, causing fetal distress)
- breech position (baby's feet or buttocks presenting instead of the head)
- increased risk of a C-section, or use of medical instruments to help get the baby out
- hypertension or high blood pressure
- abnormal genes in the baby
- growth retardation
- meconium-stained amniotic fluid (if the fetus excretes feces or stool before it is born, it could inhale it from the amniotic fluid, blocking its airways and damaging its lungs)
- premature labor
- prolonged labor
- fetal distress
- stillbirth
- low birth weight
- low Apgar scores
- difficulties for the baby after birth
- difficult maternal recovery after birth

Worried? Don't be. As you continue to read, you will begin to realize that these myths are not only unfounded, but that the reverse of each myth is usually true. It's as if Mother Nature supplied us with this incredible safety blanket to ensure the safety and health of the growing fetus. Although it is important to be cautious at all times, remember that exercise *promotes* the health of your growing fetus, rather than *endangering* it.

Being pregnant can be hard enough, but by being fit and healthy you can make it much easier on yourself. You will feel stronger; have more energy; experience fewer aches, pains, and discomforts; decrease your risk of complications; and cope better throughout the nine months of pregnancy. You'll also give yourself a head start on bouncing back into shape postpartum. These positive results are not just confined to the time of your pregnancy, labor, and postpartum, they also extend to your child—children born of fit pregnancies are leaner, healthier, and more intelligent.

Old-fashioned myths, beliefs, and medical guidelines were very restrictive for pregnant women wanting to exercise. They advised limiting sessions to fifteen minutes and keeping your heart rate under 140 bpm (beats per minute). When you're pregnant, your resting heart rate increases by about ten to twenty bpm, so just walking around could bring it up that high. Most prenatal fitness research done in the past was performed on animals. Not surprisingly, scientists have discovered that those findings often do not quite correlate to human pregnancies.

Recent research, performed over the last ten to fifteen years, has proven that exercise is not just okay for a healthy pregnant woman, it is actually beneficial, and not just to the mother but to the baby as well. We can thank two American gynecologists—Raul Artal, M.D., and James F. Clapp III, M.D., for most of this research. Dr. Clapp, professor of the Department of Obstetrics and Gynecology at Metro Health and Medical Center in Cleveland, states, "Pregnancy is a normal physiological state, not a disease, and the benefits of exercise appear to be substantial for both the woman and the pregnancy."

"Pregnancy is a normal physiological state, not a disease, and the benefits of exercise appear to be substantial for both the woman and the pregnancy."

If you have decided to work out through your pregnancy, be consistent—irregular workouts can do more harm than good. Sporadic workouts can cause injuries and muscle fatigue. Regularity is the key. Your level of fitness is defined by the frequency, intensity, and duration of your workout, as well as the type of exercise. A good program consists of at least three weekly workouts, each of at least twenty minutes duration (this can be split up into two ten-minute sessions in one day, not counting the warmup and cool-down periods). Unless you are extremely fit, it is wise to limit aerobic activity to forty-five minutes at a time, listen to your body, and not overexert yourself. If you were previously inactive or overweight, start with five minutes a day and gradually work your way up to twenty minutes over a two-week period.

Your program should be individualized for your specific circumstances, preferably with the help of your doctor, caregiver, and/or someone with expertise in prenatal fitness. This book can also guide you in designing your own exercise program—how to pick what suits you, what activities to avoid, and how to keep it interesting and fun. Remember that taking a walk, playing with your children, gardening, or doing housework can be quite a workout, too. Before you commence, clear what you intend to do with your OB/GYN. It is your physician's responsibility to help you make decisions about physical activities.

There are going to be times when you don't feel like working out. You may feel down, fatigued, or suffer from morning sickness. When this happens, listen to your body, take a day off, relax, and work out the next day—it's okay. You are pregnant, you are not supposed to bubble with energy every day.

never too late to start

Being fit, or planning to become fit before conceiving is of course preferable. Your body will adapt more quickly to the pregnancy, and exercising while pregnant is easier if you are already fit. The healthier and stronger your muscles are, the better you will cope with pregnancy and labor. But it is never too late to embark on an exercise program, even if you are reading this in the maternity ward.

If you're anxious to get started *now*, you're probably wondering how much you can or should exercise through the different stages of your pregnancy, and what kind of activities are suitable. This segment will explain what exercise does to you and your baby while pregnant, as well as what your pregnancy does to your exercise program. There are some limitations to what you can and should do. You will learn how to modify your workouts and why. You'll also learn not to be afraid of exercise.

changing pace

Mother Nature has seen to it that you do not need to exercise as hard to reap the same results as when you are not pregnant. We could only wish that exercise would work as efficiently when we are not pregnant! Add to that the physical changes in your body, and you will quite naturally and automatically modify and slow down your activities and workout program for the different stages of pregnancy.

Even though you can carry more oxygen with all the extra blood that is produced when you are pregnant, which in a sense makes you fitter just by being pregnant, you may not be able to perform as well, particularly in the first trimester. At this time, your body is adjusting to being pregnant, the fetus is grabbing all of the carbohydrates that it can, and your body is storing fat for the baby's needs at the end of the pregnancy and for nursing. Therefore, there may not be much energy left for you. All of this may slow down your workout intensity 10 to 20 percent, which is a "feto-protective" combination, reducing any negative risks and boosting the positive results of exercise.

By the second trimester your body has more or less adjusted to its new condition. You are not storing much fat at this time, so you will be more energetic. Some women may be able to work out as hard or even harder than they did before they became pregnant, depending on their previous strength and fitness level.

You can't be Super Woman and be pregnant at the same time. It's okay to slow down.

The last trimester is a different story. With blood pooling, rapid breathing, big belly, and loss of balance and stability, most exercising moms slow down about 30 to 45 percent. This is completely normal; don't push yourself too hard. You can't be Super Woman and be pregnant at the same time. It's okay to slow down. In fact, Mother Nature helps ensure that you will slow down in the last trimester, by allowing less blood (cardiovascular output) to be available for exercise. So listen to your body—it knows what's best for you and the baby.

Your endurance level will pick up again postpartum—twelve to twenty weeks after delivery you will be able to work out much harder, particularly if you exercised throughout your pregnancy.

the effects of exercise on your pregnant body

When you exercise, or exert your body, it affects different bodily systems. Working out changes hormonal activity, activates muscles, raises body heat, increases heat dissipation, changes mineral and fluid balance, speeds up metabolism, and uses up stored energy reserves. Your body readily adapts to these alterations, because the human body wants to be fit and healthy—it likes to feel good. How easily it adapts depends on your age, weight, diet, health, and fitness level; the type, intensity, and duration of the exercise; and the altitude, weather, and environment.

Exercise causes you to use more oxygen, which makes your energy systems more efficient. With this extra oxygen your body will utilize stored fat and carbohydrates better, both during exercise and when you are at rest. You can take in more oxygen, burn more stored fat, and increase lean weight (muscles, bones, organs) in your body if you are fit. Yes, not just the muscles, but the bones will get stronger and denser as well. Your heart will get bigger and stronger, just like any other muscle, and more blood will be available for your heart to pump, bringing your blood pressure and resting heart rate down. Your cooling system will become more efficient by letting you dissipate heat more easily, meaning you will sweat more. The result of all this is that you will be able to do the same amount of work with much less effort.

CARDIOVASCULAR SYSTEM

When you exercise, the primary targets for your blood to flow to are your muscles. Pregnancy itself increases your blood volume by 40 to 45 percent—it increases the amount of red cells that carry oxygen, and allows blood vessels to carry more blood at once. Exercise increases your blood volume another 10 percent. Put all of this together, and you have an abundance of blood, ensuring that there is always plenty to go around, protecting the fetus and serving the needs of your other organs. With more hemoglobin in the blood transporting oxygen during exercise, the fetus draws more blood and oxygen than usual through the placenta, and more blood is being pumped with each beat of the mother's heart. A sufficient oxygen supply to the fetus is thus ensured.

This safety mechanism might have something to do with the fact that pregnancy improves your metabolism to compensate for your weight gain. Therefore, you won't need as much oxygen to do the same amount of exercise. This faster metabolism, combined with extra blood and increased oxygen intake, gives pregnancy a "training effect," making you more fit.

With all this extra blood, your body may at times have trouble moving it around. If you lie on your back or sit in the same position for a long time, the circulation slows down, and blood pools in your legs, preventing it from returning to the heart or flowing to the fetus. This makes you tired and dizzy. This is called "supine hypotension," and is another safety mechanism of the pregnant body. If this happens when you are in a standing position and the blood doesn't get back to the heart, your blood pressure falls and you need to lay down to enable the blood to rapidly return to the heart—so you faint and fall. Amazing how it all works—who knew fainting could, in a way, be "good for you."

Exercising and moving your body will keep your blood circulating properly. When exercising, keep your legs moving as much as you can. If you are doing certain seated, standing, or lying exercises, make sure to walk around a little between sets, to prevent blood pooling in your legs. It is probably this blood pooling that accentuates varicose veins, which is why exercise helps to alleviate them. Sitting for a long time can also add to pressure in the pelvis, so you're not going to be comfortable in any position for very long. In order to keep your blood circulating efficiently, it is almost as if pregnancy makes your body say, "Get up and move."

When exercising, keep your legs moving as much as you can.

Another supine hypotension problem can occur when you lie on your back after about the fourth month. The uterus by this time is so heavy that in this position it puts pressure on the vena cava (vein returning blood from the legs to the heart), causing dizziness even though you are lying down. This also slows blood flow to the fetus. If you must lie on your back, moving the legs and/or torso a little will help circulation. However, raising your feet to a vertical position when supine may hamper blood return. Some women seem to be able to do supine exercises without problems, but our medical guidelines advise against exercising on your back after the sixteenth week. There are many other ways of doing chest and abdominal work. Lie either in a semi-recumbent position with plenty of pillows behind you or on your side. The left side is usually best, because the vena cava is more to the right, and the growing uterus rotates to the right side of your body.

RESPIRATORY SYSTEM

The further your pregnancy progresses, the harder it will become to breathe, and more so when you exercise. The uterus is pressing up on the diaphragm, giving your lungs less space to expand. But your lungs have their own safety blanket, too. Your rib cage becomes pliable in pregnancy due to the hormone relaxin. It stretches out and expands sideways and backward, enabling more air to come in, improving your lung capacity. You will also breathe more often—your lungs will process 40 percent more oxygen during pregnancy.

Exercise may not increase lung function at this time, but it will improve oxygen transportation and delivery. Fit women can breathe less air to get equivalent oxygen during moderate or higher intensity exercise.

You may feel tired in the beginning of an exercise, or for the first ten minutes, because your lungs can't quite get oxygen to the working muscles fast enough. But don't give up. If you can make it past the first ten minutes, the respiratory system will adapt, and the exercise will become easier. You need to exercise aerobically for at least twenty minutes a day, three to six days a week, to take advantage of its beneficial effects. These twenty minutes can be split into two ten-minute sessions (not including the warmup and cool down) in one day.

Caution: Hyperventilation (very, very fast breathing or breathlessness) in pregnancy could harm your baby. If you begin to hyperventilate, discontinue exercise. Sit down, take slower, deeper breaths, and call your caregiver.

Your Metabolism

In a non-pregnant state, for every quart of oxygen that is used by the body, your body burns five calories. When you are resting, you burn only one calorie per minute, but you can burn up to fifteen calories a minute with high-intensity activity or exercise. For a non-pregnant woman who is trying to lose weight, this of course means that the more oxygen she can take in, the more calories she will burn. The only way to take in more oxygen is to expand the lung capacity, which happens when you get more fit through continuous exercise. The more fit you are, the more oxygen you can take in with every breath. Fitness and exercise are the only things that will naturally speed up your metabolism (besides being pregnant). Dieting will slow your metabolism down, but that's another book!

BODY TEMPERATURE

Overheating can put your fetus in distress. In the beginning of the pregnancy, particularly around the twenty-first to twenty-seventh day, overheating can cause neural tube and central nervous system defects. Many women do not know that they are pregnant this early. If you even suspect you may be pregnant, avoid hot tubs, Jacuzzis, saunas, steam rooms, and exerting yourself in hot, humid weather.

A fetus does not have its own means of sweating or dissipating heat. In the old days, there was an unfounded concern about exercise during pregnancy, because exercise elevates your body temperature. But we know better now. Both exercise and pregnancy very conveniently make you sweat more quickly and more easily. During pregnancy, blood will flow more rapidly to the skin to get rid of heat caused by a faster metabolism and exercise. This raises skin temperature and gives you that "glow" of pregnancy. Add the fact that there is more blood in your body (10 percent is added by exercise and 40 percent by the pregnancy), more oxygen, and more skin (your bigger belly) for the blood to go to, and your cooling system is actually much more efficient during pregnancy. So much so that you may find you have to turn up the heater to stay warm when not exercising.

Your temperature will not rise as high or as fast as when not pregnant. A pregnant woman's core body temperature will actually fall slightly as soon as she is on her feet and moving around. The exercise and the pregnancy will complement each other to help the heat dissipation. Resting body temperature continues to fall throughout pregnancy. A fit mom will have 30 percent less heat stress in early pregnancy, and 70 percent less in late pregnancy, if she keeps working out to the end. Professional athletes and very fit women also have better natural thermal adaptation, which allows them to eliminate heat more efficiently than less fit women.

However, be cautious and avoid exercising in hot and humid weather. If you can, stay indoors on hot days, in an air-conditioned environment, or exercise in the early morning or late afternoon. If you must exercise in hot weather, modify your workout—reduce the intensity and go a little longer instead. Periods of exercise longer than one hour are not advisable if you're very warm or sweating. Wear exercise clothes that breathe, such as cotton or Supplex®.

Drink water, water, and more water!

Drink water, water, and more water! Dehydration can reduce blood flow thereby limiting nutritional flow to your baby. It can predispose you to premature labor. Drink water all day—even if you are not thirsty, your baby is. Drink water before, during, and after a workout—you lose a lot of fluid when you perspire. Being well-hydrated also helps keep you cool.

Avoid exercise if you have a fever or are ill. Be aware of overheating during exercise; you may feel dizzy, nauseous, get a headache, or lose your coordination. If you feel too warm during an aerobic exercise or activity, discontinue any arm movement. Using arms and legs at the same time may increase your temperature, blood pressure, and heart rate, more than just using your legs would.

On the other side of the coin, cold temperatures increase the need to deliver energy to your muscles. Exercising will help speed your metabolism and raise your body temperature on cold days.

HORMONAL CHANGES

There are no significant changes in your hormonal balance during exercise; what changes do occur recover rapidly afterward. However, just like in non-pregnant people, exercise does cause a reduction in blood sugar. You can easily compensate for this by consuming some fruit or fruit juice prior to and during your workout. To exercise, your muscles need glucose from your blood, preferably coming from the liver and stored fat. This reduces the need for insulin—it normalizes your blood sugar, preventing pregnancy-induced diabetes.

Exercise also increases certain hormones (catecholamines, endorphins, and opioids) that were once thought to reduce blood flow and possibly make the uterus contract prematurely, but instead they compensate for everything else that may be pulling you down during pregnancy. These hormones stimulate alertness and reduce perception (feeling) of pain, such as pregnancy discomforts and labor pain. These "feel good" hormones help you feel better about yourself. As your self-image improves, you become proud of your body and its achievements. You believe in yourself more and feel that you can handle anything that may come your way. This is great when you are preparing yourself for labor—thinking of it more like an exciting experience, rather than dreading or fearing it. These hormones help relieve stress and tension, and temporarily relieve depression. This relief will be welcomed because pregnancy may cause a lot of tension, anxiety, and stress, depending on how you feel about yourself and your pregnancy. Fit moms tend to be better off emotionally after delivery; they suffer less from postpartum depression.

METABOLISM

When you exercise, your body starts to burn more fat than sugar for energy, both when you are active and at rest. Your body stores and utilizes sugar (glycogen) more easily, so that you do not need as much insulin, which helps maintain blood sugar levels. In the first trimester of a pregnancy, your body will store fat, saving it for the baby's needs later in the pregnancy. During mid- and late pregnancy, your fat use increases, saving even more sugar for your baby. As another precaution when you are pregnant, exercise will not burn quite as many calories as when you are not pregnant, saving additional glucose for the baby. Our bodies are pretty amazing.

Unfit women need a lot more exercise than fit women to modify their weight gain and fat accumulation during pregnancy, and to burn the same amount of calories.

Hypoglycemia

Because the baby needs a lot of glucose, your own blood sugar may at times get a little low, and you might crave sweets for extra energy. Please resist the temptation. Sugary foods will only raise your blood sugar rapidly, just to drop it as rapidly, maybe even lower than before you ate the snack. Symptoms of hypoglycemia include feeling weak, shaky, nervous, hungry, disoriented, faint, and having clammy skin. In a worst case scenario, you could go into a coma. To prevent hypoglycemia, before and after you exercise, snack on a high fiber, complex carbohydrate food like fruit, whole wheat breads and muffins, or low sugar granola bars. Whole grain carbohydrates tend to stabilize the blood sugar for a longer time than refined sugar products. Stay away from snacks that are high in fat, they will only make you feel more sluggish.

Weight gain is a must during pregnancy.

Hyperglycemia

Hyperglycemia or diabetes occur when there is too much sugar in your blood. Pregnancy sometimes induces a diabetic condition, which usually goes away postpartum. The condition is called gestational diabetes. It can be anywhere from mild to severe. Severe cases need insulin therapy, but a milder form may be kept under control with a special diet and exercise. Exercise is recommended because the muscles utilize the excess blood sugar as fuel, lowering the need for insulin. It works better than just changing the diet, and it may even make insulin therapy unnecessary for many women.

A workout session will affect your blood sugar levels for about two days or forty-eight hours straight. Therefore, frequent exercise at least every other day is important. If a diabetic mother does not eat before a workout, the exercise can make her hypoglycemic. To be on the safe side, she should check her blood sugar levels before and after exercise. She should never exercise by herself, or change her workout in any way without consulting her OB/GYN. She should always drink water and eat something light before and after a workout.

BODY COMPOSITION AND WEIGHT GAIN

Your body composition is determined by your sex, age, race, height, genetic factors, nutritional habits, your mother's nutritional habits during pregnancy and nursing, and your level of activity and exercise. Our bodies are mostly made up of water (70 percent) and protein (muscles and organs).

Weight gain is a must during pregnancy as a nutritional support for the baby in late pregnancy and lactation. The recommended weight gain during pregnancy for an average-sized woman is 25 to 35 pounds. Exercise reduces weight gain and fat deposition throughout pregnancy, and more so in late pregnancy. But you must already be fit and continue to exercise until delivery.

If you gain too much weight during your pregnancy, it may be very difficult to lose it postpartum.

If you were previously inactive and begin exercising for the first time during pregnancy, you need to exercise more than someone who is continuing an exercise program in order to reap the same benefits. If you quit working out halfway through your pregnancy, you will gain approximately five pounds more than a woman who never exercised, as your reduced activity level slows your metabolism. Exercising moms gain about eight pounds less than non-exercising moms. If you gain too much weight during your pregnancy, it may be very difficult to lose it postpartum.

The fat that you need to gain during a pregnancy is usually deposited in and around your hips and on your arms. Most of it will be collected in the first trimester. The rest of the maternal body, including the belly, seems to stay fairly lean. There is unfortunately not yet any accurate method of measuring maternal body fat because most of the fat deposits are internal, within the pelvic region and abdominal cavity, making them too difficult to measure. These fat deposits protect the fetus both nutritionally during pregnancy and lactation, and physically during pregnancy and labor. Exercise during pregnancy will improve your muscular function but does not seem to increase any muscular lean body mass.

Fluid retention caused by your pregnancy can decrease your ability to move ankles, feet, fingers, and wrists. Drinking lots of water, and exercising, especially in water, can lessen these problems.

YOUR CHANGING BIOMECHANICS

The mechanical workings of your body (how your joints move and which muscles are doing what work during a movement), are definitely affected by both your pregnancy and any physical training you may do.

The physical changes that you will experience from pregnancy—increased size, weight, changing shape and center of gravity, swelling tissues, and softer joints—affect the way you walk and perform everyday tasks. You are carrying more weight around, on top of softer, less stable joints, which makes you more susceptible to injuries, sprains, and lower back pain. Exercise, when done properly, strengthens your body, reducing this risk of injury and strain.

After the fifth month, your hips won't move as well and your range of motion will be restricted. A simple movement such as getting up from a chair becomes not so simple. Leg strengthening exercises for the outer and front thighs (quadriceps), and front lower legs (tibia), will help, and thereby reduce the risk of injury to your knees. Pressing yourself up with the help of your arms will also alleviate the strain on your legs, which means that you should strengthen your arms and upper body, too. It's hard to imagine that just getting out of a chair could get so complicated, but when you are pregnant and your body doesn't move as well, you have to become more aware of your posture, body position, situation, and surroundings. You need to come up with ways to reduce the stress on your body. Instead of sitting on a low chair or sofa, try sitting on a higher chair or bar stool.

You need to come up with ways to reduce the stress on your body. Instead of sitting on a low chair or sofa, try sitting on a higher chair or bar stool.

Stair climbing is another movement that puts a lot of strain on hips and knees. By the end of a pregnancy you have doubled this stress, stress that could lead to joint instability and arthritis later on. It only makes sense that you would be better off strengthening your lower body. However, exercises that involve fast moves, turns, jumps, and changes in direction should be avoided to prevent falls, dizziness, and muscle injuries.

Supported squats help strengthen your thighs by almost mimicking the labor position. The abdominal and the pelvic floor muscles need to be strong during labor contractions. Be very careful with lateral, inner, and outer thigh exercises if you're not used to them. They can put a lot of strain on the pelvis and pubic bone, which can separate during pregnancy. This is a rare occurrence, but if it happens, you will be on strict bed-rest until delivery. The inner thigh muscles or "adductors" are attached to the pubic bone. Lateral exercises are any sideways activities such as skating, slide aerobics, running sideways, and the "grapevine." If you didn't do them before conceiving, don't do them during your pregnancy. However, if you're well trained in these activities, they may be okay to continue.

Your shoulders and upper back will ache and feel tired from having to carry your bigger breasts and belly. They need strengthening, while your chest needs stretching. Your lower back also needs to be stretched, because it is in a perpetually flexed position during at least the latter half of pregnancy. Strengthen the lower back muscles while it is still comfortable—preferably before you conceive, and for the first two months of pregnancy or so. It becomes difficult to do so in late pregnancy.

There are different kinds of low back pain. Sciatic pain that runs down your buttock and leg is a common complaint. Sometimes your baby moves and puts pressure on your back, either temporarily or for the duration of

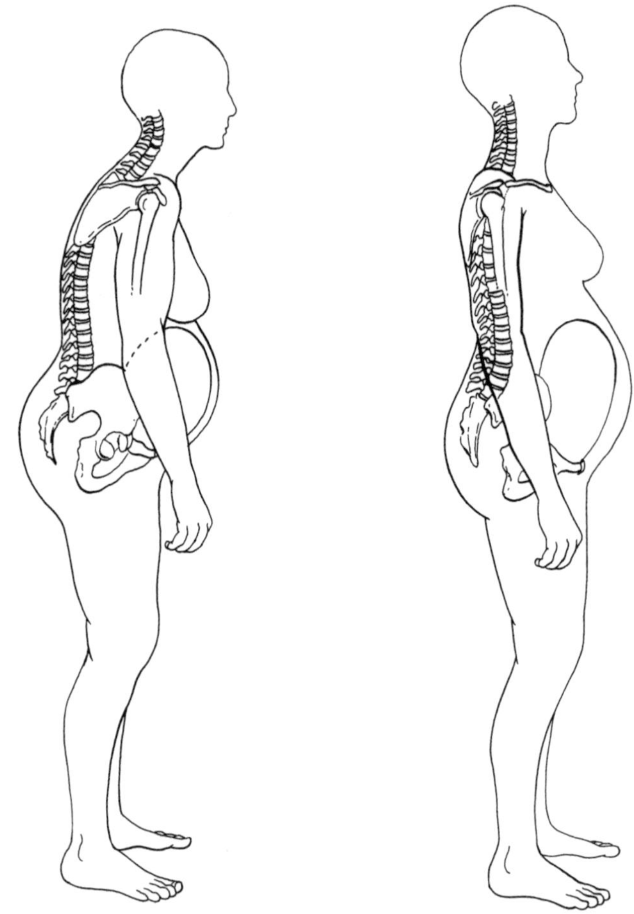

incorrect posture (left) and correct posture (right)

the pregnancy. Some women confuse posterior pelvic pain with a backache. It is important to know the difference, but both types of pain can be alleviated by a proper exercise program. Wearing a maternity belt may temporarily alleviate low back strain, but don't wear it all the time—it could weaken the abdominals and lower back muscles by giving you false support. Unless ordered by your doctor, wear a maternity belt only during exercise, housework, or other strenuous activity.

effects of exercise on the placenta

Moderate exercise seems to promote growth and function of the placenta in mid-pregnancy, which both improves its ability to transport blood and nutrients to the baby and prevents fetal oxygen deprivation. This may even have protective benefits to the fetus during a difficult labor. The placenta will keep growing as you continue to exercise. A healthier placenta, combined with higher blood volume during pregnancy, provides additional protection for the baby's nutrient flow. Studies have shown that the placentas of mothers who quit exercising in the middle of their pregnancies decrease to the size of an inactive mother's placenta.

the effects of exercise on the length of pregnancy and labor

The information in this section comes primarily from studies conducted by James F. Clapp III. Through his research, as well as my own personal experience, I have gained an understanding of the benefits of exercise during pregnancy. These benefits not only affect the length of labor, but also the growing fetus and its development beyond the uterus.

The length of your pregnancy is not significantly affected by exercise. If you continue to exercise until the day you go into labor, you are most likely to go into labor about a week earlier than planned, but it is not unusual for some exercising moms to go overtime by a week or so. However, the length of your *labor* is definitely affected by exercise. In a recent study, Dr. Clapp discovered that moms who exercise until the last day will have a shorter labor—by more than 30 percent. He also found that 65 percent of exercising moms will deliver in less than four hours. Moms who work out only in the beginning of their pregnancy will not change the length of their labor.

Also, moms who exercise throughout their pregnancies have a better chance of a natural vaginal delivery; and the likelihood of needing medical interventions like forceps, drugs, and C-sections is reduced by 50 to 75 percent. They will also experience a less painful labor (by as much as one-third), which may be due to the combination of strong muscles and a higher pain tolerance. The endorphins created by exercise work as natural painkillers.

the effects of exercise on the baby

The interactive connections and dependent active links between the mother and the fetus are amazing and fascinating, though even today, still not fully understood. So far, medical findings concerning the effects of exercise on a pregnant woman's fetus all point to the positive. Even studies that were initially intended to prove that exercise during pregnancy was harmful ended up proving that the reverse is true, making believers out of nonbelievers.

Fetal distress and complications from exercise were previously a concern, but research has proven the opposite. Mothers who exercise regularly throughout their entire pregnancies have fewer complications than those who either exercise sporadically, quit halfway through, or remain sedentary. These complications include meconium stained amniotic fluid (fetus's feces in the amniotic sac), umbilical cord entanglement (cord wrapped around the baby's neck or body), abnormally fast fetal heart rate (fetal tachycardia), gestational diabetes, hypertension, C-section, and low Apgar scores.

Other complications, such as rupture and displacement of the placenta, premature labor, and breech position (the baby coming out feet or buttocks first) occur with the same frequency, whether or not the mother exercises. It was thought that running and bouncy or ballistic movement could cause some of these problems, but so long as these movements were practiced by the mother prior to conceiving, she can continue them as long as she feels comfortable doing so. Most exercising moms will naturally slow down or modify their exercise routine after the fifth or sixth month.

Breech position is not caused by exercise, bouncy or not, except *possibly* by inverted (upside down) exercises, such as some yoga positions. I suggest you avoid any exercise where your head is positioned below your stomach. It has not yet been studied, but it is possible that being turned upside down may confuse the baby, as far as when to "drop" and turn head down. Some women who had breech births think that their inverted exercises may have been the cause. If nothing else, these positions will probably make you dizzy, so it is best to avoid them.

There was concern that exercise could lower the fetal heart rate too much (a condition called bradycardia), but this happens only if a sedentary, unfit mother exercises extremely strenuously, or possibly in the case of very high-risk pregnancies with high blood pressure/hypertension. Fetal bradycardia is usually caused by complications like fetal heart disease, umbilical cord compression, or a contracting/hyperactive uterus. If for any reason you suspect that your baby is not moving enough, especially right after an exercise session, call your caregiver. Depending on the gestational age of the fetus, your caregiver will perform either a nonstress test, which observes the fetal heart rate for a twenty-minute period, or a biophysical profile, which evaluates the amniotic fluid level, fetal breathing, tone, and movement.

Another concern was that the uterus may start contracting from exercise, causing preterm labor, but this has not happened in studies in which participants exercised between 60 and 85 percent of their maximum exercise intensity. The notion that hypoxemia (oxygen deficiency in the fetus) could be caused by high-intensity exercise has also been disproved.

WHAT *DOES* HAPPEN

The fetal heart rate will increase after about ten minutes into the mother's workout. The baby's heart will beat faster the harder and longer that you exercise, and the further you are into your pregnancy. Mild to moderate exercise will keep its heart rate up for five to fifteen minutes after you have stopped the exercise. More strenuous exercise can keep the fetal heart rate up for thirty minutes after a workout before it returns to normal. This is a normal response to exercise and does not change fetal behavioral patterns nor cause fetal distress. Just as we deliberately increase our heart rate by exercising because it's good for us, it is also good for the baby, so long as the increase in heart rate is not caused by stress or adrenaline.

Studies have shown no compromising oxygen or nutrient deprivation in fetal brains, organs, or muscles due to exercise. "Fit" babies seem to be just that, fit—tougher and better able to handle potential problems. They appear more relaxed during labor and adapt more readily to life on the outside.

"Fit" babies seem to be just that, fit—tougher and better able to handle potential problems. They appear more relaxed during labor and adapt more readily to life on the outside.

Birth weight is an important factor of the baby's health. If the baby weighs in at less than five and one-half pounds, it has a higher likelihood of experiencing health problems. Naturally, the concern that exercise may reduce the baby's birth weight is valid. However, it's important to distinguish between fat levels and lean tissue weight.

Moderate intensity workouts continued throughout the entire pregnancy will not cause significant changes to the baby's birth weight. However, frequent exercise and exercise intensities over 50 percent, particularly in the third trimester, will cause a 5 percent, or 300 gram, weight reduction in the baby, but this reduction is all in body-fat content. Most babies have a 14 percent body-fat level at birth, but "fit" babies have only a 9 percent body-fat level. Everything else—including body length, size of the baby's head, and lean tissue weight—are comparable.

The nervous systems of "fit" babies also seem to work better. At five days old they are more calm, more content, and more alert.

If a pregnant woman stops her exercise routine in the third trimester, her baby will weigh about 200 grams more than average in fat weight, with no change in the lean tissue weight (muscles, bones, organs) of the baby. This may be due to the mother's unchanged eating habits, combined with a slower metabolism after cessation of exercise, and the fact that the baby's fat cells start multiplying in the last trimester.

In short, continuous exercise will result in a baby with less body fat. This is good. Common sense tells us that these children will most likely grow up without a weight problem. Ongoing long-term studies are examining the outcome of these children and their weight in later stages of life. Some studies have already shown that "fit" babies are leaner children at five years of age. By exercising during your pregnancy you can prevent your child from becoming part of the new statistics that show that more than twice as many children and adolescents in the United States are overweight today compared with ten years ago (according to the National Center for Health Statistics). Leaner children will likely have a lower risk of developing cardiovascular and metabolic disease in later life.

The nervous systems of "fit" babies also seem to work better. At five days old they are more calm, more content, and more alert. They adapt more easily to their environment. They seem to be more independent and require less attention. They sleep through the night earlier and have less colic. Their mental development is accelerated and they may begin to talk earlier. A five-year-old "fit" child has better speech, oral abilities, and a higher intelligence level than children whose mothers did not exercise during pregnancy.

The reasons for these findings are presently being studied. The author's theory is that it may have to do with the combination of a more efficient placenta and improved blood and nutrient supply to the baby, as well as the endorphins (the "feel good" hormone) produced by exercise, which make you feel better and more alert. Furthermore, sound and movement stimulation during pregnancy may accelerate the baby's mental development.

special considerations for professional athletes

Being a professional athlete is very commendable (I was one for ten years), but it's an obsessive lifestyle in which priorities are centered around peak performance. When you are pregnant, your baby needs to be your main priority. It is not the time to set goals in speed, strength, agility, or balance. Improving fitness and an overall sense of well-being is more important.

Elite and professional athletes, or anyone who exercises excessively (more than ten hours a week), should be under medical supervision to prevent any possible risks. This is important even though athletes have little risk of overuse or accidental injury. Athletes' joints become softer just like all other mothers' joints. Most athletes take some kind of nutritional supplements. During pregnancy, consult a professional dietician or nutritionist before you take any supplements, as excessive amounts of certain supplements during certain stages of pregnancy could cause birth defects.

When you are pregnant, your baby needs to be your main priority.

Preferably, athletes should not plan to compete in any event during pregnancy at all, and definitely not after the sixteenth week. Professional competition, particularly at higher levels, requires more intense exercise than is "healthy" for anybody, particularly a growing baby. If you must compete, do not exceed your normal level of intensity. Postpartum, schedule competitions no closer than ten to twelve weeks after delivery. By then, if you train properly, your fitness level may be even higher than before you become pregnant, due to the training effect that pregnancy has on you.

Some sports that could be particularly dangerous are water- or snow skiing, diving, scuba diving, mountain climbing, ball or contact sports, ice- or rollerskating, car racing, and horseback riding, because of the potential trauma that a fall or blow may cause. If you must participate in these sports, they will require serious modification.

This does not mean that you can't keep up your present peak level of training, or close to it, through at least the first half of your pregnancy. After twenty weeks your added weight, loose joints, loss of balance and coordination, and change in center of gravity may slow you down. Listen to your body; it is important that you slow down when your body is telling you to. Your regimen should include a variety of cardio, strength, and flexibility training.

Pregnant athletes tend to gain less weight; their babies tend to be born at least one week early and weigh about one pound (500 grams) less than the average baby (in fat weight). Many athletes deliver even smaller babies, at or near six pounds. This could be caused by too much exercise, but it is more likely due to inadequate nutritional intake. Some athletes are concerned with their weight gain, and may not increase their food intake as much as they should (or even worse, they may reduce their food intake). A non-active woman needs approximately 300 extra calories a day during her pregnancy, an active woman needs up to 500 extra calories, and a professional athlete may need an extra 800 calories a day to deliver a healthy baby.

Amenorrhea (cessation of menstruation) in athletes will affect their ability to become pregnant. Too much training, nutritional deficiencies, and below-recommended body-fat levels (less than 14 percent) change your thyroid function and hormonal balance, which stops your reproductive cycle. Without ovulation you will not be able to conceive. If you suffer from amenorrhea and want to become pregnant, you need to modify and reduce your activity, and possibly increase your food intake and body-fat levels to get your period back. Depending on the severity, it could take at least two to three months to get your period back, perhaps more.

Amenorrhea can also be detrimental later in life. It causes estrogen levels to be abnormally low, mimicking the symptoms of menopause. Without estrogen, your body can't absorb calcium very well, which could weaken your bones and lead to osteoporosis, especially if your athletic activities are exclusively aerobic, non-weight bearing activities such as cycling or swimming. Weight training promotes bone strength along with muscle strength, thereby increasing calcium absorption, even with a loss of estrogen.

some yet unanswered questions

Previously restrictive and conservative guidelines slowed down researchers trying to study the effects of exercise on pregnant women. There are still many unanswered questions that we need to study. We still need to find out the exact effect that exercise during and after pregnancy has on pregnancy-related diseases such as hypertension and macrosomia (very big baby), and on preexisting diseases in the mother, such as heart disease. We need to find out how exercise during pregnancy affects you and your baby on a long-term basis. Issues currently being studied include the effects on the child from different maternal diets, weight training during pregnancy, maternal cardiovascular response from exercise during pregnancy, and whether exercise can prevent premature delivery and poor fetal growth in teens and older mothers. Studies that are now underway will take as long as twenty years before they are completed. Ask your doctor to keep you abreast of the latest medical findings and watch for revised editions of this book.

summary

Hopefully this has convinced you that being fit and pregnant isn't just okay, it is beneficial for both you and your baby. There is no evidence to support any of the myths listed at the opening of this chapter. To the contrary, studies demonstrate how well the woman's body adapts to pregnancy and exercise, and best of all, they work together and complement each other to protect the fetus. Even studies researching pregnant women who exercise well above the guidelines showed positive results. As exercise prevents you from illness and disease, it also protects your fetus from complications. Exercise is one of the most important things you can do during pregnancy, for yourself and your baby.

Being fit and pregnant isn't just okay, it is beneficial for both you and your baby.

Chapter Two

pregnancy basics and Q&As

IN THIS CHAPTER

- *What to do before you conceive*
- *How each bodily system changes during pregnancy*
- *How to relieve typical pregnancy-related discomforts*

During pregnancy every bodily system is very much dependent on every other bodily system, to very delicately accomplish the miracle of growing life into a new human being. As this life is growing, it is coexisting and sharing an interactive existence with its mother. This chapter describes the changes you can expect to experience during your pregnancy. We begin with the steps you should take *before* you become pregnant, if possible. Next, we'll take you through typical changes during each trimester, broken down by bodily system. Even though no two pregnancies are exactly the same, there are similar things that most pregnant women will experience. The end of the chapter provides answers to commonly asked questions about pregnancy and fitness.

preconceptional care

Having a healthy baby doesn't just involve taking care of yourself during the pregnancy. Giving birth to a healthy child is a process that should start before the child is even conceived. Unfortunately, 60 percent of all pregnancies are unplanned. Even 40 percent of children born to married couples are not planned. In addition, many women don't discover they're pregnant until it's too late to rectify certain developmental problems (problems that may happen in the first month if your body is not prepared for conception). Therefore, a large percentage of babies do not get the head start that proper preconceptional care can provide. The importance of pregnancy planning and preconceptional care cannot be overemphasized: the health and well-being of our children is at stake.

Steps to Take One Month before Conception

STOP taking birth control pills
STOP taking extra vitamin A
STOP using alcohol, cigarettes, and illicit drugs
STOP douching

START taking folic acid and a prenatal vitamin supplement to decrease risk of neural tube defects
START a workout program
START washing the pesticides off of fruits and vegetables

AVOID X-rays
AVOID second-hand smoke

If you are overweight, you should consider trying to take the weight off before you become pregnant. Obesity in pregnancy increases your risk of heart disease, diabetes, and fetal distress. Pregnancy is not a time to diet, so if you want to make this change, it is important to do so before you become pregnant. Overweight women will increase their chances of becoming pregnant if they lose weight by exercise and diet.

Preconceptional care includes having your risk factors checked by your doctor at least a month prior to trying to conceive. Your doctor should screen your family health history for possible genetic problems, evaluate your reproductive health to ensure that everything is working properly, and check your medical health and history to ensure that you and the fetus will be able to go through the pregnancy safely. You should also undergo nutritional counseling and have blood tests performed to check your glucose and iron levels. If you are deficient in iron or other essential nutrients, you can begin "stocking up" before you conceive. Blood tests can also reveal your blood type and check if you've been exposed to Rubella (German measles).

Also discuss with your doctor any medications that you may be using, to be sure they won't be harmful to a growing fetus. If you have any medical conditions such as diabetes, asthma, hypertension, or a thyroid imbalance, it's crucial to have them under control to minimize problems in your pregnancy. If possible, start exercising months before a planned pregnancy. Not only will it condition your body for the changes ahead, but exercise increases fertility and can help control diabetes and hypertension.

the first trimester—weeks one to twelve

For the first four weeks you may not know that you're pregnant, but your body is already manufacturing hormones that will maintain the pregnancy.

As your body is trying to adjust to being pregnant, fatigue and mood swings may set in, making it very difficult to find energy and motivation for your exercise program. Growing a baby requires a lot of energy, and as far as your body is concerned, your baby is priority number one. You get whatever energy is left over. If you are tired, you may need to rest more. Some women get so fatigued they can't exercise at all. Morning sickness also appears in the first month, as do food cravings and/or aversions. Moderate exercise and small but frequent meals can usually alleviate these problems.

By the second month, you will probably have figured out that you're pregnant and begun making modifications to your lifestyle. You should have your first prenatal checkup by the eighth week. Fatigue will probably last into the middle of the second trimester. Depending on your own individual condition, you may need to modify your exercise program on a daily basis. If you're having a bad day, so be it, exercise tomorrow. But keep in mind that exercise in general will work wonders in keeping your energy levels up. If you feel fine, continue your regular routine as long as you are considered a normal, healthy pregnancy. If you are a high-risk pregnancy, your doctor may prohibit exercise altogether until the second trimester, when your pregnancy is more secure.

Your growing uterus will put pressure on your bladder, making you run to the bathroom frequently. Go before, during, and after your workout if possible. Your bowels may slow down, making you constipated. This can be alleviated by exercise, eating more fruit and bran, taking a stool softener, and drinking more water. Do not use laxatives or mineral oils.

Take extra care to ensure that your meals are nutritionally balanced. In addition, you should be taking special prenatal vitamin and folic acid supplements. Drink lots of water and juice. Avoid tea, coffee, and anything else containing caffeine. If you need to follow a special diet (not for weight loss)—due to allergies, diabetes, or maternal obesity, for example—see a registered dietitian. Make sure he or she understands your needs, not just as a pregnant woman, but as an exercising pregnant woman.

You may experience headaches, which can be alleviated by exercise, meditation, and relaxation techniques. At times, you may also feel dizzy or faint. Be careful not to make any sudden moves or perform exercises that require balance and coordination.

Picking the Best Time for Conception

You are more likely to conceive in the fall between September and November and at the end of March. The highest number of births during the year occur in August and at Christmas time. Conception is more likely when the temperature is between 40° and 70° Fahrenheit on the day of ovulation and five days before. Another tidbit: Women have more orgasms in the middle of their cycle, around ovulation.

the second trimester—
weeks thirteen to twenty-eight

As your body is finally adapting to being pregnant, you will start to feel more energetic. You should enjoy your workout much more now. If you experienced morning sickness, it should be on the wane, and your appetite should return. As your uterus is growing bigger and heavier, it will put more pressure on the vena cava (the vein that returns blood from your legs back to the heart) when you lie on your back. It is best to avoid lying still on your back, because this may make you dizzy, cause hypotension, and decrease the flow of oxygen to your baby. Lying on your left side will keep the weight of the pregnancy off the inferior vena cava. Although some women may feel fine exercising on their backs, if you feel at all dizzy while supine, roll onto your left side.

Your belly should be quite large by now, and your heart is probably beating a lot faster because it has to work harder. Even so, you should be feeling more energetic. This is a great time to exercise and participate in all kinds of activities. If you participate in any sports, be careful to avoid activities that could cause accident or injury, such as blows to the abdomen. Due to your faster heartbeat, you cannot quite rely on the old "target heart rate scales" to monitor your workout intensity any longer. If you get tired during the day take a break and rest. You may find that you will need more sleep at night, too. If you are experiencing leg cramps, you may not be getting enough calcium in your diet.

Your uterus is now so big that it is crowding your intestines and colon. As in the first trimester some women experience constipation. Drink lots of fluids, eat high-fiber foods, and exercise regularly. Do not use laxatives or diuretics. Your energy level should still be very good. If you get overheated from working out too hard, slow down and cool down.

Blood pressure usually goes down during the second trimester of pregnancy, but if yours should go up, reduce or avoid doing any arm movements (especially overhead arm movements) during cardiovascular exercise and practice relaxation exercises. Proper exercise will also help lessen the pain of backaches and the severity of stretch marks, water retention, and varicose veins.

At twenty-six to twenty-eight weeks, your doctor should do a blood test for gestational diabetes. Exercise usually minimizes the risk of becoming

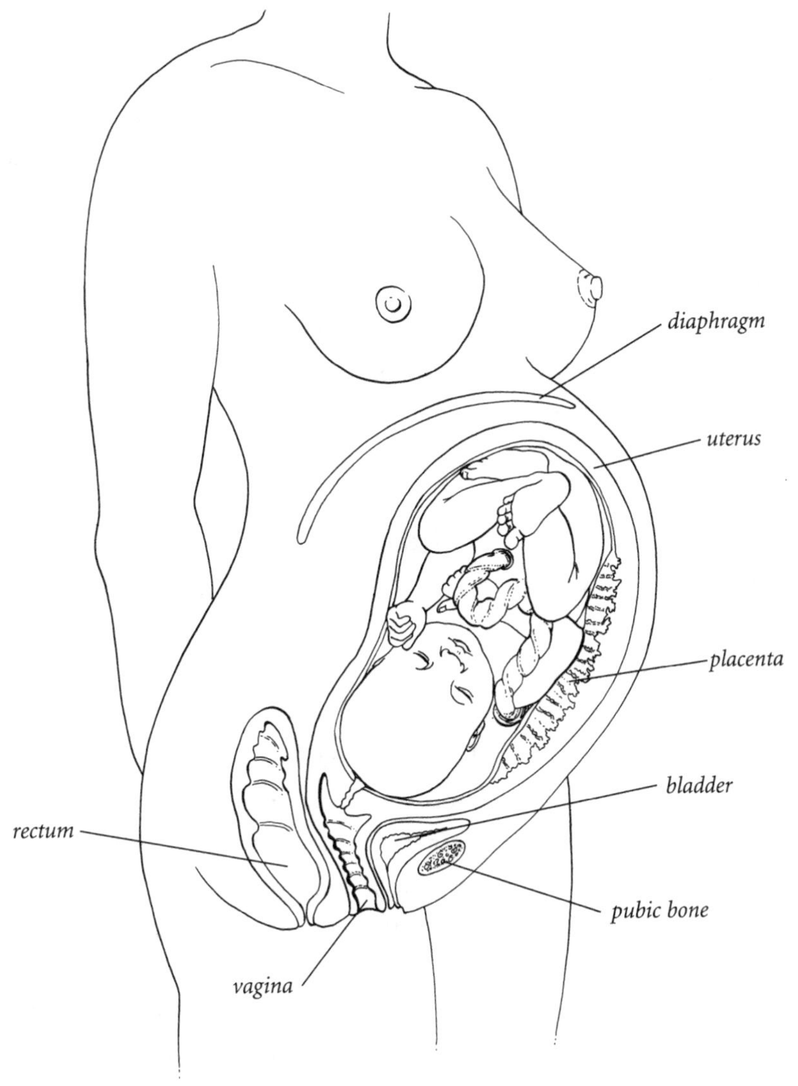

inside view of a nine-month pregnancy

diabetic, by normalizing your blood sugar. If you test positive, you will have to change your eating habits. Gestational diabetes usually disappears after the birth of your baby.

the third trimester—weeks twenty-nine to delivery

You're probably so big that you're having difficulty moving around. (Of course, the more fit you are, the less difficulty you should have.) You may not be able to get comfortable, no matter what you do. Even eating may be difficult, because the baby is crowding your stomach and intestines. Eating smaller meals helps. Your uterus has grown all the way up to your rib cage, crowding your lungs and making breathing a lot harder. This will probably slow down the pace of your workouts. This is normal. You will still be able to exercise until the day of labor; just listen to your body and rest a lot.

After the baby drops into your pelvis and settles head down, breathing will be easier because the baby has moved away from your lungs. However, more pressure will be exerted on your bladder instead, making you run for the bathroom more often. Wearing a maternity belt during exercise may help to alleviate this problem.

labor

The dictionary defines *labor* as "the progressive dilation of the cervix, with repetitive uterine contractions." This is the time when relaxation exercise and techniques (discussed in chapter 7) are so important.

The fact that you have exercised throughout your pregnancy will not only shorten and ease your labor, lessen the chance of complications and the need for medical intervention, it will also increase your stamina and lung capacity, making them better able to handle the stress of labor. If you have maintained a healthy diet and followed a proper fitness routine, you are now the mother of a beautiful little miracle—your healthy baby.

Are you starting to see how incredible your body is, and how everything happens for a reason? All of these idiosyncrasies are part of a very finely tuned machine called the female body. Let's take a quick tour of each of the body systems and how they are affected by pregnancy.

reproductive anatomy

PELVIS

The female pelvis is shaped like a bowl to carry and protect a fetus in the uterus during pregnancy, as well as to permit safe passage for a baby through the birth canal. The tops of your thigh bones support the pelvic bone. The hip joints, which don't easily dislocate, provide a large, flexible circular range of motion. During pregnancy the pelvic ligaments soften due to hormonal changes. As a result, your balance and coordination will be less stable. You should avoid excessive repetitive flexing, such as unsupported squats, turns, and fast changes in direction. The pubic bone normally can separate 3 to 4 millimeters, especially in late pregnancy. Relaxation of the pelvic ligaments and joints and a growing uterus can lead to an unsteady gait and pelvic pain. If pelvic pain intensifies be sure to contact your caregiver—it could represent a significant separation of the pubic bone.

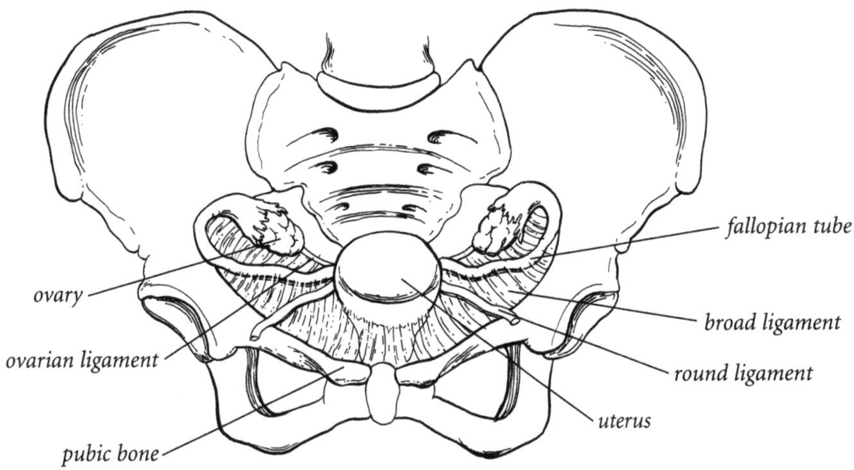

pelvic bones and reproductive organs

The entire pelvis can move as a unit sideways, up and down, forward and backward, and in circles. With a proper exercise program that promotes hip agility and strengthens and stretches the inner and outer thighs, you can develop a comfortable walking stride during your pregnancy, avoid the "pregnancy waddle," and have more agile hip joints during labor.

PELVIC FLOOR MUSCLES

The pelvic floor muscles stretch from the sacrum and coccyx (tailbone) to the pubic bone. They are like a support net for the vagina and the rectum. These muscles also form the sphincters, or circular pelvic floor muscles,

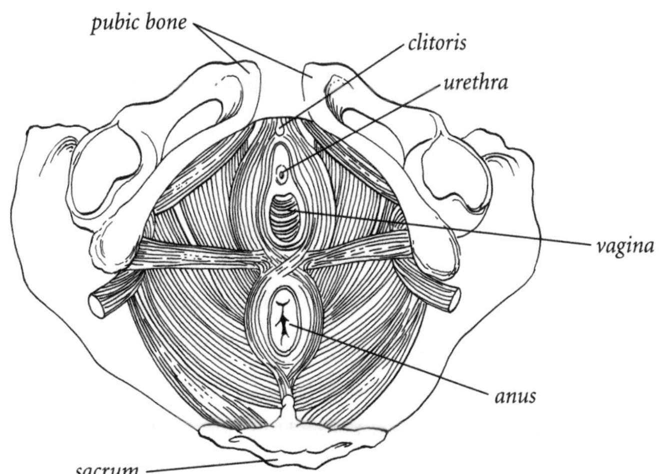

pelvic floor muscles

around your vagina and anus. During labor, the vaginal muscles must stretch to allow for your baby's head to emerge. When the muscles and skin around the vagina are stretched too tightly an episiotomy, or incision of these muscles, may be done to prevent tearing. To lessen the chance of tearing and decrease the risk of needing an episiotomy, Kegels—exercises to strengthen the pelvic floor muscles—should be performed throughout pregnancy. These exercises are described in chapter 5.

UTERUS

The uterus is the core of your reproductive tract. It will grow several times its original size by the end of the pregnancy. This expansion pushes your intestines, stomach, lungs, and heart out of place, and exerts pressure on your bladder, rectum, and abdominal wall. After twelve weeks, the uterus actually outgrows being a pelvic organ, and becomes an abdominal organ.

The broad and round ligaments brace and support the uterus. Pregnancy would be a lot more comfortable if we walked on our hands and knees, because these ligaments do not brace the uterus as well when you are standing upright as when you are on all fours. Most women find exercising on all fours to be a comfortable position during pregnancy.

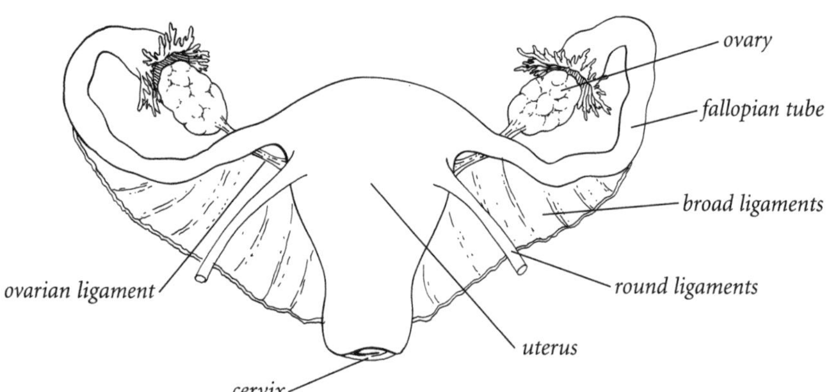

the uterus

other body systems

Your reproductive system isn't the only part of your body that goes through a transformation during pregnancy. The influx of hormones and the growth of the fetus will have an impact on nearly every part of your body. Here is an overview of the changes your body will go through, by system.

MUSCULOSKELETAL SYSTEM

Your hormones will affect your fitness level, strength, endurance, coordination, range of motion, flexibility, balance, and the amount of control you have over your body. The hormone relaxin, which is only produced when you are pregnant, softens your joints and increases the amount of fluid in them. This makes your joints, particularly your hips and pelvis, more flexible—and also less stable. Theoretically you should feel more flexible, but most women actually feel less flexible, which could have something to do with water retention. (Edema also lessens muscle definition.)

As your uterus enlarges, it throws off your center of gravity, by rotating the pelvis, giving you lumbar lordosis (sway back) and rounded shoulders. Your growing breasts also affect your balance. A heavier body, combined with softening joints and ligaments, can result in that off-balance "waddling" many women experience in the last trimester. Strengthening your hips and thigh muscles will help.

Pregnancy speeds up your metabolism, so you have to eat more than usual.

NEUROLOGICAL SYSTEM

Your reaction time will change, along with your sleep patterns, stress levels, moods, and mental proficiency. These changes make it important to execute exercises slowly, with control, caution, and proper posture and alignment.

METABOLIC SYSTEM

Pregnancy speeds up your metabolism, so you have to eat more than usual. During pregnancy, you should consume approximately 300 extra calories a day (that's around 80,000 for the entire pregnancy)—more if you exercise: 500 extra calories are needed to make up for moderate exercise, and up to 800 extra calories a day are needed for professional athletes.

In addition to speeding up, your metabolism changes dramatically during pregnancy as its priority shifts from you to the growing baby. Carbohydrates, protein, and fats all fuel the baby's growth. All reserves will go to the baby first. This is why you need to eat more, so that there is something left for you to live on, too.

The body begins to store fat in the first trimester and almost completely ceases halfway through the pregnancy. At that time, the fetus begins to use the stored fat, while the other half of its fat comes from the mother.

In the last trimester, nutrients are no longer stored or deposited as fat, unless you overeat. Instead, most are used for fetal growth and energy, with the rest going to the mother. This is the time when the fetus accumulates its body fat. In the very last stage of the pregnancy, carnitine (an amino acid) production will increase to break down any excess fat that may have accumulated. Premature babies that are born before this process occurs do not benefit from carnitine's "fat-burning" effects.

GASTROINTESTINAL SYSTEM

Your digestion will slow down during pregnancy. The food you eat will travel more slowly through the intestines to allow for better absorption. This can result in drier feces and constipation. Exercise and drinking lots of water will help reduce this problem.

Heartburn is very common in pregnancy. It is the result of relaxation of the esophageal sphincter (the lid that separates the esophagus from the stomach), and the uterus pushing up on the stomach, causing acidic food in the stomach to be pushed back up into the esophagus. Exercising and eating foods high in calcium and fiber will reduce stomach problems by stimulating digestion and bowel movement. If symptoms persist, try a calcium supplement, because calcium neutralizes acids naturally. If that doesn't help, liquid antacids may be needed to relieve the symptoms. Avoid overeating, mixing too many different types of foods (makes the digestive process more difficult), eating "junk food" and spicy foods, and eating immediately before lying down. Using pillows to elevate your head above your stomach at bedtime may also help.

RESPIRATORY SYSTEM

Oxygen is life's most important ingredient. All of our cells need oxygen. The oxygen that you inhale flows through your system, reaching the fetus through the placenta and the umbilical cord, and enables the cells of the developing fetus to multiply and grow.

Although your lung function improves during pregnancy by 40 to 50 percent, the actual space available in your lungs is diminished by the growing uterus, so you will have to breathe more often to compensate. You may feel flushed or short of breath, as if you just worked out or ran a flight of stairs, even if you didn't. Relaxation and breathing techniques can help.

If you feel short of breath while exercising, slow down, catch your breath, and do not resume your exercise until you can breathe normally again. Your lungs do have the ability to increase their capacity, particularly during exercise or severe stress.

The chest cavity, which houses your lungs, is separated from the abdominal cavity by a muscle called the diaphragm. The diaphragm stretches downward when you inhale, to allow the lungs to fill up with oxygen, and rises back up when you exhale, to expel the now carbon dioxide–rich air out again. As your uterus grows, it pushes up on the diaphragm, reducing its capacity to stretch downward. But the female pregnant body has an incredible adaptive mechanism—it can flare the rib cage out sideways and backward to make room for your lungs to expand. This is helped along by the pregnancy hormone relaxin, which softens the muscles between the ribs. You can practice expanding the rib cage by lifting your arms out to the side or over your head. Breathing will become easier again after your baby "drops" and settles head down toward the end of your pregnancy.

CARDIOVASCULAR SYSTEM

Your heart and blood vessels go through quite a change. They have to transport more oxygen, not just to the fetus, but also to all of the involved organs that are now working a lot harder. Your cardiac output (the amount of blood pumped by your heart) increases 40 to 50 percent, so that there is always enough blood to carry nutrients and oxygen to the fetus, no matter what you are doing. Your resting heart rate may be up to twenty beats per minute higher than normal, which in turn throws your training heart rate off. Your maximum training heart rate will not change, but you will reach it faster with less work. Your heart rate can also vary depending on the time of day, eating habits, stress levels, sleep patterns, and age. A forty-year-old woman's training heart rate can be ten to twenty beats slower than a twenty-year-old's. Drinking lots of water can help keep your heart rate down.

To do all this, your heart grows a little bigger as well. It's normal for pregnant women to have lower blood pressure and faster heart rates. Blood pressure is the force of pressure with which your heart pumps the blood. The higher the blood pressure, the harder the heart is pumping.

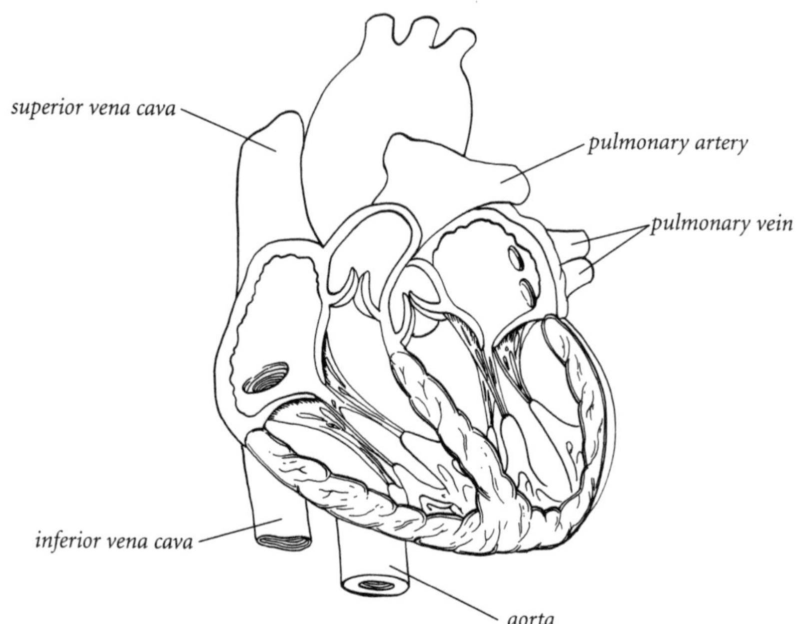

the heart

With extra blood and relaxed arteries during pregnancy, your heart pumps more often but does not have to work quite so hard with each beat. The end result is usually lower blood pressure.

You should have your blood pressure checked every month during pregnancy. Should your blood pressure go up, you will need to choose your exercises carefully, and only exercise with supervision. You may even have to stop exercising altogether, depending on the severity of your condition. Gestationally induced high blood pressure could cause growth retardation and other complications for the fetus.

Your body position can also alter cardiovascular output. Certain body positions affect the venous return (blood going back to the heart). When you stand upright, the uterus shifts the pelvis forward, which is okay as long as you are moving. Moving your legs helps circulation, keeping the blood from pooling in your legs. Avoid standing still for a long time. Also avoid lying still on your back after the sixteenth week. In a supine position (on your back), the uterus falls back and puts pressure on the vena cava (the main blood returning vein), reducing blood flow. This makes you feel dizzy and may put your baby's health in jeopardy. Lie on your left side instead. Exercise in general will help your circulation and venous return.

DISPOSAL SYSTEM

Waste disposal includes heat dissipation. Your body transmits heat to the skin, where it radiates and evaporates, aided by dilated blood vessels near the skin's surface. During pregnancy this process works faster because of all the extra blood, harder working sweat glands, and increased surface area of the skin. As a result, you don't have to worry about overheating from exercise during pregnancy, unless it is very hot or humid.

Overheating can be harmful to the fetus. The fetus has no way of sweating by itself, so your body has to get rid of excess heat. When you are too hot, your baby is too hot. In the very early stages of pregnancy, overheating can cause birth defects; toward the end, excessive heat may cause fetal distress. Overheating also causes dehydration, which may predispose you to premature labor.

In the summer months, exercise early in the morning, in the evening, or in an air-conditioned room. If it is hot, modify your exercise program to a shorter or less strenuous workout. Drink lots of water. Always wear clothes made of natural cotton or special breathing materials, such as Supplex or Coolmax®. Layer your clothes so that you can remove them as you warmup.

Exercising throughout a pregnancy increases the size of the placenta. This growth should help increase blood supply to the fetus.

ENDOCRINE SYSTEM

The glands that produce and secrete hormones (the pineal, thyroid, parathyroid, hypothalamus, pituitary, adrenals, and pancreas) get very involved in the pregnancy. For the first two months, a cyst on the ovaries produces the pregnancy hormones. After that, you will have a new hormonal gland, the placenta. It will take over and become the main hormonal organ for the rest of your pregnancy. Your baby will depend on it to deliver oxygen, nutrients, and hormones, and to dispose of its wastes. Unfortunately, anything else that you may consume will go through the placenta to the fetus as well, including toxins, drugs, cigarette smoke, and medication.

Exercising throughout a pregnancy increases the size of the placenta. This growth should help increase blood supply to the fetus.

PREGNANCY HORMONES

Hormones are the reason for just about everything that happens during pregnancy, and to understand how exercise relates to pregnancy and vice versa you need to understand what these hormones are and what they do. The hormones that are produced during pregnancy are relaxin, androgen, progesterone, estrogen, hCG, and insulin. The following is an overview of their functions.

Relaxin

Relaxin relaxes and softens the cartilage and ligaments that support your joints to prepare your body for an easier delivery. This makes your joints looser, but increases your risk for injury because your balance and coordination are diminished. Exercise prevents injury by improving joint stability and body awareness.

Androgen

Androgen is a male hormone that gives you energy and strength during your pregnancy, as well as a higher libido. If you are carrying a girl, the placenta will convert most of the androgen into estrogen to prevent any male characteristics from developing in the female fetus.

Progesterone

Progesterone is the hormone that maintains the pregnancy. It supports the growth of the fetus, uterus, and breasts, and speeds up the metabolism. It will reduce your muscle tone, relax your bowel muscles, and make your heart and lungs work harder.

It is also responsible for causing your body to accumulate fat in the first and second trimester. These fat deposits cushion the uterus and are used for storage for the last trimester when the fetus needs fat for brain development. Do not try to lose this extra weight, gaining a little fat is normal and necessary. Progesterone increases your appetite, so that you will gain enough weight.

Progesterone also makes you retain fluid, up to 8.5 liters (2.2 gallons) of water during your pregnancy. You will lose approximately 6.5 liters during labor, the rest remains in your bodily tissues for a while postpartum.

At the end of pregnancy, a decrease in progesterone helps initiate labor.

Estrogen

Estrogen, like progesterone, maintains the pregnancy. Both of these hormones are essential for normal development and functioning of the female reproductive system. If you're too skinny or undernourished, estrogen production is reduced, often resulting in irregular periods or amenorrhea (absence of menstruation), which affect your ability to become pregnant. In pregnancy, estrogen makes the uterus more elastic, allowing it to stretch and grow. It helps the uterus contract at labor. Estrogen also contributes to softening of the joints, fluid retention, and growth of the breasts and uterus. High levels of estrogen are possibly responsible, together with hCG, for "morning sickness."

Obese women have the highest risk of becoming diabetic during pregnancy.

hCG

hCG, human chorionic gonadotropin, is produced by the placenta in early pregnancy. It stimulates the ovaries to produce estrogen and progesterone.

Insulin

Insulin is a hormone that permits blood sugar to enter muscle cells, where it is converted into energy. In a diabetic person, the pancreas produces too little insulin, resulting in high blood sugar levels or hyperglycemia. Symptoms include extreme thirst and hunger, weight loss, and frequent urination. If this condition is not controlled it can cause blindness and kidney failure. In pregnancy, gestational diabetes can increase your chance of having a very large baby and pregnancy-induced hypertension.

The reverse condition, having too much insulin and too little blood sugar, is known as hypoglycemia. Hypoglycemia can occur in athletes or anybody exercising a lot, because exercise causes your muscles to use glucose better. Symptoms may include blurry vision, sweating, disorientation, dizziness, weakness, shakiness, and headache. This is easier to remedy. If you experience any of these symptoms, eat something containing carbohydrates, and you should feel better almost instantly. Report any such symptoms to your physician.

GESTATIONAL DIABETES

A small number of women (about 3 percent) who did not have diabetes prior to becoming pregnant will develop diabetes during pregnancy, a phenomenon called gestational diabetes. Onset is most likely after the twenty-fourth week. Obese women have the highest risk of becoming diabetic during pregnancy. Pregnancy-induced diabetes can be controlled

Always wear a good support bra or jog bra.

with exercise and a special diet designed to control blood sugar levels. Exercise makes your muscles more efficient at utilizing blood sugar for energy, thereby lowering your blood sugar levels. Careful monitoring by your doctor is very important.

Gestational diabetes usually goes away after delivery. However, long-term follow-up has shown that 50 percent of gestational diabetics will become diabetic again within fifteen years after pregnancy. Maintaining good exercise and nutritional habits can help prevent this from happening.

Nearly all women with established diabetes can have a normal pregnancy, provided the diabetes is well controlled before conception and throughout the pregnancy. If you are diabetic before becoming pregnant, it is essential to exercise and normalize your blood sugar levels prior to becoming pregnant and for the first eight weeks of pregnancy, when the fetus's organs are developing. Preconceptional diabetes education and control are of paramount importance in minimizing complications.

typical pregnancy discomforts

Upper back and shoulder ache

Upper back and shoulder ache can result when the increased weight of your enlarged breasts and belly pull your upper back and shoulders forward, causing poor posture. Strengthening your upper back and stretching your chest muscles will help. Always wear a good support bra or jog bra. Try sleeping on a firmer mattress. Sleep on your side, support your back and leg with pillows, and get someone to massage any sore areas.

Lower back and pelvic pain

Lower back and pelvic pain are sometimes confused as the same. Lower back pain is related to posture—the change in your center of gravity—and softer ligaments. The more children you have had or the older you are, the more pain you are likely to have. Excessive weight gain also increases your risk of lower back pain.

Sometimes you may feel a pain going down the back of your buttock and leg. This could be caused by the uterus putting pressure on the sciatic nerve or possibly a herniated disk. It may persist throughout your pregnancy. To alleviate this pain, stretch the lower back, hip rotators, and hip flexors, and strengthen the abdominals, buttocks, and hamstrings. Do pelvic tilts and other postural exercises. Wearing a special pelvic girdle may also give you some relief, but don't rely on this too much because your abdominals will weaken from this "cheating" support. Wear flat shoes—high heels will only further aggravate the problem. If pain persists, inform your caregiver.

Hip pain

Hip pain can be related to your back or pelvic pain and is often caused by the same factors. If you sit too much, your hips will get very tight. Stretching and increasing the range of motion of your hip joint will help.

Pubic pain

Pubic pain can feel like tenderness or pressure on the pubic bone. It could be caused by softer ligaments. If you experience pubic pain, avoid lateral moving exercises such as walking/running sideways, the grapevine (an aerobic/dance side step), ice- and rollerskating, and especially "slide aerobics," and gym equipment that works the inner and outer thigh muscles. Mild pain can be treated with ice and rest. Avoid straining or using your inner thigh muscles in a stretched-out V position (legs apart), as this could aggravate the pain. If you have a significant separation in the pubic bone, even walking will be painful. See your doctor immediately. You may be ordered on bed-rest or have restricted activities throughout the remainder of your pregnancy.

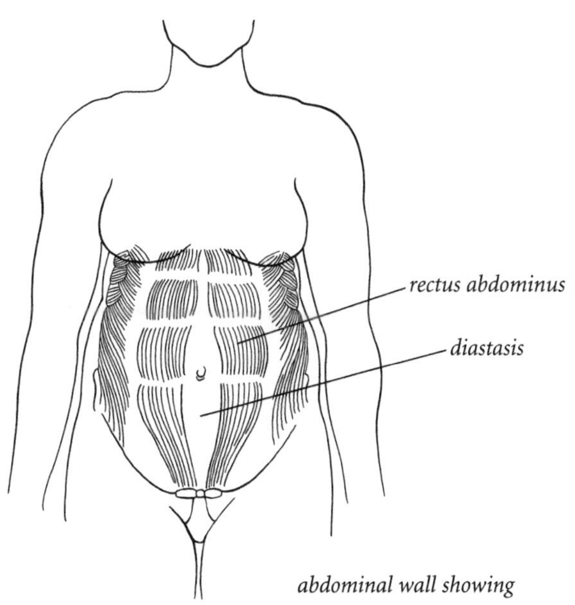

abdominal wall showing diastasis recti

Diastasis recti

Abdominal separation, or diastasis recti, can occur when the abdominals are stretched out, as in pregnancy. The vertical midline of the abdominal wall is called the linea alba. It softens, along with everything else during pregnancy, as it stretches around your growing belly. It also weakens and may even separate. If this happens, you will feel a hole under your skin near your belly button. Your chance of separation is higher if you are carrying more than one baby.

The muscles in your legs, particularly your calves, may cramp at times. This is usually an indication that you are not consuming enough calcium.

This separation usually happens in the second or third trimester. It is painless, so if you do not feel for it, you may not know it is there. You should check for diastasis recti before every workout. If you feel a separation, you need to change your workout to put less strain on the abdominals, and do your abdominal exercises differently to prevent a larger separation. This is not a reason to stop all abdominal exercises, only to modify them. However, if the separation is wider than two and one-half inches, seek medical advice.

Most of the time the separation mends by itself after delivery and does not require any treatment. However, depending on the extent of the separation, it can take years before it is perfectly healed.

The linea alba is very thin, and in some pregnant women it may turn dark brown. This pigmentation is called linea negra, and it usually goes away after delivery. During an abdominal exercise, this brown line may protrude like a hard ridge all the way down the middle of your belly, making your midsection look like the Swiss Alps. Do not worry, this is normal.

Knee pain

Knee pain can be the combined result of softer ligaments and extra weight bearing down on the knee joint. Strengthen your knees with exercises such as leg extensions and isometric wall squats. Avoid bending your knees too much, whether you are sitting or standing.

Leg cramps

Leg cramps are a common complaint. The muscles in your legs, particularly your calves, may cramp at times. This is usually an indication that you are not consuming enough calcium. Add calcium supplements to your diet. Avoid pointing your toes, as this will often initiate a leg cramp. Flex the foot by pulling the toes toward you to stretch the calf muscles and alleviate cramps. Massages and warm baths may also help.

Foot pain

Foot and ankle pain have several causes. Your feet and ankles may swell from edema (water retention) or bad circulation. Your shoes may have become too small, worn out, or no longer support your feet properly due to your changing posture and weight. Exercise will help to alleviate these pains. Put all of your high heels away until after you have delivered your baby, and invest in a pair of good comfortable shoes or sneakers. Put your feet up when you are seated whenever possible. When seated, do foot circles, flex your feet, and massage them. Treat yourself to a professional manicure or reflexology session once in a while.

Swelling

Edema, swelling in your legs and feet due to water retention, is normal. Lying on your side and elevating your feet can help ease the swelling. Exercising in water can also reduce water retention.

Carpal tunnel syndrome

CTS is a compression of the median nerve, which goes through the carpal tunnel in your wrist. In your last trimester, tendons and soft tissue in your carpal tunnel may swell, causing your thumb and first two fingers to feel numb and tingle. This is similar to Repetitive Strain Injury caused by typing, piano playing, and other repetitive activities. Flexing your hand down for thirty to forty-five seconds at a time and applying ice may help. Wearing wrist splints at night can also be helpful. Should you suffer from carpal tunnel syndrome, avoid exercises such as push-ups or triceps bench dips, which will put additional pressure on your wrists.

Posterior tibial nerve compression

Numbness may result from squatting for too long (as in labor). This nerve runs down the back of your leg, from the knee to the heel. If the nerve becomes compressed, your inner foot will feel numb and tingle, and your toes may feel weak. Apply ice and limit your ankle movements until the symptoms pass.

Fatigue and anxiety

When you are pregnant, fatigue and anxiety are quite natural. Fatigue is your body's way of telling you that you need to slow down and conserve energy. You may also feel overwhelmed about your pregnancy, which could bring about feelings of stress and anxiety. You may be boundlessly happy one day and terrified of motherhood the next. You may not feel comfortable with the way your body is changing, or you may worry about losing your shape and fitness for good. These feelings are all normal. This is a monumental event in your life, and hopefully a happy one. I'm not going to tell you not to worry or to deny your feelings. Instead, try to reduce tension by exercising, or by trying some of the relaxation or yoga exercises in chapter 7. Treat yourself to a massage or get your partner to give you one. If you are severely fatigued or anxious, seek medical help. Fatigue could be an indicator of anemia or other disorders. Normal pregnancy-related fatigue usually abates spontaneously by the fourth month of pregnancy.

The goal of exercise in pregnancy is not to lose weight, it is to condition the muscles, improve circulation, increase blood and oxygen flow, speed metabolism, and regulate blood sugar levels.

Feeling faint or dizzy

Feeling faint or dizzy usually means that your blood is not circulating well. It may have pooled in your legs, particularly if you have been lying on your back or standing still for a long time. After sixteen weeks, do not lie on your back or stand in the same position for too long, you could cut off the fetus's oxygen supply. Move around—use your legs to help pump your blood around. Also eat often—do not go more than four hours without food.

pregnancy Q&As

If I'm considered "obese," can I still exercise?

Yes. Obese women may be classified as high-risk pregnancies, but they definitely can and should still exercise on a supervised and modified program, to prevent and minimize pregnancy discomforts and complications during labor. An obese pregnant woman has a higher risk of heart disease, diabetes, and fetal distress (excess fat places pressure on the uterus). C-sections are more prevalent with obese women. Obesity is defined as being 20 percent heavier than your ideal weight, or weighing more than 200 pounds at the end of your pregnancy. The goal of exercise in pregnancy is not to lose weight, it is to condition the muscles, improve circulation, increase blood and oxygen flow, speed metabolism, and regulate blood sugar levels.

If you are obese or overweight, you should not diet or restrict your food intake during pregnancy. Your diet should be monitored by a nutritionist to ensure that you are getting the proper balance of nutrients. Your expected weight gain during pregnancy will be less than that of most pregnant women.

Is water exercise during pregnancy as good as they say?

Doing your workout in the pool isn't just a lot of fun, it can also make it easier for you to move, as it puts less strain on your joints than land exercise. In addition to reducing your risk of injury, water exercise can be very rehabilitative. Athletes exercise in the pool to heal injuries faster. Immersing yourself in water can also help reduce fluid retention.

The buoyancy properties of water work like magic, supporting your body and absorbing most of any impact—50 to 60 percent when immersed to the sternum, and 90 percent to the neck. This makes the exercise seem easier, even though your body is working harder to move through all that water. Yet water exercise doesn't raise your heart rate as high as the same exercises on land, nor do your muscles need as much blood flow. Keep in mind, however, that water exercise is a "non-weight-bearing" form of exercise. Weight-bearing exercise seems to produce more health benefits during pregnancy. So make sure that you supplement aquatic exercise with some type of weight-bearing exercise, such as walking or weight training.

Weight-bearing exercise seems to produce more health benefits during pregnancy.

The temperature of the water is very important: The best temperature to exercise in is about 82° to 87° Fahrenheit; higher than 89° is too hot.

As an older mom, will my pregnancy be different?

Women older than the age of forty usually have normal and healthy pregnancies, but they are at an increased risk for complications, including diabetes, hypertension, and C-section. Unfit women older than forty will experience more severe pregnancy discomforts than unfit younger women. Exercise during pregnancy at this age is even more important, to prevent or decrease the incidence of pregnancy-related discomfort and complications, speed delivery time, and ease labor pain.

Do higher altitudes affect my pregnancy and ability to exercise?

Yes. Pregnant women in higher altitudes need to adapt to less oxygen in the air. Because oxygen is *the* most vital fuel for growth of the fetus, this can be difficult, especially for an exercising mom. People who live at high altitudes seem to adapt quite well to less oxygen-rich air. Those who are not accustomed to it may suffer adverse affects when traveling to such a location. You may feel fatigued or dizzy, and suffer from headaches, vomiting, or loss of appetite for the first four days. Exercise will be difficult, as your lungs must adapt to the reduced oxygen supply.

It is not a good idea for a pregnant woman to go on a short trip to the mountains or other high altitude locale for less than four days, such as a long ski weekend. The combination of high altitude and exercise (such as skiing, hiking, or mountain climbing) produces the most stress in the first three to four days.

It may take your body about four days to adapt to the changes in heart rate, blood pressure, and cardiac output that the higher altitude causes. It adapts by improving the way it transports oxygen. Different people's adjustment times will vary. People who are very fit with great lung capacity may not even feel the change in altitude.

So long as you are not smoking, anemic, or fearful of flying (an adrenaline rush may reduce blood flow), flying is not harmful to you or your baby. However, you should avoid altitudes higher than 10,000 feet (3,000 meters) on land altogether, exercising at higher altitudes than 8,000 feet (2,500 meters), and exercising for the first three to four days if you are higher than 6,500 feet (2,000 meters). When you do exercise, do so at a slower pace and intensity, and beware of mountain sickness, which may occur after the first twelve hours. Altitudes of higher than 9,000 feet (2,750 meters) have 45 percent oxygen in the air, and approximately 30 percent less humidity than at sea level, making it very difficult to breathe.

Some women who live in high altitudes have reproductive problems, such as delayed onset of menstruation, low fertility rate, repeat miscarriages, pregnancy complications, lower birth weight, premature labor, and more infants dying in the first month. If a pregnant woman living in high altitudes smokes, her baby's birth weight will be even lower than it would be if she smoked at sea level. This is all due to a lack of oxygen.

What is hyperventilating?

Hyperventilating occurs when your breathing speeds up excessively. You may be taking shorter, faster, shallower breaths. Hyperventilation causes an abnormal loss of carbon dioxide from the blood and can cause you to feel faint. If you experience this, slow down, sit down, and breathe as slowly and deeply as you can to replenish some oxygen. If this becomes a recurrent problem, consult your caregiver. You may need to modify your workout program. Exercise helps your circulation and oxygen uptake. Fit women will probably not experience hyperventilation as often as less fit women.

What should I do if I get a stitch?

A stitch is a temporary, sudden, sharp pain in the side, which may result from uneven breathing during aerobic exercise. If you get a stitch, slow down and concentrate on your breathing. Unless it's severe, don't stop exercising completely; an instant drop in heart rate and temperature can be harmful. Instead, continue at a lesser intensity until the pain subsides.

What is hypotension?

Hypotension occurs when blood pressure falls to the extent that blood flow to the heart and brain is reduced, causing dizziness or fainting. Whatever you do, don't ever hold your breath during pregnancy. Holding your breath while bearing down, pushing, or exercising (especially weight lifting), is called the Valsalva maneuver. It puts pressure on the vena cava, preventing blood from circulating and returning to your heart and brain. This hypotension makes you dizzy, but worst of all, it decreases blood and oxygen flow to your baby. Lying on your back may also give you hypotension, because a pregnant uterus will compress the vena cava in this position.

What is ketosis?

Ketosis is a chemical reaction that occurs due to the burning of your body's stored fat or protein from tissues and organs. It would happen only if you are not getting enough nutrients in your diet, due to dieting or severe morning sickness. When your body doesn't have enough glucose to burn for energy, it turns to fat or muscle instead (it literally *eats up* muscles and other tissues), and ketones (an acidic substance) are formed. Ketones are chemically related to acetone (found in solvents like nail polish remover). Ketones will travel through the placenta to the fetus and could severely harm your baby if exposure is prolonged. Therefore, dieting or restricting food intake during pregnancy could be disastrous for your baby's well-being.

Can varicose veins be alleviated?

Yes. Varicose veins are veins that do not pump the blood back the way they should. Varicose veins in the legs are the best known type. (Hemorrhoids are varicose veins in the rectum.) Pools of blood collect in the veins just under the surface of the skin, resulting in swelling. Varicose veins tend to be an inherited problem, so if your mother had them, you probably will too. Exercise can prevent, or at least minimize, varicose veins. If you are prone to varicose veins, make sure your exercise regimen includes leg exercises such as stair climbing, squats, and lunges, so long as they are not contraindicated by your pregnancy. (But avoid calf raises, which can cause leg cramps.) These leg exercises will make your veins pump better, improving your circulation.

Existing varicosities will become more prominent as pregnancy advances because your weight increases and the length of time spent upright is prolonged. Wearing support hose may help severe problems. (However, never wear support hose while exercising because doing so could cause you to overheat.) Rest with your legs elevated periodically and avoid standing still for long. If you have to stand for housework or other chores, wear wooden shoes such as clogs. To alleviate and prevent hemorrhoids, practice your Kegels, take a stool softener, avoid constipation, soak in a warm bath, and dab on some witch hazel.

Why do I feel so hot all the time?

Feeling hot means that your cooling system is working better, which it does during pregnancy. Your faster metabolism creates more heat, so your body becomes more efficient at dispersing heat, to keep the fetus cool. However, if you are sweating heavily, your blood sugar may be low, and you'll need to eat more carbohydrate-rich foods. To stay cool, avoid wearing body lotion, which traps heat and perspiration under your skin. Wear only natural fiber clothing such as cotton, to allow your skin to breathe. Drink plenty of water, as overheating could cause dehydration, which may lead to premature labor.

I often feel short of breath. What can I do to breathe easier?

Feeling breathless is caused by your growing uterus pushing up on the diaphragm, leaving less room for your lungs. You now have to breathe more often to take in the same amount of oxygen. However, you can create more space for your lungs by lifting your arms up and out to the sides, flaring and lifting up the rib cage. Keep breathing and practice deeper or slower breathing.

My heartbeat seems so much faster, is this okay when I exercise?
Yes. Your heart rate can be up to twenty beats per minute faster when pregnant. And younger women have faster training heart rates than older women. However, an extremely rapid heartbeat or heart palpitations associated with chest pain, faintness, or shortness of breath should be reported to your obstetrician. You don't want to overexert yourself when pregnant, so it is important to warmup slowly before a workout and cool down afterward. To monitor your intensity, you can check your pulse before, during, and after your workout, or use the Rate of Perceived Exertion method described in chapter 3.

When you lift anything off the floor or move objects around, use your legs, keep the object as close to you as you can, and stay as upright as you can when bending your knees to prevent straining your back.

Why does my pregnant body feel and move so differently?
Because of biomechanical changes. Your changing size, shape, and weight shifts your center of gravity, changing the way you walk, run, and perform other activities. These changes can be controlled to a certain extent by a good exercise program.

Your bones and joints may feel less stable than you are used to. When you are pregnant, the additional estrogen and the new hormone relaxin soften your ligaments, cartilage, tendons, tissues, and joints. These changes increase your risk for injuries unless you exercise.

About twenty weeks into your pregnancy, your belly has grown big enough to limit how far you can move in the hip joint. Because of this you can't lean forward as far as before. This overextension of your hip joint when standing up or sitting down can strain your knees, front thighs, and lower leg muscles. You can strengthen your legs to prevent an injury. You will probably start using your arms to help you get up from a chair or a couch, so your arms will also need some strength training to make this easier.

Become aware of your posture. You can lessen backaches and strains by controlling your pelvic tilt. Be aware of how different positions put pressure on your body. For example, a tall chair may be easier to get out of than a regular chair or sofa. Putting a box under one foot when doing standing housework may alleviate strain on your back. When you lift anything off the floor or move objects around, use your legs, keep the object as close to you as you can, and stay as upright as you can when bending your knees to prevent straining your back.

Strengthening and toning your muscles all over will make moving around in the latter part of pregnancy easier. It will also help your balance, coordination, and stability. In your workout, make sure that you include strengthening exercises for the upper back, shoulders, arms, abdominals, buttocks, and hamstrings, and stretching exercises for the chest, hip flexors, thighs, and lower back muscles.

Are there times when I should reduce my level of exercise?
Yes. If you suffer from chronic fatigue, aches, pains, heart palpitations, or respiratory problems (including cold, flu, bronchitis) you should reduce your exercise intensity temporarily. Also, if your baby doesn't move much, particularly after an exercise session, it may be an indication that you are overtraining. Your baby should move two to three times within thirty minutes. If it doesn't, you need to undergo medical evaluation of fetal behavior and growth, and reduce exercise levels by 10 to 25 percent.

Chapter Three

guidelines for exercising during pregnancy

Hundreds of years ago, pregnant women would give birth and then go back to working in the fields the next day. Although the advent of early twentieth-century medicine disproved the wisdom of such grueling practices, the new mindset was only slightly better.

According to Raul Artal, M.D., "The prevalence of the Victorian view, fear of malpractice, and a lot of unscientific assumptions encouraged doctors for many years to advise women to put their feet up for nine months. But with the exercise boom of the 1980s, questions started coming up about working out while expecting." Dr. Artal, professor and chairman of the department of obstetrics and gynecology at SUNY Health Science Center at Syracuse, initiated and heads some of the foremost prenatal fitness research.

Back in the 1980s, active and athletic women became very impatient with the restrictive levels of exercise that were imposed upon them. Some of the rules, such as keeping workouts to less than fifteen minutes a day and maintaining a heart rate below 140 beats per minute are, in retrospect, ridiculous. Years of research have led to revised guidelines that acknowledge exercise as a top priority for pregnant women.

IN THIS CHAPTER

- *Exercise guidelines from the American College of Obstetrics and Gynecology*
- *Before you begin—assessing your readiness and fitness level*
- *Designing a safe pregnancy workout*

Dr. James F. Clapp III, a pioneer in this field of research, says, "I'm finding that women can continue a very vigorous regimen of exercise that is much higher than recommended by college guidelines, without any evidence of harm, and with some evidence of benefit. Both women and babies tend to tolerate labor better, and the mothers have a higher rate of quick labor, and spontaneous birth, and recover faster." He cautions, however, that pregnancy is not the time to *start* a vigorous exercise regime: "My rationale is that if you continue to do what the body is used to, you won't interfere with reproductive factors. If you increase it very much, you might."

ACOG guidelines

The American College of Obstetricians and Gynecologists (ACOG), with the help of Raul Artal, M.D., published a new set of guidelines in February of 1994. Following are some of ACOG's recommendations for pregnant women, adapted with permission from their Technical Bulletin No. 189, *Exercise During Pregnancy and the Postpartum Period*:

- Limit exercise intensity and lower target heart rate only if the woman has risk factors that could compromise her pregnancy. She should have a health assessment and an individualized exercise program.
- Regular exercise (at least three times a week) at mild to moderate intensities is better than sporadic exercise.
- The supine position after the first trimester is not advisable. Neither is standing still for a long time.
- Exercise should be halted if the woman is fatigued, because she has less available oxygen with which to do aerobic exercise. It is also not recommended to exercise to exhaustion.
- Weight-bearing exercises, such as walking, running, and yoga may be continued throughout pregnancy, but with caution. Non-weight-bearing exercises, such as cycling and swimming, minimize the risk of injury and can be continued throughout pregnancy.
- Exercises that compromise a woman's balance, or have the potential of causing abdominal trauma, should be avoided. This is especially true for the third trimester.

- Eating more than the 300 extra calories a day that the pregnancy needs is advisable if the woman exercises regularly.
- Drinking a lot of water, wearing clothes that breathe, and avoiding hot, humid weather when exercising are advisable.

CONTRAINDICATIONS TO EXERCISE

According to the ACOG, regular exercise programs are not recommended if a pregnant woman has certain conditions or risk factors. These factors include cardiac, vascular, pulmonary, or thyroid diseases. Other medical barriers include diabetes, seizure disorder, obesity, hypertension (whether chronic or caused by the pregnancy), anemia or other blood disorders, and problems with the back, joints, or muscles.

Leading a sedentary lifestyle, being very underweight, having an incompetent or weak cervix, and having a history of premature labor or of growth retardation within the uterus are also warning signs not to exercise regularly.

If you suffer from persistent bleeding in the second or third trimester, if your baby is in the breech position in the last trimester, or if your water has broken (a ruptured membrane), do not attempt any form of exercise.

If you have had three or more miscarriages, you should not exercise until your pregnancy is secure in the second trimester. In this case, a highly modified program including pelvic floor exercises is best. See chapter 6 for more details.

You should be able to continue a modified exercise program if you are carrying twins. However, remember that premature labor is very common with multiple births. If you were not fit prior to conceiving or are carrying triplets, do not start a new regular exercise program. Instead, you should do some special exercises for "high-risk" pregnancies to maintain your strength, as well as the abdominal, lower back, and pelvic floor exercises after the first trimester when your pregnancy is secure. See chapter 6 for more information.

Finally, if the placenta is covering the cervix (placenta previa), or has broken away from the uterus (placenta abruption), you should not do any exercises other than Kegels and lower back stretches.

Even if you fall into a high-risk category, you can still do some form of modified, supervised exercise. I have worked with women suffering from several of the aforementioned conditions, including incompetent cervix. With proper instruction, monitoring, and modifications, it is amazing what a pregnant woman can safely do.

If there are no medical complications, a pregnant woman can continue to exercise without fear. If you were healthy before becoming pregnant, you can maintain your fitness level, but you may need to modify your program due to the inevitable body changes.

Pregnancy is a time to maintain fitness and strength.

Most of the physical changes caused by pregnancy last for about twelve weeks postpartum, but they can vary from woman to woman and may last up to six months. This means that after delivery you should resume your exercise routine slowly and gradually increase the frequency and intensity, depending upon your condition. See chapter 10 on postpartum exercise for specifics.

before you begin

The 1994 ACOG guidelines, a godsend at the time, are seen by many experts today to still be a tad conservative. Due to more recent research, these guidelines may be revised within a few years. The guidelines in this chapter combine the ACOG guidelines with safety recommendations from the American College of Sports Medicine (ACSM), and tips I've learned from my many years of experience. Regardless of whether you are a beginner or a seasoned athlete, pregnancy is a time to maintain fitness and strength. It is not an opportunity for an all-out physical challenge. Pregnancy is a challenge in itself and you will get more fit in the process anyway.

Make sure to get a complete physical before you start your own program or join any exercise class. Your physician will want to monitor your progress and may advise you to modify your program as your pregnancy advances or if previously unknown risk factors develop. If you have a healthy, normal, low-risk pregnancy, but your doctor advises against exercise, ask why. If you are not satisfied with the answer, get a second opinion. There are still some medical practitioners who advise their patients against exercise during pregnancy, because they are either overly cautious or uninformed about the latest research. Make sure you are comfortable with your doctor's advice.

If you want to take an organized group aerobics or prenatal class, or even hire a personal trainer, you will need to obtain written permission from your doctor. The health club or instructor will also usually make you sign a waiver.

Find a fitness instructor with special knowledge in pre- and postnatal fitness. This may be easier said than done. He or she should be a certified instructor, preferably with prenatal certification or a degree in a related subject and practical experience. Fitness instructors come in all forms, from certified aerobics instructors, personal trainers, exercise physiologists, physical therapists, physical education Ph.D.s, athletic trainers, and nurses, to those with no other training or experience but their own workout.

If you have any doubts, check with your doctor first before undertaking any exercise program.

Your instructor should give you a health and physical evaluation. He or she should also consult with your doctor. The more informed the instructor is about your condition and special considerations, the better and more individualized your training program will be. In addition to surveying your general health and fitness level, your instructor should ask special pregnancy-related questions, including the questions in the self-assessment that follows.

PRENATAL FITNESS ASSESSMENT

The following list of questions will help you to gauge your readiness to begin an exercise program. *This self-assessment is in no way meant to substitute for a doctor's or instructor's consultation.* As always, if you have any doubts, check with your doctor first before undertaking any exercise program.

Has your water broken?
If so, stop all activities and call your doctor.

Do you have a placenta abruption (placenta has broken away from the uterus) or placenta previa (placenta is covering the cervix)?
Have you experienced any bleeding?
If you answered yes to either question, call your doctor before proceeding with any type of exercise. You may be able to practice your Kegels and lower back stretches, but that's about it.

Is your cervix weak or incompetent?
Are you carrying three or more babies?
Are you carrying twins and have not previously exercised?
Have you ever gone into premature labor?
Are there any signs of growth retardation in the fetus?

If you answered yes to any of these questions, then you are an extremely high-risk pregnancy and may require bed-rest. You should do no exercise except for Kegels and possibly a few bed-rest exercises (see chapter 6 for instructions).

Do you suffer from pregnancy-induced hypertension?
Is your baby in a breech position in the last trimester?
If you answered yes to either of these questions, you are a high-risk pregnancy, and should not participate in a regular exercise program. However, some light exercises and slow-to-moderate walks may be enjoyed, and you should still perform abdominal and lower back exercises, as well as your essential Kegels (see chapter 6 for more information).

Have you had three or more miscarriages?
If so, you are a high-risk pregnancy and should wait until your pregnancy is secure in the second trimester before you exercise.

Are you a fit mother carrying twins?
Do you suffer from chronic hypertension (not pregnancy-induced) or diseases of the thyroid, heart, or lungs?
If so, you are also in a high-risk group and will need to carefully modify your current workout program and be monitored by your doctor and a knowledgeable instructor. Unless you experience complications, you should be able to exercise through the entire pregnancy. If you have any of these conditions and have not previously exercised, your program may need to be limited to Kegels, abdominal, lower-back, and some bed-rest exercises.

Do you have anemia, diabetes, or any blood disorder?
Do you have a seizure disorder?
Are you obese or overweight?
Are you very underweight?
Do you have a very sedentary lifestyle?
Do you have any joint, back, or muscle problems?
Answering yes to any of these questions means that you are in a high-risk category and your condition warrants special care. As long as you modify your workouts along with your bodily changes, and are monitored by a

doctor and knowledgeable instructor, you should be able to exercise for the full nine months. Even if you have not exercised previously, you should walk regularly, do Kegel exercises, abdominal and lower back work, and other exercises designed for your high-risk condition (see chapter 6).

If none of these conditions apply to you, your pregnancy is healthy and you may continue almost any exercise program. If you want to embark on a new exercise program, consult with your doctor and instructor, and refer to pages 91–92 on how to design your program.

This self-assessment, along with a general health evaluation and fitness test, will help you, your doctor, and your instructor design the perfect workout program for you.

fitness testing

As shown, pregnancy affects all of your bodily systems. Therefore, the standard methods of testing fitness levels won't always work when you're pregnant.

Your *resting heart rate* will be about ten to twenty beats per minute higher than normal, which will throw off your *training heart rate.* A better way to measure and monitor your exercise intensity during pregnancy is the Rate of Perceived Exertion (RPE) method, described on pages 84–85.

It will be practically impossible to accurately measure your *cardiovascular capacity or fitness level.* During pregnancy, your cardiovascular and lung capacity increase, along with your heart rate and body weight. Together, these elements will make your fitness level measurements seem low, when in fact you are more fit just by virtue of being pregnant. During pregnancy, you should not work yourself to exhaustion, so any kind of stress or intense cardiovascular fitness test is not recommended.

Your *blood pressure* will probably go down while you are pregnant, especially during the second and early third trimester, due to the extra blood in your body. If you develop hypertension due to your pregnancy, certain exercises may exacerbate your condition such as overhead weight lifting, isometric muscle contractions, and high-intensity anaerobic exercise.

Your girth measurements can be interesting to record monthly, but do not obsess over them. You are supposed to get bigger when you're pregnant.

Your *lung capacity* may increase, but breathing will be more difficult as your pregnancy progresses. Lung capacity is usually measured using a spirometer, a device in which you blow forcefully into a tube. This can make you dizzy during pregnancy. Instead, you can estimate your lung capacity using a simple tape measure. On exhalation, measure the smallest circumference of your chest (in inches), and on inhalation, measure the largest circumference. Divide the smallest measurement by the difference, and you will get a number between one and ten. A normal healthy non-pregnant rate should be five or more, but it may measure much less during a pregnancy.

Your *body fat* cannot be accurately measured due to the internal fat deposits that support the pregnancy. However, it can be fun or interesting, depending on how you feel about it, to take your skin fold measurements every month to see how they change. Whether you exercise or not, your fat deposits in the first and second trimester will not be affected. If you do exercise, your body will deposit less fat in the last trimester, which is perfectly okay.

Your *girth measurements* can be interesting to record monthly, but do not obsess over them. You are supposed to get bigger when you're pregnant.

A *postural assessment* can be a valuable tool in modifying and designing your workout. Your posture will change as your pregnancy progresses, but you can counteract these changes to a certain degree with the right exercises and stretches.

Your *strength* is not important to measure, nor is strength testing recommended at this time.

Your *flexibility* can be tested as long as each stretch is not taken to maximum. Theoretically, because the pregnancy hormone relaxin softens your joints, you should be more flexible when you are pregnant. However, in reality, most women do not experience a change in their flexibility; some even notice a decrease.

rate of perceived exertion

Because the resting heart rate of a pregnant woman can rise up to twenty beats per minute over normal levels, your heart rate will also be much higher than normal during any activity. As a result, measuring exercise intensity with your heart rate will not work. Forget the Target Heart Rate charts on the wall in your gym—you are off the chart. The "old" guidelines (1984) for exercise during pregnancy were very conservative, recommending that pregnant women keep their heart rates lower than 140 beats per minute during exercise. Due to new research, however, this rule has now been abolished, making way for a more realistic approach to measuring your fitness intensity—you.

A better way of measuring how hard you are working is the Rate of Perceived Exertion (RPE) method. (For this book, I modified and simplified Borg's 20-point RPE scale.) On a scale of one to ten, you rate how hard you feel you are working during an exercise session. If you are not pregnant, a 6.5 to 8.5 rate means that you are working hard enough to increase your fitness level. During pregnancy, a rate of anywhere from 5 to 8.5 will be beneficial, and 9 or higher can be harmful. Be aware that listening to music makes exercise feel easier, and you may not realize how hard you are working. Remember that when you are pregnant you do not have to work as hard to reach your maximum exercise capacity.

The Rate of Perceived Exertion chart should be your main method of gauging your exercise intensity. However, it is still a good idea to check your heart rate once in a while, especially on a hot day. To check your heart rate, feel the pulse on the inside of your wrist or at the side of your neck under your jaw. Count for ten seconds. Multiply this count by six to get the number of beats per minute.

RPE Scale

1. *Sleeping*
2. *Being awake*
3. *Light exertion: typing, eating*
4. *Strolling*
5. *Moderate walking or exercise*
6. *Moderately intense walking or exercise*
7. *Intense walking or exercise*
8. *Very intense exercise, speed-walking, or jogging*
9. *Extremely intense anaerobic exercise*
10. *Adrenaline-driven action (running from a burning building)*

monitoring

All pregnant women who exercise should monitor their progress. You can use the Prenatal Fitness Diary on the next page to record your weight gain and exercise performance on a regular basis, either daily or weekly. (Professional athletes require more specialized monitoring, including glucose and lactate levels, and fetal heart rate.) Pay particular attention to weight gain. If you are losing weight, it could be a sign of dehydration. Some of the measurements, such as well-being, are not scientific but are subject to your own personal interpretation. Because you can't "feel" fat deposits, have your body fat or skin folds measured once a month by a fitness instructor. It will give you a record of your pregnancy to look back on later.

PRENATAL FITNESS DIARY

	weight	*exercise type*	*length of workout*	*intensity RPE**	*training heart rate*	*strength*	*flexibility*	*well-being*	*body fat***
date: **9/17** *time:* **9 A.M.**	**139**	**walking & stretching**	**40 min.**	**7**	**156**	**feeling strong**	**muscles are less supple**	**good energy**	
date: *time:*									
date: *time:*									
date: *time:*									
date: *time:*									
date: *time:*									
date: *time:*									
date: *time:*									

* *see pages 84–85*

** *sum of skinfolds (optional for athletes)*

precautions

Not every place is a good place to exercise. For example, the higher your altitude, the less you should exercise because of the oxygen deficit. It is okay to work out at up to 6,500 feet above sea level, but not until you are four to five days into your routine. Do not exercise at higher than 8,000 feet, and avoid altitudes of 10,000 feet or higher altogether.

Exercising to exhaustion, lifting very heavy weights, or participating in athletic competition does not mix well with pregnancy. Exercises calling for prone (on your stomach) positions or exercises that crowd your abdomen should not be a part of your program.

Because of your softer joints, avoid deep flexion (bending your knees or elbows to less than a 90-degree angle), quick changes in movement or direction, and toe touches from a standing or seated position. You should also abstain from unsupported squats, forward bends, lunges, and the hurdler's stretch.

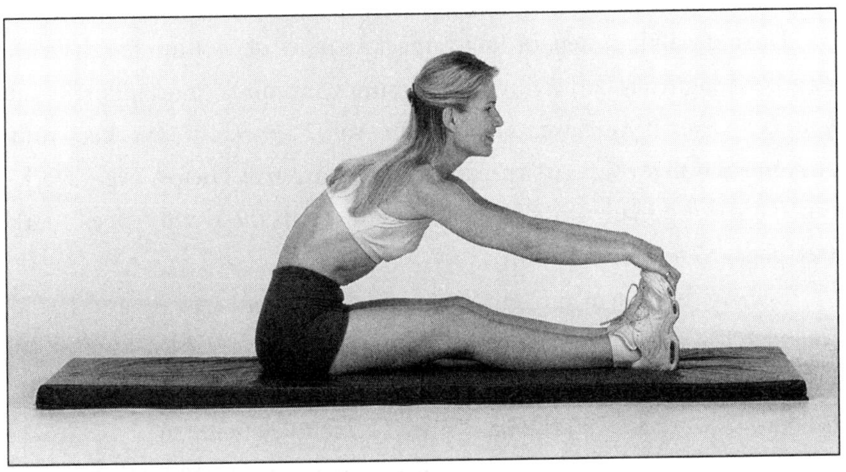

Birgitta demonstrates a seated toe touch or forward bend. Avoid this stretch during pregnancy.

Due to your reduced sense of balance and coordination, avoid difficult dance steps, aerobic choreography, and plyometric moves (jumps or lifts off the ground with both feet). Inverted (upside down) positions such as shoulder-, head-, or handstands can be hazardous. Hanging from your feet or hips, as on some types of gym equipment, and certain yoga positions such as "the plow" and "the up or down dog" are also not advised. Finally, if it causes you discomfort, do not hyperextend (arch backward) your back.

When you rise from the floor or a seated position, do so slowly. Moving your legs or walking around between each exercise will improve circulation.

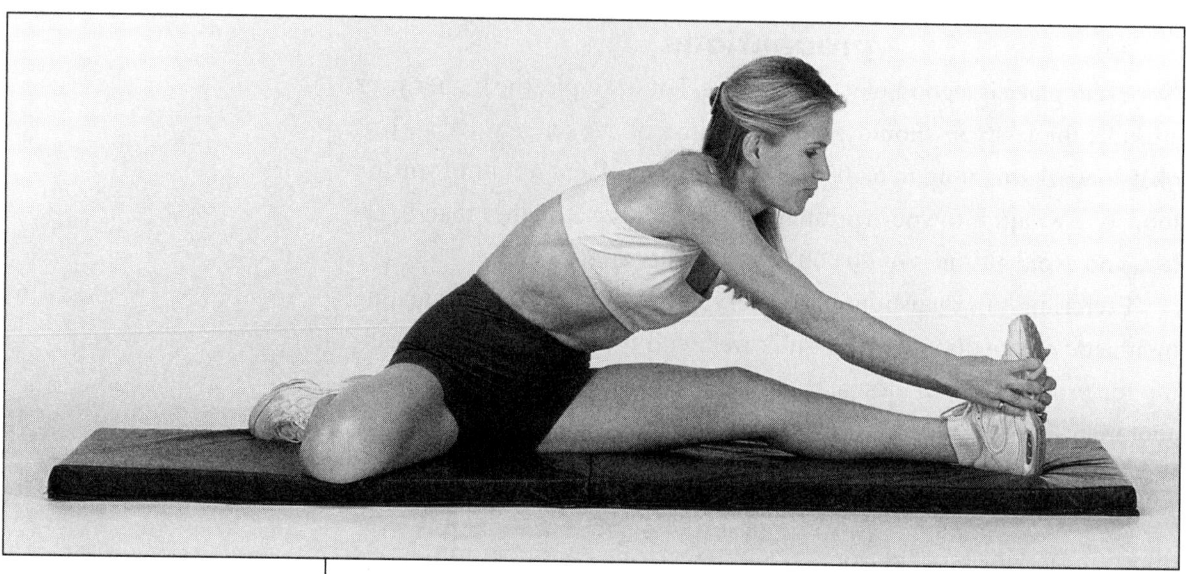

Birgitta doing a hurdler's stretch—another position that should be avoided in pregnancy.

Check your heart rate and use the Rate of Perceived Exertion to determine how hard you are working. A good pace is between 50 to 85 percent of your capacity, depending on your fitness level.

During walking, step, or low-impact aerobics do not use hand, wrist, or ankle weights. A bad swing could injure your joints or accidentally hit your belly. Even if you never directly injure your stomach, always check your abdominal wall for signs of a separation (diastasis recti) before every workout. This is especially important when you reach the twenty-week mark (see pages 67–68 for details).

Because high arm movements can raise your heart rate and blood pressure, avoid doing overhead arm exercises during aerobics. By the way, the myth that stretching your arms over your head will cause the umbilical cord to wrap around the baby's neck is completely untrue.

Cool down properly for at least five to ten minutes. Although you may feel like lying down, don't—positioning your head lower than your heart level right after any aerobic activity may throw off your equilibrium, making you feel dizzy.

Stretch after a workout, when your muscles are warm. Your joints may feel more flexible since they have softened, but if a stretch is taken too far beyond comfort, it can damage your ligaments or other soft tissue.

If your heart beats too rapidly or irregularly, stop exercising. Sit down, keeping your head higher than your heart. Until your heart rate has dropped, do not bend over. Instead, drink water and relax.

Sit down if you feel faint or dizzy, but don't bend over or put your head between your legs. Put something cool on your forehead, drink water, and eat something light.

If you experience any of the following problems, stop whatever you are doing, lie down on your left side, and call your doctor:

- you feel extreme pressure or pain in the pubic bone
- you notice vaginal bleeding
- your water breaks
- you experience strong, regular contractions (every five to ten minutes), or you experience irregular contractions and you are less than thirty-seven weeks pregnant
- you suspect that your baby has stopped moving
- you fall onto your abdomen
- you feel any pain

Call your doctor in the event of any injury.

In Case of Injury

If you hurt a body part other than your abdomen, use the RICE *method on the injured body part:*

R*est*
I*ce the injured part for twenty minutes*
C*ompress and wrap the injured part*
E*levate the injured part, but not higher than your heart*

workout guidelines for pregnancy

- If you're a beginner, start slowly and increase gradually. Remember, pregnancy is a time to maintain strength and fitness.
- Get a complete physical before you join any exercise class or start your own program. Have your exercise program periodically evaluated by your physician and/or trainer. Your program may need to be modified or discontinued due to your advancing pregnancy or a previously unknown risk factor.
- Get written permission from your doctor before enrolling in any aerobic or prenatal class or hire a personal trainer. The class organizer, health club, or instructor will also have you sign a waiver.
- Do not exercise at altitudes higher than 8,000 feet, and do not exercise for the first three to four days at higher than 6,500 feet. The higher you travel, the less you should exercise, due to decreased oxygen at high altitudes.
- Eat a light snack about thirty minutes to an hour before your workout to prevent low blood sugar. Fruit, juice, or other high carbohydrate foods are perfect.

- Check your exercise equipment to make sure it is in proper working condition.
- Drink plenty of water before, during, and after your workout.
- Wear comfortable, appropriate clothing for the activity and weather. A well-supporting sports bra is a must. If you suffer from varicose veins, do not wear support hose when you exercise. Such clothing can cause you to overheat. If it is cold, wear several layers of clothing that can be removed as your temperature rises. If it is warm, wear loose cotton or breathable fabrics such as Supplex to stay cool and dry.
- Do not exercise in hot or humid weather. An air-conditioned room is often the perfect setting for a workout.
- When you are pregnant, steady, low-impact exercise is better than interval training, which alternates high and low intensities. To prevent boredom, you can cross train (alternate sports or activities), but try to choose activities of roughly the same intensity.
- Always warmup slowly and thoroughly to loosen your muscles, increase your heart rate, and prevent injuries.
- Prevent accidents by practicing proper posture, alignment, and muscle control, and by avoiding quick changes in movement or direction.
- Rise slowly from the floor or a seated position to avoid getting dizzy.
- Check your heart rate and use the Rate of Perceived Exertion chart to determine how hard you are working.
- Move your legs or walk around between exercises; do not stand or sit still for long periods.
- Do not exercise to exhaustion or lift very heavy weights.
- Do not participate in athletic competition.
- Do not use hand, wrist, or ankle weights during walking, step, or low-impact aerobics. You could injure your joints or accidentally hit your belly.
- Always be aware of your abdominals, checking for a possible separation in the abdominal wall (diastasis recti) before every workout.
- If you feel your chest pounding, or if you feel sick or hot and sweaty during a workout—stop, sit down, and keep your head higher than your heart level. If you have an injury, seek medical attention.

- After every workout, cool down properly and stretch slowly and carefully.
- Listen to your body and modify your workout as you see fit. Slow down if you are not feeling well. If you feel terrific and full of energy, take advantage of it, stay active, and have a great workout.

TYPICAL WORKOUT

You can use the following guideline when planning your own exercise routine. Modify as necessary according to your lifestyle, stage of pregnancy, and special considerations.

Warmup

At least five minutes before every exercise session. Perform movements similar to what you will do in your workout, or do smooth, full-range dynamic stretches. Warm up with dynamic stretches and long, smooth movements such as arm circles. Dynamic stretching involves moving parts of your body and gradually increasing your reach. Static stretches (stretching a muscle or group of muscles and holding that position) are not a good way to warmup; this type of stretching is best performed after your workout, when your muscles are already warm. Take more time warming up if you are exercising early in the morning, have an injury, or it is just plain cold.

Aerobic exercise

Twenty to forty-five minutes a day, three to six days a week. Your daily aerobic exercise can be divided into separate ten-minute sessions, not including warmups and cool downs.

Toning exercises

Twenty to sixty minutes a day, two to three days a week. Stretch every muscle group except your abdominals after every workout, with emphasis on your legs, upper back, and abdominal muscles.

Kegels

Include Kegel exercises in your workout or cool down. Make sure you also fit them in on days you don't work out. Do them at home, in your car, while out dining, while working at your computer, or whenever.

Cool down

Ten-plus minutes after every exercise session. Avoid lying down or positioning your head below your heart level immediately after aerobic activity as this could cause dizziness.

Stretching

Ten to thirty minutes after every workout. Stretching can be part of your cool down. Do at least one stretch per muscle or body part, with more for the lower back, chest, and hips. Do not stretch the abdominals.

Now it's up to you and your caregiver to design a suitable and appropriate exercise program for you. These guidelines should give you enough flexibility. There are a lot of precautions to keep in mind, but as you will see as you read on, there are more things that you *can* do than you *can't* do, and there are ways of modifying most activities to suit your changing needs.

Chapter Four

how to modify sports and activities for pregnancy

There is no single activity, exercise, or workout that suits every woman, and every exercise will affect your body differently. Even the different stages of your pregnancy will probably cause you to change activities, or at least intensities. Furthermore, you could be in a different mood each day, so a strict program won't work. Take each day as it comes. If you planned a weight workout, but do not feel like it, go for a walk. If you are very tired, take a nap and do your workout later, or even tomorrow. Do not overexert yourself. Avoid outdoor activities in hot weather, especially during the first trimester.

Previous chapters have given you basic guidelines on how to listen to your body and customize your workout program during pregnancy. This chapter contains instructions on how to modify specific sports and activities. The list is extensive but not exhaustive. If your favorite exercise is not covered, compare it to a similar listed activity. Then decide whether to continue, modify, or eliminate it. If it feels good, you can probably continue, and if it causes discomfort, you should quit or modify it. Definitely quit any activity that causes pain or injury. Some sports and activities are inherently dangerous to pregnant women, and they are designated as

IN THIS CHAPTER

- *An alphabetized guide to sports and activities and special considerations during pregnancy*
- *Cross-referencing of similar sports and activities for ease in comparison*
- *A quick-reference chart of activities to be continued, modified, or avoided altogether*

such. If you feel you absolutely must participate in one of these activities, take all possible precautions.

Some guidelines instruct you to stretch or strengthen particular muscle groups before or after an activity. These strengthening and stretching exercises are described in later chapters. See chapter 5 for strength training and chapter 7 for stretching.

aerobics and prenatal classes

(Including hip-hop and funk aerobics) Participating in an aerobics class is a great way to exercise and socialize at the same time. However, many instructors are not trained in prenatal fitness and do not know basic pregnancy physiology. Choose a certified instructor who has prenatal fitness training. If you can, pick a special prenatal class, preferably one recommended by a friend, caregiver, or childbirth education center. There are many different types of aerobics classes. Funk and hip-hop aerobics can be a fun alternative to traditional aerobics, and they're a great way for you to let loose and have some laughs while still getting the benefits of a good cardio workout.

If there are no prenatal aerobics classes in your area, or you would like to stick with a regular aerobics class that you like, there are a few things you should know. If you are a beginner, start in a low-impact or toning class. If you are accustomed to a high impact program, you may continue for as long as you feel comfortable, but with a few modifications.

Exercise only on soft floors, such as wood or special aerobic flooring, to lessen the impact on your joints. Always warmup and cool down properly, taking care to stretch all of your muscles carefully, but never as far as you did prior to pregnancy. Stretching to the point of pain means that you are close to straining your joints or pulling a muscle.

The change in your center of gravity and your diminished sense of balance make it important for you to avoid quick changes in direction, mid-air propulsions (hops), circular movements, and complicated choreography. Don't worry about keeping up with the rest of the class. Modify any movement that doesn't feel comfortable. Walk, improvise your own steps, or just practice your Kegels.

Remember that you may do just about anything while lying on your side, on your knees, or seated. Floor exercises on your back are okay as long as you do not feel dizzy. Avoid arching or extending your back, and forget about any inverted or upside down positions. Also avoid deep forward lunges, side lunges, or deep unsupported squats, unless you are used to them. You may do half squats or half lunges (don't bend below a 90-degree angle) if they feel okay. Unless you are very experienced and in the early stage of your pregnancy, avoid plyometric moves (lifting both feet off the ground simultaneously), such as hops, skips, and jumps incorporated into the choreography. Instead, walk through them as the rest of the class leaps.

As always, keep a water bottle handy and do not overexert or overheat.

You may find that lateral (side-to-side) stepping increases your heart rate more so than any other stepping. If at any time you feel the need to slow down, first eliminate the arm movements. If that is insufficient, slow down to a walk. Do not completely stop at any time unless you get dizzy or feel pain.

Because high arm movements will raise your heart rate and blood pressure unnecessarily high, avoid raising your arms overhead. Keep your arms below shoulder level or do not move them at all. These exercises will not significantly tone your arms anyway. If a segment of the class is devoted to toning, keep your legs moving between sets with half squats, half lunges, or stepping exercises to prevent blood from pooling in your legs.

Aerobic means "with oxygen." Aerobic exercise conditions the heart and lungs by increasing the efficiency of oxygen intake to the body. Increasing your oxygen intake doesn't mean you should be out of breath. If you are huffing and puffing, you need to slow down.

As always, keep a water bottle handy and do not overexert or overheat. Keep your doctor's phone number available should you have an emergency.

See also Stairs, Step Aerobics, and Step Machines.

aquatic exercise and sports

(Including pool aerobics) Aquatic exercise is fun and safe during pregnancy. With the water supporting most of the body's weight, less stress is placed on the knees and ankles, making this type of exercise particularly well suited for pregnant women of all fitness levels. However, you should supplement aquatic exercise with weight-bearing activities (such as walking), which provides greater prenatal fitness benefits.

Several exercises incorporate running and walking in the pool. You can use a floating device, tread in deep water, or use a sprint leash hooked to the pool edge for resistance. You can also run or walk through the shallow end of the pool forward, backward, sideways, and in circles. You can actually do just about anything in the pool that you can do on land. Try imitating your specific sport's moves in the water. Volleyball, step aerobics, high hurdles, boxing, dancing, tennis, and even golf may be mimicked in the water as part of your workout.

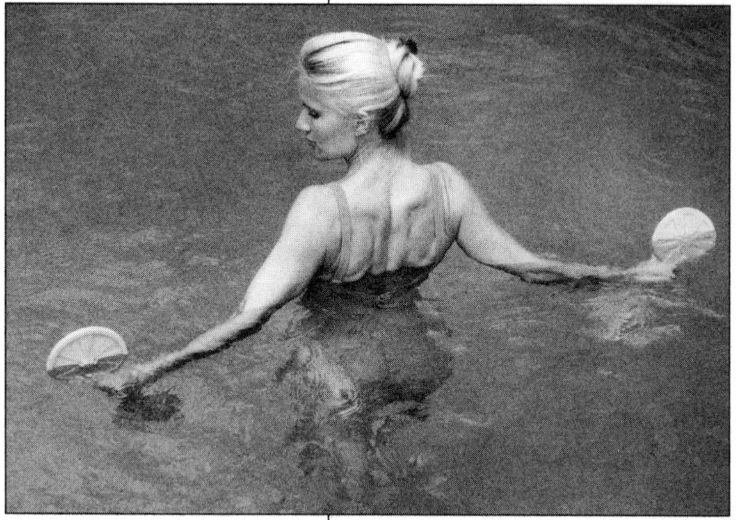

Birgitta using pool accessories

Pool aerobics can provide a fun, refreshing workout. You can safely participate in any pool aerobics class that has calisthenics, running, jogging, walking, and jumping. You can also do toning and strength training by using either the resistance of the water or various pool toys.

There is a variety of pool equipment available that simulates regular weight training movements in the water. Foam dumbbells, barbells, ankle weights, paddles, balls, and webbed gloves are just some of the devices you can try. Kicking-boards are also great if you are not comfortable swimming without support. Deep water exercises are also fine.

Competitive water sports such as water polo should be avoided in late pregnancy due to the risk of sustaining a blow to the abdomen or being forced underwater. Even though the water will support the weight of your body and reduce the impact, such an accident could still be dangerous. *See also* Swimming.

bicycling

(Including stationary and recumbent bikes) Early in your pregnancy it is okay to ride a bike outdoors, so long as the weather isn't too hot. Avoid rough terrain and steep inclines after sixteen weeks (that means no mountain biking!). Use a bike on which you can sit up straight. The aerodynamic forward lean on speed bikes may strain your back and crowd the uterus.

Unless you are a seasoned athlete, I don't recommend outdoor bicycling after the first trimester—it is too easy to lose your balance and fall.

Also, even if you never stumble, riding outside exposes you to traffic and smog, which can harm both you and your baby. For these reasons, you may want to stick with an indoor stationary bike.

Recumbent bikes are built so that you ride from a reclined position. This takes pressure off your pelvis and reduces the risk of lower back pain. Recumbent seats are larger and you sit *in* the seat rather than perching on top of a narrow saddle. These bikes are very comfortable, particularly during pregnancy. The bigger your belly gets though, the greater the odds of you crowding your uterus with your knees. Regardless of the bike you use, stretch your quadriceps, hip flexors and rotators, hamstrings, buttocks, and calf muscles afterward. *See also* Spinning®.

bowling

Bowling is a calm, non-stressful sport that is safe for a pregnant woman to continue. As your belly grows larger, you will need to be more aware of your posture, balance, and muscle control when releasing the ball to avoid a fall.

calisthenics

Calisthenics is a system of exercise movements, without equipment, for the building of strength, flexibility, and physical grace. The term is derived from the Greek *kalos* (beautiful) and *sthenos* (strength). It is an anaerobic (non-aerobic) form of strength training that helps condition your heart and tone your muscles. This form of exercise is not recommended for beginners or anyone suffering from chronic or gestational high blood pressure or arthritis. Otherwise, you can continue calisthenics throughout pregnancy, with some modifications due to your changing shape and shift in center of gravity. Avoid supine (on your back), prone (on your stomach), or inverted (upside down) positions, and exercises that crowd the uterus or otherwise feel uncomfortable.

car and motorcycle racing

This type of sport should be avoided altogether by any pregnant woman. The dangers of crashes and abrupt stops are obvious. The impact of the steering wheel, seatbelt, or a deployed airbag could strike a devastating blow to your belly. If you absolutely have to continue this dangerous sport, stop by week twenty of your pregnancy.

dancing

Dancing is a great way to get your exercise, whether the moves are ballet, modern, jazz, tap, salsa, Afro-Caribbean, hip-hop, or ballroom. Even a beginner can start dancing and continue through to the end of pregnancy. As always, however, there are a few guidelines to follow.

Avoid fast turns, pivoting movements, and quick changes of direction. Dancing on your toes or in high heels could cause your calves to cramp unless you are well trained. In ballet, be aware of your knees if you have to do pliés (knee bends performed with the legs turned out). It is best to avoid grand pliés (deep bends) altogether, and stick to demi-pliés (half-bent). Press down through your heels, not through your toes. Doing relevés (raising the heels of both feet) is not a good idea unless you are a professional dancer.

Dancing can vary in intensity from very slow to strenuous. Use your best judgment to modify your program. If practiced enough, dancing can have a great toning effect on the entire body, but it can always be complemented with some strength training. Stretch your entire body after a dance session or class.

exercise videos

The viability of exercise videos depends on the type of program they describe. Avoid any video that was not specially designed for pre- or postnatal women, unless you have used it many times and know how to modify the exercises to suit your changing biomechanics.

There are not many prenatal videos available, and they vary in quality. There will surely be many more made available in the future. Ideally, pick a video that incorporates the new pregnancy exercise guidelines from 1994. If you can, rent the videos first so you can test them out before buying. You want something that will motivate you. Older videos with high ratings and recommendations from fitness magazines are Kathy Smith's *Pregnancy Workout* and *Buns of Steel: Pregnancy Workout.*

golf

Golf, a very low intensity and non-impact sport, is relatively safe to participate in during your pregnancy whether you are a pro or a beginner. However, if you are considering making this your main form of exercise, walk the course. Just swinging a golf club and driving a cart is not sufficient exercise.

The slightly bent over position requires good posture and proper alignment to prevent back strain. Keep your back as straight as possible and keep both abdominals and lower back muscles tight for support. Golfers often end up with back pain or injured rotator cuff muscles from the unnatural rotating body movement.

To counteract postural weaknesses caused by the golf stance and swing, work out your upper back, rear shoulder muscles, and triceps. To prevent injuries, strengthen the quadriceps, hamstrings, abdominals, lower back, and rotator cuff muscles.

Swing carefully, don't come down too hard on the ball, and watch out for your belly. Halfway through your pregnancy, the golf stance may crowd your belly somewhat, and your swing will definitely be affected by your size, but these are game concerns, not health problems.

Play at least three days a week if this is your only exercise. Do not carry your golf bag yourself. Instead, wheel it around on a pulley-cart or have someone else carry it for you. Bring water and some snacks with you, and do not be afraid to run to the nearest restroom whenever you can.

An eighteen-hole golf game can take four to six hours if the course is very busy. You may want to stick with a shorter nine-hole game. Do not play at all on hot or humid days. When you feel uncomfortable, or are just too big to swing a golf club, switch to walking or to pool exercises. (You can practice your swing in the pool.)

As always, do not forget to warmup first. Twisting, stretching, or hitting balls on the driving range are all good warmups. After the game, stretch your hip flexors, chest, shoulders, and arms.

gymnastics

(Including balance beam, parallel and uneven bars, ring work, vaulting, and floor exercises) Gymnastics require enormous strength, endurance, agility, flexibility, speed, balance, and precision. Landing and dismounting can be risky if not executed perfectly. Handsprings, cartwheels, twists, somersaults, and similar movements can be dangerous. Though it hasn't been scientifically proven, many believe that inverted exercises increase the risk of breech birth by confusing the baby's sense of direction.

Even if you are an Olympic gymnast, until more research has been conducted, avoid any of these activities as soon as you know that you are pregnant. The risk of injury is just too high. You can, of course, continue stretching to stay flexible. However, stretch statically or use the PNF method (passive stretching by a partner or coach) and don't bounce. You can also practice some plyometrics in the pool to stay agile.

hiking

Naturally, hiking uphill is harder than walking on a flat surface. However, it is a good low-impact activity to continue throughout your pregnancy. Hiking strengthens the back of your legs and buttocks. If you are a beginner, begin a regular walking program before attempting hills or mountains.

Use the same techniques described in Walking, but keep your arm movements smaller and bend your knees more. Lean forward from your ankles, not your waist. Your body should be in a straight line from the back of your heels to the top of your head.

The higher the altitude, the more slowly you should climb. Do not exercise at higher than 8,000 feet above sea level. It may be okay to hike at up to 6,500 feet above sea level if your body has adjusted to the altitude (wait four or five days if you are on vacation).

When walking downhill, do not rush along or just let your toes slap down. Make sure to always place your heel down first when walking, and control your gait from the heel to the ball of your foot by using the shin muscles (tibialis). Be sure to stretch your quadriceps, hamstrings, hip flexors, glutes, shins, and calves afterward. Avoid rock climbing completely while pregnant.

horseback riding

If you do not ride on at least a weekly basis, stop once you become pregnant. Riding requires very good balance, and even if you are a good rider, you cannot always predict what the horse is going to do.

Only if you are a very experienced rider and know your horse very well should you continue riding for a while. But avoid hills, aggressive riding like cantering, galloping, and jumping, or anything that may cause you to fall off the horse. Trotting is fine, unless it makes you uncomfortable. I do not recommended any type of riding past the first trimester. Polo should be avoided completely.

Sprinting—running at top speeds for short distances—is too strenuous for any pregnant woman to do safely after the sixteenth week.

ice skating and rollerskating

These exercises can be very risky and unpredictable. If you are a professional athlete or are very proficient at these sports, you can probably continue at least throughout the first trimester. However, they are definitely out for pregnant novices.

If you do continue with these sports, modify and slow down your activity. Skate on a smooth, even surface. Do it regularly, not sporadically, so you will stay well trained. Wear all of the protective gear available. In the third trimester, you should stop altogether due to the increased risk of falling.

Substitute your skating with slide or lateral training. You may do this on a smooth surface or in the pool. You can keep your thighs strong with adductor and abductor exercises (only if you are already experienced at these), leg curls, supported squats, and lunges. Stretch the hip flexors, external rotators, abductors, adductors, and the lower back afterward.

jogging, running, and sprinting

Jogging or running should be fine so long as you ran before you became pregnant. Some women who begin a walking program in pregnancy may feel fine advancing to a light jog. Sprinting—running at top speeds for short distances—is too strenuous for any pregnant woman to do safely after the sixteenth week. If you smoke, are asthmatic or hypertensive, or are a high-risk pregnancy, avoid any form of running.

A good supportive running shoe and a sturdy sports bra or two are a must. To reduce the impact on your joints, run on a soft surface like grass, sand, or an electric treadmill. Manual treadmills are unreliable, and when your balance is a bit off, that could be positively dangerous.

Because of softer joints, you may not have proper control over your feet and ankles, so make sure that the running surface is level. Don't be surprised if you are not able to run as far, or for as long, as you are used to. When you find that running no longer works for you, switch to speed walking or running in the pool.

If bouncing becomes uncomfortable, wear a maternity belt during your run. If your belly hurts, you feel short of breath, get dizzy, or have a headache, stop jogging altogether. Your body is giving you a not-so-subtle hint that conditions are too strenuous for you to continue.

Even if you feel fine, be careful not to overexert or overheat. Drink lots of water. As with walking or hiking, exercise with a friend or stay close to a phone. After running, stretch all your other leg muscles, particularly the hip flexors, hamstrings, and calves.

jump rope and plyometrics

A plyometric move is any movement that requires you to lift both of your feet off the ground at the same time. This category includes jumping rope, running hurdles, or doing any forward, backward, or lateral jumps either on a flat surface or on and off boxes and platforms. These moves are not for pregnant beginners.

You may, depending on your fitness level continue plyometrics for a little while. Just reduce the intensity as your pregnancy progresses. When the jumps become uncomfortable, eliminate them from your program. You may then either practice plyometrics in a pool or choose another exercise. After a plyometric workout, strengthen the hamstrings and stretch all muscle groups.

martial arts and contact sports

(Including kickboxing, karate, judo, tae-bo, tae kwon do, t'ai chi, and judo) Martial arts can help you develop better muscle control, breathing techniques, relaxation methods, and concentration skills. All of these can decrease tension, which could be very beneficial during labor. Martial arts also teaches self-esteem and inner strength, which are important during pregnancy. However, contact forms of martial arts—including karate, judo, tae kwon do, fencing, and kickboxing—are dangerous during pregnancy. The jarring effect of hitting somebody or striking a boxing bag may become uncomfortable after the first trimester. Worse yet is the potential of getting hit by somebody else, especially in your stomach. Only experienced martial artists should continue this form of exercise. Beginners should not attempt to start a martial arts program, with the possible exception of t'ai chi.

T'ai chi is a slow, meditative form of exercise, known for its relaxation and strengthening benefits. T'ai chi includes balancing movements that require standing on one leg. You may want to avoid those positions, but otherwise you may practice this activity without fear of strain or injury. However, you should complement t'ai chi with some kind of cardiovascular exercise.

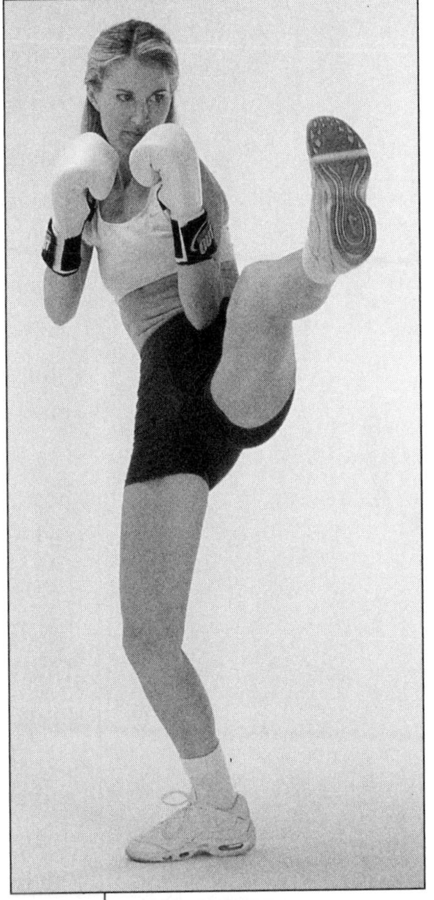

Birgitta kickboxing

For experienced athletes continuing with more strenuous forms of martial arts, the following guidelines will help you modify for pregnancy. Practice your kicks, punches, and jabs without a partner. After the first trimester, practice without a bag. Avoid sparring, jumping, and mid-air turning kicks.

You may be able to continue shadow-boxing or kicking (without a bag) through the second trimester, but always be aware of fetal movements and any pubic pain or contractions. The martial arts are very intense activities, so slow down as you see fit. Until there has been more research, stop and choose another activity in the third trimester or simulate your moves in the pool.

For kickboxing, follow the same guidelines as for martial arts and boxing programs. Avoid the competitive version of this sport. Cardio-kickboxing is the aerobic form, which usually doesn't involve sparring. Kickboxing requires punches and kicks in every direction imaginable, and therefore strengthens and tones the entire body. The kicks require a lot of agility, balance, and coordination. Hold on to a ballet bar along the wall or something else that is stable while practicing kicks. Tae-Bo, which combines tae kwon do movements with dance, involves similar moves; you can adapt it as you would kickboxing.

The dangers of wrestling to pregnant women are obvious. Eliminate it from your program.

For boxing, follow the same guidelines as for martial arts programs. Boxing strengthens and tones the upper body very well, but the typical boxing stance tends to round the upper back and shoulders. Add rear shoulder, trapezius, and leg strengthening exercises to your workout. Stretch your chest, arms, and lower back to straighten out your posture.

For all of these activities, avoid overexertion, and drink plenty of water before, during, and after your workout. Make sure to warmup thoroughly before exercising and stretch your muscles afterward. Most martial arts classes do not include a stretching session after class.

pilates

Pilates, which is enjoying a resurgence in popularity lately, is an exercise program developed by Joseph Pilates in Germany more than eighty years ago. It involves controlled movements usually performed using a special apparatus. Its pulleys, springs, and sliding bench system create non-impact exercises that are beneficial to pregnant women. The Pilates machine offers superior methods over regular weight training during pregnancy, as most of the upper body exercises are performed seated.

Pilates exercises develop balance, control, strength, flexibility, alignment, posture, and most important for a pregnant woman, trunk strength and stability. With modifications and proper supervision, even a novice may start Pilates during pregnancy. Because the cost of Pilates equipment can be prohibitive, this is probably not an activity you will undertake at home. Find a Pilates studio or a gym that offers Pilates, and make sure your instructor is knowledgeable about modifications for pregnancy.

Do not do any of the unsupported, inverted, or prone position exercises, and avoid supine positions if they make you dizzy. After the first trimester, many of the footwork exercises can be done seated by propping the bench up sideways behind your back or using a special C-curve spine supporter. You can also lie on your side for certain exercises. Unless you are very well trained, the footwork should be done with the heels, instead of the toes, on the foot bar. Avoid full relevés up on your toes to prevent leg cramps.

Be careful with some of the abdominal exercises that do not offer back support. These are probably best avoided after the first trimester. Even if you are well trained, do not lift your hips higher than your chest.

The lateral breathing technique practiced in Pilates can be very beneficial to any pregnant woman. Instead of trying to fill your lungs in a downward fashion, which becomes almost impossible in the later stages of pregnancy, lateral breathing lets the rib cage flare out sideways and backward for additional space. Mastering this technique requires practice. Please see Breathing Techniques in chapter 7 for more details.

racquet sports

(Including tennis, racquetball, squash, badminton, ping pong) Racquet sports demand speed, agility, technique, balance, coordination, and endurance. Though they can be very strenuous, they are not purely aerobic because of the stop-and-start nature of the action. Depending on how you play, these sports can be considered anything from low to high impact, and low to high intensity.

Pregnant beginners or sporadic players are not encouraged to continue racquet sports, with the exception of ping pong. If you are an avid or professional player, you should be able to keep going for at least a few months. Most tennis players stop by the fifth month due to a loss of balance or coordination. If you need to give it up, try playing toy-racquetball games in the pool. If you continue, and if anyone dares to play with you, you may need to slow down your game or play doubles instead of singles. Avoid active competition after the first trimester. There is not only the risk of you taking a fall, but also a chance that the ball will hit your belly. Keep it light and easy—there will be plenty of time to beat your opponent after you have your baby.

You will have to modify many of your moves if you want to continue playing throughout pregnancy. Some positions, like the ready stance in tennis, may crowd the uterus, while others may strain your back. Be careful not to lunge at the ball, as overstretching or fast moves can strain your joints. Your knees will be especially vulnerable, but you can prevent injuries by strengthening your quadriceps, hamstrings, calves, and inner thighs, and by wearing elastic knee supports. To prevent any shoulder problems such as rotator cuff strains, strengthen this area with shoulder and special rotator cuff exercises.

Be very aware of heat stress. It can get very hot out on a tennis court or in a badly ventilated indoor racquetball court. Keep lots of water handy and take a break if you feel overheated. Warm up before playing, and stretch and cool down afterward.

Ping pong, with its hollow plastic ball and smaller playing area, poses fewer risks to the pregnant woman. This game is acceptable throughout pregnancy, but try to avoid jumping and fast turns.

Rowing machines provide a good low-impact, non-weight-bearing form of exercise, which especially works the upper back muscles.

rowing and rowing machines

If you are experienced at rowing a boat or a canoe, you can probably continue for as long as you feel comfortable. However, halfway through your pregnancy, you may want to switch to an indoor rowing machine, as the change in your center of gravity and the accompanying loss of balance increase your risk of falling into the water. Whitewater rafting shouldn't be considered at all during pregnancy due to the risk of capsizing, and the possibility of vaginal infection if the water is dirty or contaminated.

Rowing machines provide a good low-impact, non-weight-bearing form of exercise, which especially works the upper back muscles. Rowing machines are suitable for beginners. However, they can be troublesome for pregnant women—as your belly grows, you may have difficulty pulling your elbows back far enough to properly perform this exercise. Also beware of back strain due to leaning forward to grasp the handles. After rowing, stretch your hips, hamstrings, arms, and upper back.

scuba diving, snorkeling, and diving

Snorkeling is safe as long as you can breathe properly through the snorkel. However, scuba diving below sixteen feet can be very risky. Some of the potential dangers include decompression sickness from the change in water pressure, too much oxygen supply, too much carbon dioxide in the blood, and asphyxiation. Until more research has been done, avoid scuba diving for the duration of your pregnancy.

Diving is also not recommended as it could cause a blow to the belly, or force water up through the vagina and into the uterus.

skiing

(Including downhill, cross country, ski machines, snowboarding, and waterskiing) If you are an advanced and well-trained skier, downhill skiing and snowboarding may be okay to continue at a low intensity level. However, there is always the risk of falling or colliding with something. Skiing at high altitudes is a bad idea during pregnancy.

Please put your ego and thrill-seeking tendencies aside and stay away from difficult slopes. Even a mild fall on your behind could shake things up too much after the twelfth week, and a serious tumble or loss of control could result in a blow to the abdomen and really put your pregnancy in jeopardy.

Slide training, special indoor ski-training machines, and isometric squats or plyometric ski-training exercises in the pool can all substitute for your skiing program.

Cross-country skiing, if you are used to it, should be fine to do as long as you feel comfortable. It does require keen balance and can be very strenuous, so it is probably not for beginners. Because both arms and legs are moving simultaneously, cross-country skiing can elevate your heart rate and blood pressure significantly. Listen to your body and slow down your pace as needed.

Ski machines may sound like the ideal exercise alternative for an avid cross country skier. But most cross-country ski machines require you to lean or press your hips and abdomen into a pad for support. This could get uncomfortable or even impossible after the first trimester. Instead, if you have good balance, try practicing cross-country ski moves on a slide trainer by facing the bumpers.

Water skiing, surfing, and the use of Jet-Skis and Wave-Runners are probably all best avoided. Even if you are a regular water skier or surfer, you may fall into the water. This could cause a blow to your belly, or force water into your uterus, which could have detrimental effects. Furthermore, you could inhale dangerous fumes from the motorboat pulling you or from the Jet-Ski or Wave-Runner on which you are riding. It is not worth risking your baby's health for these sports.

If you really want to practice your moves during pregnancy, you can use special water balance boards, such as the Wonder board by Sprint. Avoid balance boards for land use, unless you can hold on to something.

If you must continue water skiing or surfing, make sure to add some abdominal and hamstring strengthening exercises to your workout. Also, stretch hip flexors, piriformis, adductors, abductors, quadriceps, and the lower back afterward. As with any activity, be sure to talk to your caregiver first.

slide and lateral training

This type of exercise has been fading in popularity lately. Beginners should not perform slide aerobics during pregnancy. It may be low impact, but it can be very intense and may put pressure on your pubic bone. It has caused women unaccustomed to the lateral slide movement to go into premature delivery.

However, if you are adept at this exercise, you may continue to slide for as long as you feel comfortable doing so. Still, about halfway through your pregnancy, you may want to consider switching to something else. Sliding demands good balance, good posture, strong abdominals, and strong inner and outer thighs (adductor and abductor muscles). As your belly gets bigger, and your balance gets worse, sliding may simply become too dangerous.

Sliding strengthens muscles in all the right places, such as the inner and outer thighs, hamstrings, buttocks, lower back, abdominals, lower legs, and feet. It does have a tendency to tighten up the piriformis, however, so this needs to be stretched out after sliding.

Make sure to use correct posture. Always push off from the bumper, with your feet and knees turned out slightly. Lean forward, and squat slightly with knees bent as you slide; your knees should be in alignment with your toes. Keep your abdominals tight, and use light flowing arm movements for better balance.

Use only a slide that has adjustable bumpers angled up as well as outward, so that your feet glide gently onto the bumper. If the bumpers are fixed and straight, the outside of your foot will hit the bumper too hard. This could impact your feet, ankles, and knees. Stretch all of your leg muscles and the hip joint in all directions, after a lateral or slide training workout.

When the day comes that you cannot control the sliding movement, cannot see the slide because of your belly, or just feel unstable, stop doing this type of exercise. If you feel pressure on your pubic bone, particularly if the pressure makes walking painful, see your doctor to make sure that the bone is not separating.

spinning

Spinning is an aerobic exercise performed on a stationary bike. It provides a great workout for the legs, glutes, and cardiovascular system. The class instructor will lead you through a simulated mountain bike or road ride—up and down hills and along flat surfaces. Spinning is not for pregnant beginners or for high-risk pregnancies. If you are a healthy, experienced spinner, you should be able to continue until at least halfway through your pregnancy.

Spinning can vary in intensity from moderate to high. Each bike is equipped with a resistance knob, so you can adjust your level of difficulty if you begin to feel out of breath. If you need to rest when the class is on a high speed burst, lower your resistance and coast along for a while.

Try not to lean too far forward as it can crowd the uterus. Spin-cycles are similar to high performance bicycles, and there is a lot of contact with the saddle, which can be uncomfortable. You may want to switch to a recumbent stationary bike late in pregnancy.

Spinning is not for pregnant beginners or for high-risk pregnancies.

Drink plenty of water before, during, and after a spin class. Stretch your quadriceps, hip flexors and rotators, hamstrings, buttocks, and calf muscles afterward. *See also* Bicycling, Stationary and Recumbent Bikes.

stairs, step aerobics, and step machines

Stair machines and step classes are okay for most pregnant women, with a few caveats. Stepping is a low-impact exercise that uses your front thigh muscles (quadriceps), calf muscles, and piriformis. The sciatic nerve runs in between the piriformis. If you already have problems with sciatic pain, stepping may not be for you.

When on a step machine, avoid bending forward. Stand up straight, push down with your heels, and hold the handlebars in front of you or at your side with your fingers pointed forward. Do not lean on the bars with your wrists turned and fingers pointing backwards. You're not just cheating yourself out of burning optimum calories, you may also be placing undo strain on your wrists, elbows, shoulders, and lower back. Keep your abdominals and buttocks tight, your shoulders back, and your chest up. Lift your pelvic floor through each step to help your posture stay straight. Avoid really long or short steps, as a medium stepping motion gives you a good workout while putting less strain on the knees.

If you are a beginner, start in the manual mode on a very low level for about five minutes. As you improve, gradually increase the intensity and duration each week. Your goal is a twenty- to thirty-minute stepping workout. Due to of the nature of this exercise and its potential to cause knee strain, don't do it every day. Alternate it with walking or a similar activity.

There is a fairly new type of cardiovascular machine on the market called the EFX, which you may find in more up-to-date health clubs. This is a fabulous machine for any healthy pregnant woman. It is a non-impact combination step-bicycle-treadmill-ski movement machine, and it feels very different from any other machine you have ever used. I highly recommend it as an alternative to traditional step or stair machines.

Don't try to keep up with elaborate routines—modify by simply stepping up and down or getting off the bench-step and walking in place.

These guidelines apply to bench-stepping in a step class, but there are even more modifications for that exercise. If you are a beginner, step on the floor for a couple of weeks before advancing onto a bench. You might want to observe a class or two before trying it, to see what you are getting into.

Keep your bench-step low, preferably on no risers at all. A step higher than four inches will put too much strain on your knees. If you want to increase your intensity, put more effort into your stepping and add arm movements.

After the first half of your pregnancy, your balance may be off, so avoid any circular movements around, or any hops onto or over, the step. Whether pregnant or not, everyone should avoid the turn-step, a stepping pattern that torques the knees by rotating them in while the feet turn out. As with any aerobics class, avoid classes with complicated choreography or music that is too fast (more than 128 beats per minute) for bench-stepping. Don't try to keep up with elaborate routines—modify by simply stepping up and down or getting off the bench-step and walking in place.

Do not bench-step continuously for more than twenty minutes. If the instructor does not include intervals of floor-stepping, give your knees a break by walking. That way, you can stay for the whole class.

Do not overexert yourself, drink plenty of water, and stop if you feel dizzy, fatigued, or pained. After any kind of stepping, be sure to strengthen your hamstrings and glutes and stretch your quadriceps, calves, lower back, hamstrings, adductors, and piriformis by exercising.

strength training, toning, and weight lifting

Some type of strength, toning, or weight training should be a part of every pregnant woman's workout program. Even a beginner can start a light toning program after conceiving.

The benefits of improved muscle tone and strength are numerous. A strong body will assist you in carrying the added weight of pregnancy, improve your stability and balance, increase your energy level, and improve your sense of well-being and self-esteem. Endorphins produced when you work out will increase your pain threshold, which will be invaluable to you in the delivery room. Physical strength will give you better endurance, strength, and tolerance. After delivery, a strong body will aid you in carrying and nursing your newborn. Strength training can also help minimize your risk of injuries, stretch marks, and varicose veins.

We're not going to get into specific exercises here—chapter 5 contains instructions for a full range of strengthening and toning exercises. The following are general guidelines and safety precautions.

As with everything else, of course, moderation is the key. Do not overwork or strain your muscles. All exercises must be done with the utmost control and balance. Good form and proper breathing techniques are important, as sloppiness will only lead to injuries. Under no circumstances should you take part in powerlifting or Olympic lifting. The strain on your abdominal and pelvic cavity could have severe ramifications.

If you are a beginner, use small movements with light weights. Depending on your strength, you may be able to gradually increase your program to a moderate level. If you have been training with weights prior to getting pregnant, continue the same program but do not increase the intensity. You may even need to lessen the intensity if you find yourself getting easily fatigued.

Always be aware of your breathing. Inhale on the easy part of the exercise and exhale on the exertion. Do not ever hold your breath during any exercise. These actions can cause dizziness or fainting, and could lessen blood flow to the fetus. For the same reasons, avoid exercises that require you to lie on your back after the sixteenth week. Avoid quick, jerky lifts or extremely heavy loads. To avoid leg cramps, do not point your toes, nor should you do the top half of any calf raise exercise.

When using free weights, do not use very heavy weights that require you to strain or bear down; it can cause premature delivery. Instead, use lighter weights and do more repetitions. Check and secure all barbells, dumbbells, or other weights you may be using. There is never a good time to drop a weight on yourself, but doing so during pregnancy is the worst time possible. For safety's sake, always have a friend or instructor spot you.

Preferably, have an instructor who is certified and experienced in prenatal exercise help you design a suitable workout. Your instructor should collaborate with your doctor and use this book as a guide.

If you suffer from chronic hypertension lifting weights over shoulder level or doing any isometric exercise (holding a muscle contraction in a fixed position) is not a good idea. Such maneuvers increase your heart rate and blood pressure unnecessarily. Exercises such as unsupported rowing or unsupported squatting may put excessive strain on your lower back unless you are very well trained.

Weight machines may make it easier for you to maintain balance and controlled movements. They are also safer than free weights. However, some weight machines are not appropriate for pregnant women. Any machine with hip or waist belts, or support pads in front is not designed for you. Avoid any machine that strains your abdomen, pelvis, or lower back, requires you to lay prone or supine, or generally feels uncomfortable. Specifically, I would not recommend the use of hip-and-back machines. After the first trimester, also avoid inner and outer thigh machines if you are a novice.

stretching

Stretching after any exercise or activity should be a priority for everyone, pregnant or not. Stretching helps you to cool down, slow your breathing, and lower your heart rate after a workout. It decreases your chance of injury and delayed muscle soreness. It increases your flexibility by lengthening your muscles and making them more pliable.

When you stretch, take it only as far as you feel comfortable. Do not push into, or worse, past pain or strain. Remember that your tissues and

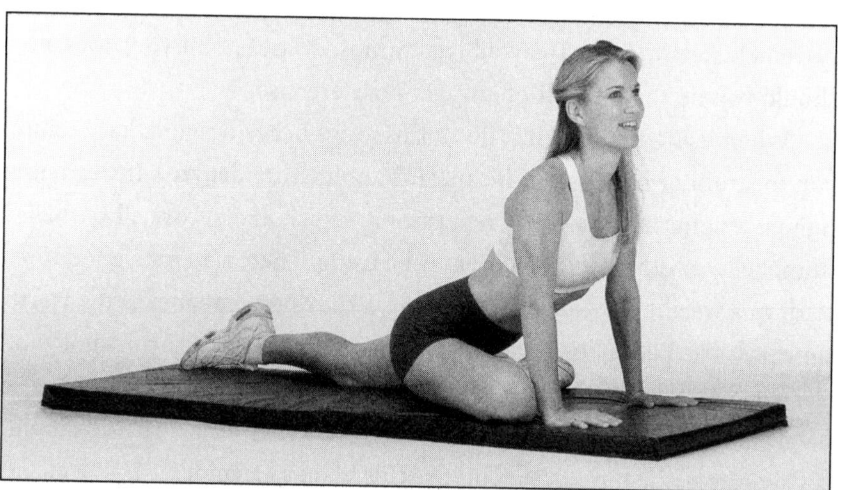

Birgitta stretching

joints are softer during pregnancy and you may tear or injure something. See chapter 7 for more detailed instructions on stretching.

swimming

Pregnant or not, swimming is a great aerobic, non-impact, low intensity exercise that helps strengthen and tone all of your muscles. The buoyancy of the water supports your body (and being pregnant makes you even more buoyant), reduces impact on your joints, and creates resistance for your muscles. It also reduces arthritis pain and is rehabilitative for injuries. As a special blessing to pregnant women, it also seems to reduce water retention.

So long as you are good swimmer, it is almost impossible to hurt yourself in the water. Just be aware of your breathing, which may become more labored because the water puts pressure on your body. Breathe in a regular pattern. During the breast stroke, take a breath on every other stroke. During a freestyle stroke, take a breath on every third stroke. Unless you are a pro, avoid the butterfly stroke during pregnancy, as it excessively arches your back. Swimming on your back is okay so long as you feel no pain or dizziness as a result.

However, never dive or jump feet first into the water. This could cause a blow to the belly, or possibly force water up through the vagina and into the uterus. These actions could cause trauma to the fetus as well as possible infection.

The water temperature should be 82° to 87° Fahrenheit. Wear a good supportive bathing suit or aerobic wear. After swimming, stretch your entire body, particularly your shoulders. *See also* Aquatic Exercise and Sports.

Your Oxygen Supply

Synchronized swimming and water ballet are safe to perform during pregnancy as long as your head remains above water. As with any type of exercise during pregnancy, you should avoid holding your breath to ensure proper oxygen supply to the fetus.

team contact sports

(Including baseball, basketball, football, ice hockey, handball, soccer, and volleyball) Because of your increased weight and shift in center of gravity, as well as the risk of falling, colliding, or getting hit in the stomach, all contact sports are dangerous and are best avoided after the twelfth week. However, a gentle non-aggressive game with your friends may be okay. If you play softball or baseball, do not slide into bases. If you have a basketball hoop at home, shooting free throws would be preferable to engaging in a game, where there is danger of falling, being elbowed, or struck with the ball. If you are a professional athlete, simulate your sport in the pool to keep the appropriate muscles in shape. Stretch all muscles afterward.

track and field and olympic sports

All track and field sports are potentially dangerous for any pregnant woman. Extremely fit and well-trained athletes may continue in the initial stages of pregnancy only. These sports can cause severe breast discomfort in late pregnancy. Sprinting, no matter the length of the track, is too high intensity to be practiced safely during pregnancy. The high jump, long jump, and pole vault are seriously jarring upon landing. Running hurdles is a high-intensity activity that crowds the uterus and also involves the risk of a nasty fall. The javelin and discus can throw off a pregnant woman's balance. However, many of these sports can be simulated in the pool.

The triathlon and decathlon involve so many intense sports that they are just too much for any pregnant woman to participate in, unless the program is severely modified for off-season training only.

walking

Whether you are fit or have never exercised in your life, walking is great exercise. If you are a beginner, start with a five-minute jaunt and slowly add more time each week. A good goal is a twenty to twenty-five minute walk, three to six days a week. Top out at forty-five to sixty minutes, however. If you walk outdoors, take a friend, a cellular phone, or at least some change for a public phone. You never know when you might need assistance. In hot weather, it is preferable to walk on an electric treadmill indoors, where it is climate-controlled and close to a phone. For information about walking on hills or inclines, *see* Hiking.

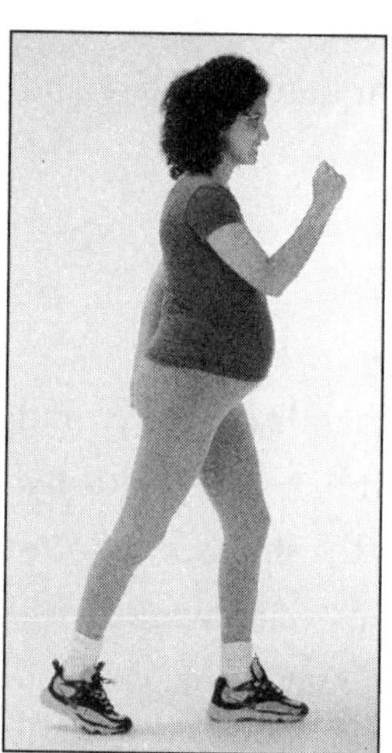

Proper walking technique

Be aware of your posture when walking. It may feel rigid at first, but you are guaranteed to have a better workout if you walk straight, with your chest and chin up, shoulders back, and abdominals and buttocks held tight. Keep your toes up and your arms pumping at a 90-degree angle. After your walk, stretch your hip flexors, quadriceps, buttocks, calves, shin muscles, biceps, and shoulders.

yoga

Yoga is terrific for any pregnant woman. It can increase or maintain muscle tone and flexibility. Yoga promotes proper breathing and alignment, calmness, relaxation, muscle control, and concentration, all of which will help you during labor. You will need to modify some of the exercises or postures with pillows, chairs, or a partner to help you balance. In my experience, inverted positions, head and shoulder stands, prone, and some supine positions should be eliminated completely. Also avoid positions that crowd your uterus, make you stand on your toes, or keep you motionless for a long time, either seated or on your feet. Be careful how far you take a stretch. If it hurts, back off slowly.

Yoga should be complemented with some type of aerobic activity. See more on yoga in chapter 7.

SPORTS AND ACTIVITIES TO AVOID DURING PREGNANCY

CONTACT SPORTS	*WATER SPORTS*	*HIGH ALTITUDE*	*MISCELLANEOUS*
*baseball**	*canoeing**	*ballooning*	*bungee jumping*
*basketball**	*diving*	*downhill skiing**	*gymnastics*
*boxing**	*scuba diving*	*hang gliding*	*horseback riding**
car racing	*water polo*	*hiking**	*ice skating**
fencing	*water skiing*	*mountain climbing*	*rollerskating**
*field hockey**	*whitewater rafting*	*sky diving*	*in-line skating**
*handball**	*synchronized swimming**	*snowshoeing**	*sprinting*
ice hockey		*snowboarding**	*track and field*
*soccer**			*triathlon**
*volleyball**			
wrestling			

* *Some possibilities for modification (with extreme caution) for the first twelve to twenty weeks.*

SPORTS AND ACTIVITIES THAT CAN BE ENJOYED DURING PREGNANCY

LAND EXERCISES	*GYM CLASSES*	*WATER SPORTS*	*RACQUET SPORTS*	*MISCELLANEOUS*
*bicycling**	*aerobics–high impact**	*pool aerobics*•	*badminton**	*bowling*
cross country skiing•	*aerobics–low impact*•	*snorkeling*•	*ping pong*	*calisthenics**
*hiking**•	*cardio-kickboxing**	*swimming*•	*racquetball**	*exercise videos**•
*jogging**	*dancing*•	*water toning*•	*squash**	*golf*
*running**	*funk aerobics*•		*tennis**	*martial arts**■
*jump rope**	*hip-hop aerobics*•			*pilates**
*plyometrics**	*prenatal classes*•			*rowing machine**•
walking•	*slide training**			*ski machine**
treadmill•	*lateral training**			*stair/step machine*•
	*spinning**			*stationary bicycle*•
	step training•			*stretching*•
				*strength and weight training**•
				*tae-bo**
				t'ai chi•
				*yoga**•

* *May need modifications throughout pregnancy. Some of these activities may need to be eliminated in late pregnancy.*

• *Can be started by a novice after becoming pregnant.*

■ *Non-contact*

Chapter Five

the exercises

IN THIS CHAPTER

- *An illustrated tour of the muscles—their function and location*
- *Essential exercises for all pregnant women*
- *Additional exercises you can add to your routine for extra benefit*

This chapter is divided into three sections. First, we'll take you on a tour of the major muscle groups you'll be working, with emphasis on the muscles that need the most work during pregnancy. Next, and perhaps most important, you'll be guided through the essential *must-do* exercises for pregnant women. These are exercises that you absolutely should not do without.

The last portion of the chapter contains a wide variety of exercises for all muscle groups. You can pick and choose from these exercises and switch them around to prevent boredom. If you are not reading this book straight through, do not jump in and start doing these exercises until you have at least read the Precautions and Workout Guidelines in chapter 3. If you are in a high-risk category or on bed-rest, you should skip ahead to chapter 6. Some exercises in this chapter suggest the use of accessories, such as Dyna-Bands, a BodyBar, or a large, inflated ball. These products can be found in most sporting goods stores. You can also modify the exercises to do them without any accessories.

Pregnancy requires you to get creative when designing your exercise program. It also creates special requirements for certain exercises. Your mantra during this time should be modify, modify, modify.

a tour of the body

Before we get to the exercises, you need to understand the location and function of the muscles we will be working, and the reasons each needs to be strengthened or toned during pregnancy.

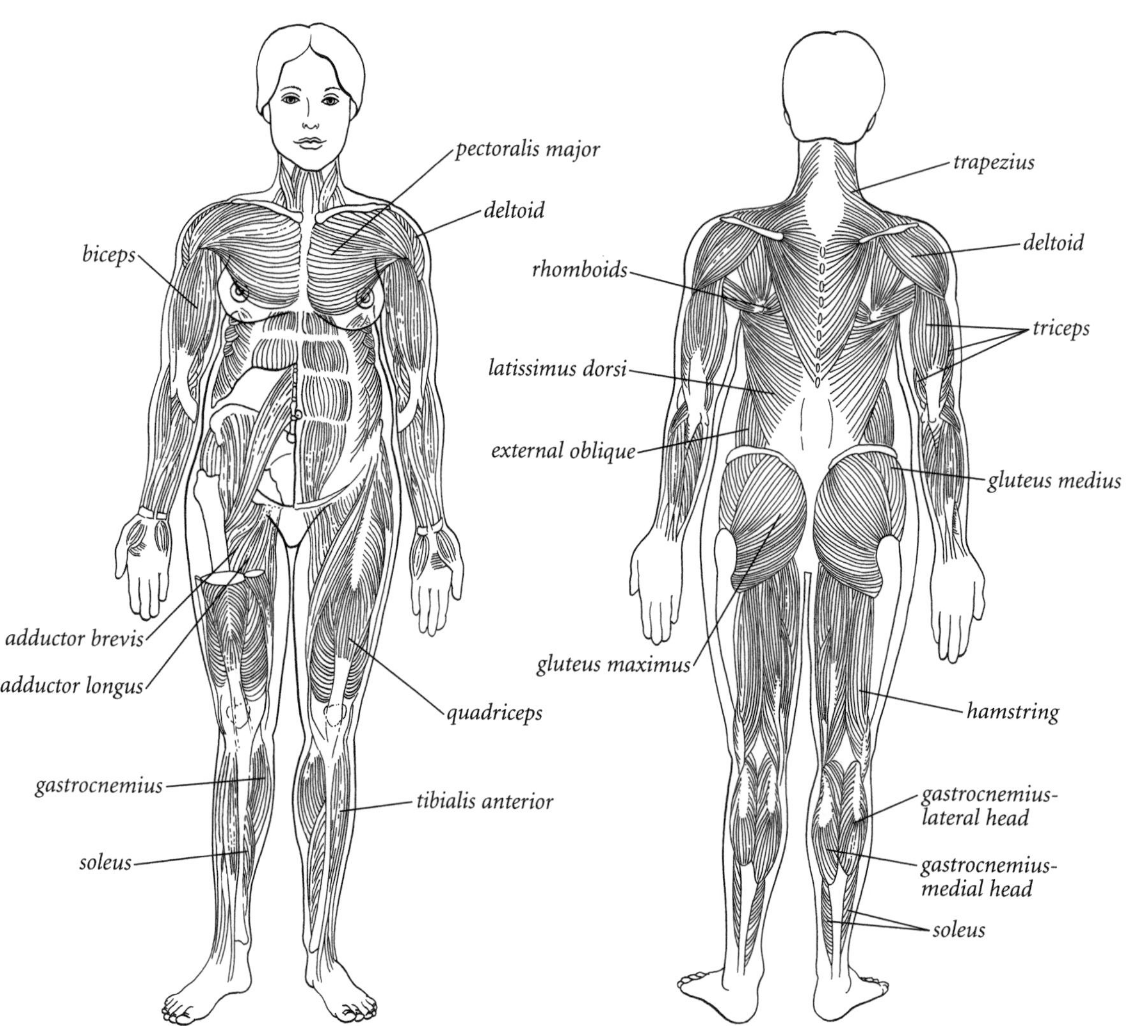

muscle chart front (left) and back (right)

PELVIC FLOOR MUSCLES

These muscles form the perineum and extend like a sling in between the tailbone and the pubic bone. They hold up the abdominal and pelvic cavity like a trampoline. These muscles surround the anus, vagina, and urethra. See page 57 for illustration.

When you are pregnant, these muscles have a much heavier workload. Imagine how hard these tiny muscles have to work, carrying an extra twenty-five to forty pounds for up to nine months. Talk about stamina! In addition, the tissue surrounding the muscles loosens in preparation for the stretching they will undergo in childbirth. This makes the muscles more susceptible to tearing or bruising, especially if you have not trained them for childbirth.

Unfortunately, most exercise programs ignore the pelvic floor muscles. Yet if these muscles are unfit, labor will be more painful, and you may need an episiotomy (an incision made to enlarge the vaginal opening). By doing the proper exercises, you will strengthen and relax the perineum, making it more supple so that you can benefit from a slower and more controlled delivery. The best way to condition the pelvic floor muscles is by performing Kegel exercises.

Kegels are absolutely essential for every pregnant woman. They can reduce labor pain and lessen the risk of tearing or the need for an episiotomy. They also reduce the incidence of hemorrhoids and can minimize or even prevent urinary incontinence.

You will need to do Kegels for the rest of your life—not just while pregnant. Fit pelvic floor muscles increase your sexual enjoyment, prevent future urinary incontinence, and decrease the incidence of other pelvic conditions such as pelvic organ prolapse. A large percentage of gynecological surgeries performed on women older than forty are done to fix a pelvic floor atrophied and weakened by inactivity and/or childbirth. These problems can be minimized or prevented by this simple exercise.

ABDOMINAL MUSCLES

Your abdominals ("abs") consist of several muscle groups, all located in the midsection, just below your chest to your pubic bone. The rectus abdominis is the large, indented muscle that runs down the front of your abdomen. This is the muscle that helps you curl your trunk when doing crunches or sitting up. For exercise purposes, we often refer to upper or lower abs, but the rectus abdominis is really just one muscle. You cannot truly exercise just the upper or lower abdominals. You can pull from different ends—either lifting the hips off the floor (hip curls) or pulling the shoulders toward the hips (crunches), but the whole muscle has to contract. In this way, the abdominal wall works very much like an accordion.

The obliques are the muscles that make up your waist. They help you twist and bend sideways. The transverse abdominals run horizontally around your body. They compress and support your internal organs, and help to hold your stomach flat (if you are in good shape and are not pregnant). They work the best when you're on all fours pulling your stomach up. That's why animals have easier labors than humans—walking on all fours keeps the transverse muscles activated all the time. Together, the obliques and the transverse abdominals balance and stabilize your torso by holding the spine up in place.

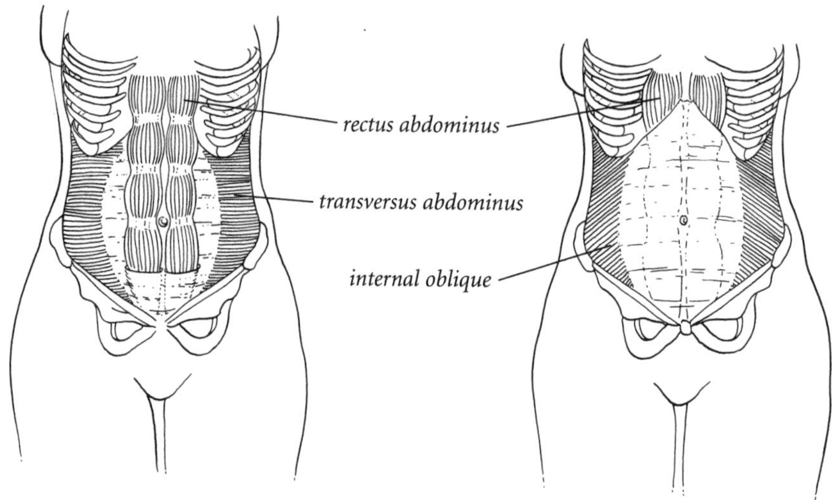

abdominal muscles

No matter how fit and strong your back is, if the abdominal muscles are not strong, you may still suffer from backaches. The abdominals help support and control the curvature of your lower lumbar spine. You can prevent or fix postural problems such as a forward pelvic tilt, sway back (abnormally pronounced sacral curve or backward pelvic tilt), or nagging back pain by strengthening the abdominals.

Labor will be easier, more efficient, and less painful if your abdominals are fit and healthy. Strong stomach muscles will prevent a saggy postpartum midsection, reduce stretch marks, speed up your recovery after delivery, and possibly prevent abdominal separation (diastasis recti).

LOWER BACK

The change in your center of gravity during pregnancy causes your spine to curve differently to counterbalance certain new compressions. Your lower back muscles (erector spinae, quadratus lumborum) will tighten up in an effort to support the new exaggerated spinal curve. Even though your back needs to be strong, strengthening your lower back during pregnancy may only tighten it further. That's probably the reason it's virtually impossible to do any regular lower back strengthening exercises while pregnant. Your spinal extensor muscles need stretching to loosen them. The exercises in this chapter will help.

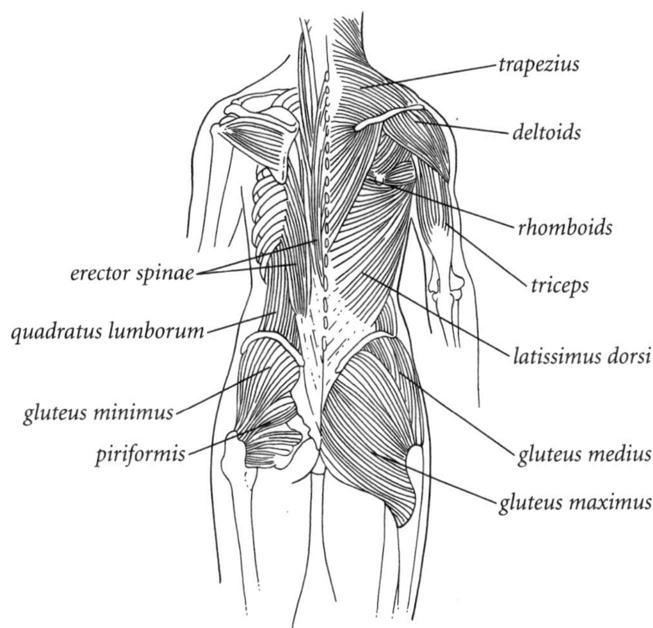

rear view of back and hip rotator muscles

Eighty percent of all backaches in men and women, pregnant or non-pregnant, are caused by inactivity. Stretching your lower back and strengthening your abdominals will give you good trunk support, the foundation for proper posture.

HIPS AND BUTTOCKS

The hip abductors (outer thigh muscles) move your legs out sideways. They include the gluteus medius and minimus, which stabilize your hips when you walk. If you keep these muscles strong when pregnant, you can prevent or minimize the "pregnancy waddle" in the last trimester. Strong outer thighs are also helpful during labor.

The hip adductors (inner thigh muscles) work to bring your legs together. They also work during lunges, stepping, and squats. You can keep them firm with ankle weights, leg lifts, or by squeezing a softball between your knees. But to help you out in labor, they need stretching.

The hip flexors start on the femur, run up through the hip joint, and hook on to the lower back vertebrae. If these muscles get too tight, you may suffer back pain. Strengthening them without stretching them will put you in a perpetually flexed forward position that can lead to a swayed back and waddling. Too much prolonged sitting can also contribute to this problem.

The hip extensor muscles include the "glutes" (gluteus maximus and minimus) and hamstring muscles. The gluteus maximus, which gives the buttocks their shape, straightens and moves your leg backward while the hamstrings bend your knees. By strengthening these muscles you will straighten out your hips and lower back, improving your posture. Working these muscles will also tighten your behind. Leg curls, pelvic tilts, hip lifts, and buttock leg lifts isolates these muscles better than lunges and squats do.

Directly underneath the buttocks, the piriformis (external hip rotators) attach the leg bone to the pelvis. Its principal job is to rotate the hip and leg outwardly, especially when you're bent at the hips. You may feel this muscle working when you do step training, lunges, or squats. Most people think that they are getting a great glute workout, when they are really getting a much greater piriformis workout. The piriformis does more work here than does the gluteus maximus, which works better when the leg is extended backward.

Your sciatic nerve, which is the nerve that goes down the back of your leg, passes through the piriformis muscle, so tightness in the piriformis may pinch on this nerve, causing sciatic pain. Pregnancy itself can contribute to sciatic pain, so you'll want to minimize your chances of developing it by not doing too many lunges or squats. Your best preventive measure is stretching out the piriformis after every workout, as well as after long periods of sitting or driving.

LEGS

Strong legs allow you to move around more easily, improve circulation, minimize varicose veins, and decrease water retention. Strong legs will also help you postpartum when it comes to carrying your baby. During pregnancy, the knee joint may ache from being softer than usual, or from carrying that extra weight. You will probably need to include some knee strengthening exercises to relieve this discomfort. Partial leg extensions, partial squats, or leg curls will do the job.

There are four primary muscle groups in the legs: quadriceps, hamstrings, calves, and tibialis. The quadriceps muscle is located at the front of the thigh, from the pelvis to the knee. The quadriceps muscles straighten the knee. The hamstring muscles (biceps femoris) are located at the back of the thigh and stretch from the buttock to the knee. They are used when you extend your leg backward or bend your knee. The calf muscles (gastrocnemius and soleus) extend from the back of the knee to the achilles tendon. The anterior tibialis is the thin muscle group on the front of your lower leg, which runs along your shins. This muscle functions to flex your foot upward.

UPPER BACK, NECK, AND SHOULDERS

Your upper back and shoulders can easily become rounded, tired, and sore from carrying the extra weight in your belly and breasts. Strengthening the upper back and shoulder muscles will help your posture tremendously and prevent backache both during your pregnancy and afterward. Postpartum, your neck and shoulders will probably get very tired from nursing. You can prevent this by strengthening the trapezius and deltoids. Remember that tired neck, shoulder, and upper back muscles are overstretched and need strengthening, not necessarily more stretching. Of course, a massage will feel pretty good, too.

The trapezius muscle is a large, diamond-shaped muscle that extends from the back of the skull, out to the shoulders, and down to the middle of the back. This is the muscle that works to shrug the shoulders and pull the shoulders back. The rhomboids run beneath the trapezius muscles. The latissimus dorsi ("lats") are the wide muscles that give the back its "V" shape. They originate at the ilium (above the buttocks) and flare from the the spinal column at the middle of the back on both sides, up and out sideways across the midback, and attach under the arms. The main job of the latissimus dorsi is to pull your arm back, down, and toward your body, and to help rotate it inwardly. You use these muscles in actions such as rowing or pulling yourself upward or forward with your arms. The deltoids form the rounded, outer part of the shoulders. These muscles are employed when you raise or twist your arm in any direction.

CHEST

The pectoral muscles ("pecs") cover much of the upper part of the front of the chest. These muscles are mainly used to draw the arm across the body. The breasts lie on top of the pectoral muscles. Even though you need to stretch your pectorals more than strengthen them, a little toning will go a long way toward preventing sagging breasts. This problem is especially common postpartum.

ARMS

Postpartum, you will be amazed at how heavy that little bundle of joy can become. However, by working out both the biceps and the triceps while pregnant, you can lessen the strain later on. The arms may not need a lot of separate work; they get a good workout during most upper back and chest exercises.

The biceps muscle runs along the front of your arm. It is the muscle you are working when you flex your arm. The triceps is the muscle at the back of the upper arm. It functions to straighten the elbow joint, the opposing action of the biceps muscle.

the essential exercises

If you don't do any other form of exercise, it is imperative that you at least do three basic exercises: Kegels, Abdominal Pulses, and Pelvic Tilts. These should be the basic building blocks for any pregnant woman's workout. This section describes these three exercises as well as others for the pelvic floor, abdominal, and lower back muscles. Whether you have a normal or high-risk pregnancy, are super fit or on total bed-rest, these muscles need to be worked to reduce pregnancy discomfort, facilitate a smoother, less complicated labor, and prevent future pregnancy-related problems.

The pelvic floor, abdominal, and lower back muscles are so vital that I have separated them into their own sections in this chapter. After you have mastered these exercises, move on to page 137 for additional exercises you can add to your routine to tone and strengthen other areas of your body.

pelvic floor exercises

KEGELS*

Kegels can be done at almost any time, in any place, and in any position—while sitting, standing, or lying down. You can practice them while working at your desk, driving your car, standing in line. Do not feel self-conscious, no one will know what you are doing. The technique can be tricky to master at first, but practice will make perfect. Do not give up—this is your most important exercise.

Visualize your pelvic floor muscles, starting at the anus. Squeeze the muscles around your anus tightly, as if you have to go to the bathroom. Then relax it. After a few times, focus on the even more important sphincters around the opening of the vagina. Squeeze them tightly and then relax.

Then squeeze and pull the perineum in and up, holding for as long as you can before relaxing. Exhale as you squeeze and pull up, and inhale as you release. Visualize the muscles as if they were on a drawstring and you could pull them in and up.

One way to check the strength of your pelvic floor sphincters is to practice with your husband. Either during lovemaking, or immediately afterward while he's still inside you, squeeze the muscles of your vagina around his penis. If he cannot feel your muscles constrict, they need more work. If he does feel it (and you will know when he does), you have done your homework. Have fun. Do not feel embarrassed: It is very important that you do your Kegels, not just during your pregnancy but every day for the rest of your life. The more children you have, the more important this exercise becomes.

Do five Kegels at a time, holding each one six to ten seconds or longer. Repeat three to four times a day. This should be your minimum target—do more if you can. They are tougher than you think. Five repetitions are about all that they can take at one time. Do your Kegels slowly to increase your perineal awareness and sensitivity. Kegels can also be incorporated into other exercises.

SUPPORTED KEGEL SQUAT**

Hold on to something sturdy for support, such as a desk or table. With your feet about shoulder width apart, squat down as far as you feel comfortable, preferably not lower than a 90-degree knee angle. Keep your back straight, your chest up, your abdominals in, and your knees behind your toes. At the bottom of the squat, do a Kegel squeeze and release before rising. Do not bear down. Use your thighs to push up, pressing through your heels. Inhale as you squat, exhale as you rise. Do two sets of ten to fifteen repetitions. This exercise is great for childbirth preparation.

PELVIC KEGEL TILT

Pull the abdominals in and squeeze your glutes together as you tilt your pelvis forward to round the lower back and exhale. Squeeze the pelvic

Key

- * *Very easy*
- ** *Easy*
- *** *Moderate*
- **X** *Contraindicated*

*Exercises denoted by * are suitable even for "high-risk" pregnancies on bed-rest, by ** are suitable for some "high-risk" category pregnancies, and by *** are not suitable for any "high-risk" pregnancy. Those denoted by an* **X** *are advanced and should be discontinued after sixteen weeks of pregnancy, even for those without risk factors.*

floor muscles at the same time. Release and inhale. Just like regular pelvic tilts, you can do these standing**, seated*, lying sideways*, or on your hands and knees**. As long as you don't feel dizzy, you can also do them while lying on your back*. Repeat ten times for two sets.

PELVIC DRAWBRIDGE**

While lying on your back, or with your shoulders on a bench, ball, or the end of a bed and your lower body on the floor, pull in your abdominals, squeeze your buttocks, lift your hips upward, and do a Kegel. Perform these motions simultaneously and very slowly. Do three levels of lifts. On the first one, lift up just slightly before you release down. On the second, raise your hips a little more. On the third, lift your hips as high as you comfortably can, or until your body is in a straight line from the shoulders to the knees. Remember to never arch your back. Repeat the sequence of three lifts ten times. When finished, gently sit down on the floor.

PELVIC LIFT AND BUTTOCK SQUEEZE**

Recline with your feet on the floor and your upper back and shoulders on a ball or bench. Keep your feet apart for balance. Place your hands on the floor if you need additional stabilization. Squeeze your buttocks and lift the pelvis upward. This is a fairly small movement. Repeat fifteen times for two sets. Prior to the sixteenth week, you may do this while lying supine on the floor.

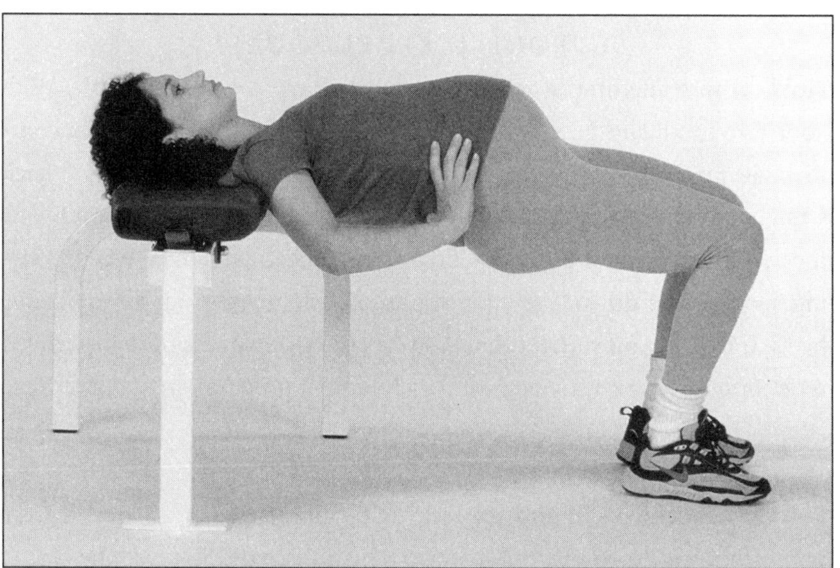

pelvic lift

abdominal exercises

Prior to doing abdominal exercises, you should check for diastasis recti, a painless abdominal separation, by feeling along the linea alba, the line that runs vertically down the center of the abdominal wall. Diastasis recti can be caused by weak abdominals being overstretched by the growing belly. If you feel a separation (it feels like a hole you can stick a finger into), you need to modify your abdominal exercises to prevent it from worsening.

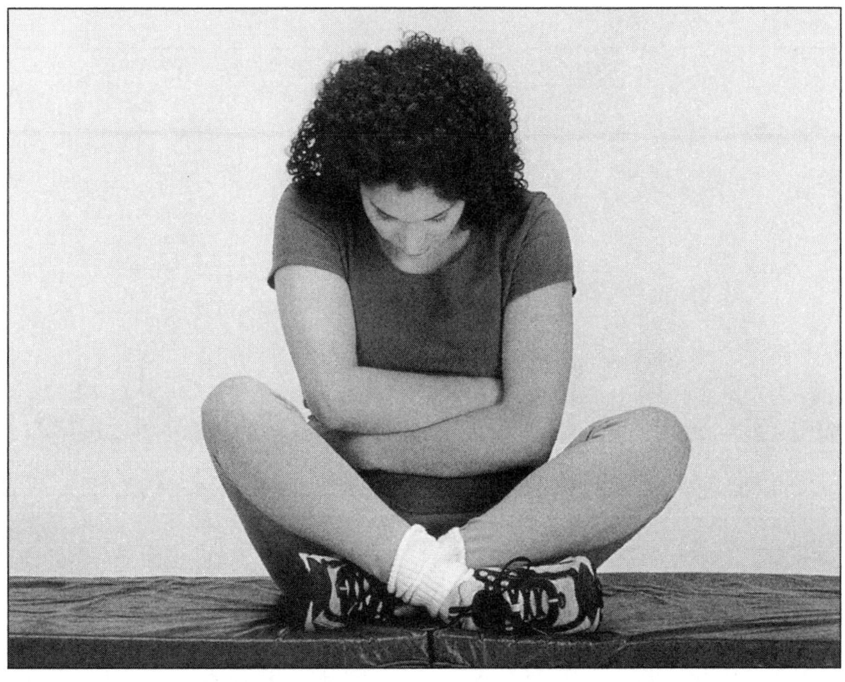

seated modified crunch

Abdominal exercises will not cause diastasis recti, but unrestricted, unmodified exercise may make it worse. In my personal opinion, working the abdominals may actually prevent diastasis recti. There is no research to confirm this theory, but none of my clients has ever had it, and many other prenatal instructors share my opinion.

To modify stomach exercises, hold or wrap your hands or a towel around the sides of your belly and pull the abdominals and obliques in toward the midline as you crunch. The stronger and healthier your abdominals are, the faster this separation will mend itself postpartum. After delivery, the same modified crunches and other abdominal exercises can speed the healing. For more information on diastasis recti, see pages 67–68.

ABDOMINAL PULSE*

Tailor-sit (on buttocks with legs crossed) against the wall or in bed. Or sit on a chair with your hands on your stomach. Inhale and let your lungs expand with air. Relax your abdominals. Exhale and contract the abdominals tightly by pulling them in. Repeat ten to fifty times for two sets. In late pregnancy, you may need to lift your arms out to the side to accomplish this. However, if practiced regularly, there is no reason why your abdominals should not be able to contract even at nine months.

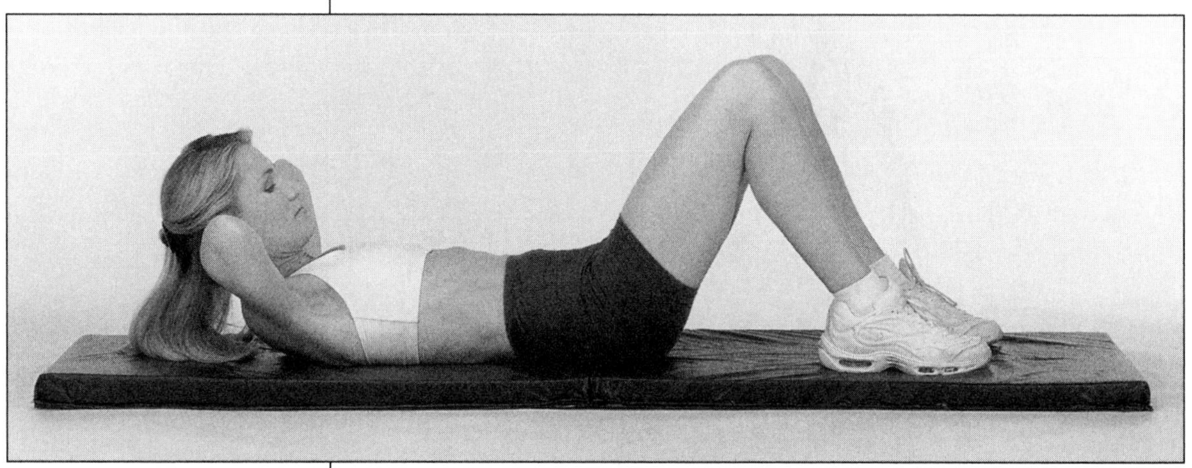

abdominal crunch

ABDOMINAL CRUNCH**

Lie on your back, with knees bent and arms forward or behind your head. Lift your shoulders off the ground toward your hips until your abdominals are tightly flexed. This is not a sit-up; do not raise more than your shoulders off the floor. Exhale as you rise, and inhale as you slowly lower back down. Repeat for two sets of ten to twenty repetitions.

This exercise will get more difficult the closer you get to your twentieth week of pregnancy. If lying on your back makes you dizzy, discontinue.

OBLIQUE CRUNCH**

Start on your back with your knees bent. Keep your left hand behind your head for support. Keeping your left shoulder down, stretch your right hand diagonally toward the inside of the left thigh, raising the right shoulder and flexing the left obliques. Exhale as you rise and inhale as you lie down. Repeat for two to three sets of ten to fifteen repetitions on each side.

HIP CURL**/**X**

Begin by lying on your back with your knees bent and raised off the floor. You can place your arms lying at your sides or put them behind your head. Contract the lower abdominals, curling the pelvis and hips up off the floor. Even if you raise your hips up only one-half inch, it will have some benefit. Make sure to keep breathing; exhale as you rise and inhale as you release slowly. Repeat this exercise for two to three sets of ten to fifteen repetitions.

After twelve to sixteen weeks of pregnancy, this exercise will crowd the uterus, leaving your back without enough support, and making blood circulation very difficult. At that time, replace this exercise with seated or side-lying knee lifts.

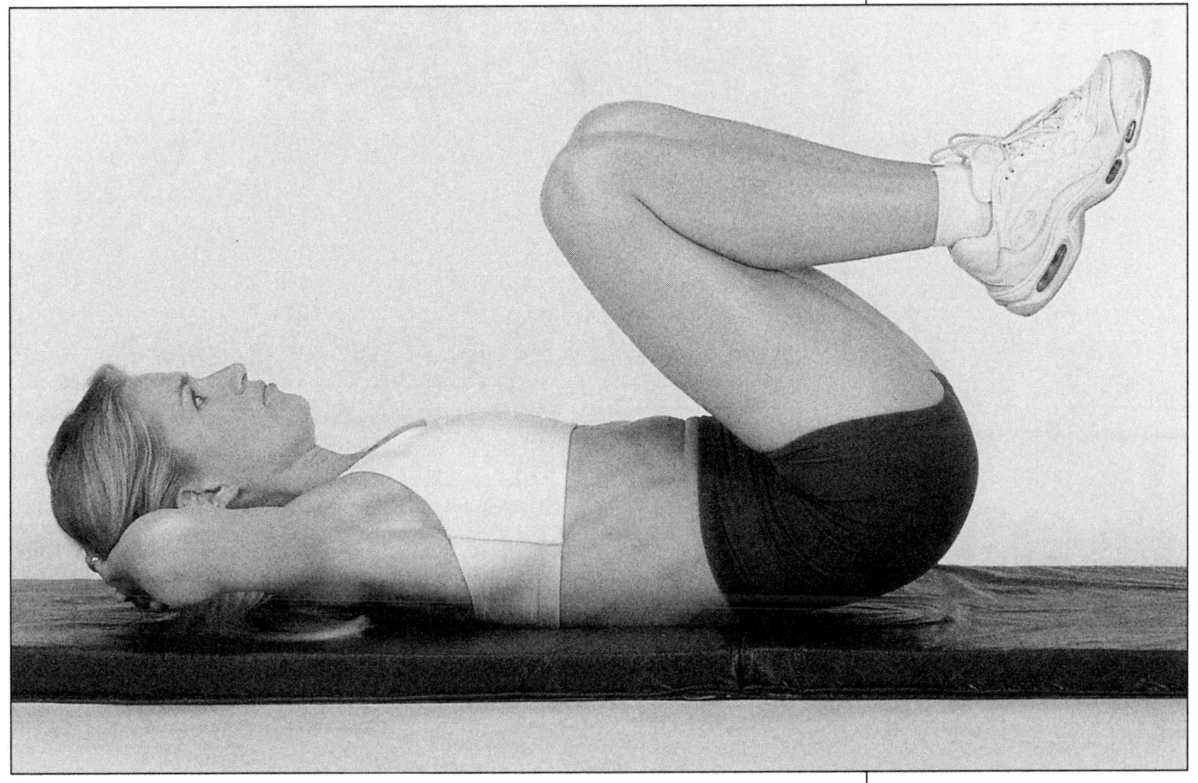

hip curl

SEATED KNEE LIFT**

Sit on a chair, bed, or bench. Pull your belly in and lift your left knee up toward your left shoulder by flexing the lower left abdominal and oblique muscles. Exhale as you lift your knee and inhale as you lower it. You should not feel this as much in your hip flexor as in the abdominals. Repeat ten to fifteen times with each leg for two sets.

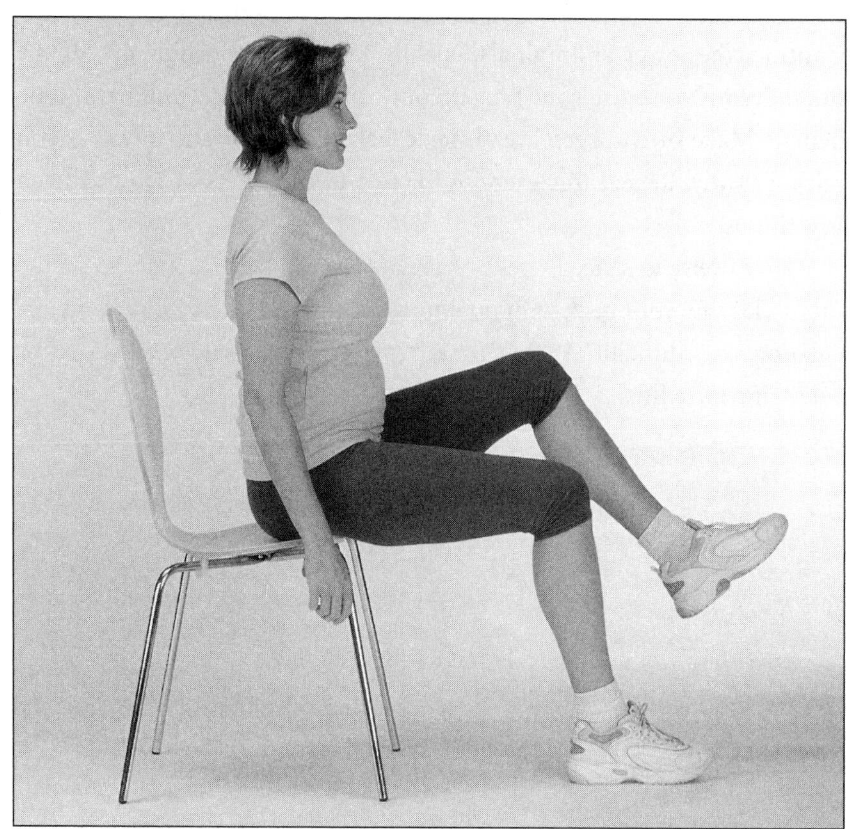
seated knee lift

SIDE-LYING KNEE LIFT*

Lie on your right side, with your right leg bent for support and your head down to keep the spine straight. You can use your right arm to support your head. Flex your left obliques, pulling your left knee toward your left shoulder. Exhale. Straighten the leg and inhale. Repeat ten to fifteen times on each side.

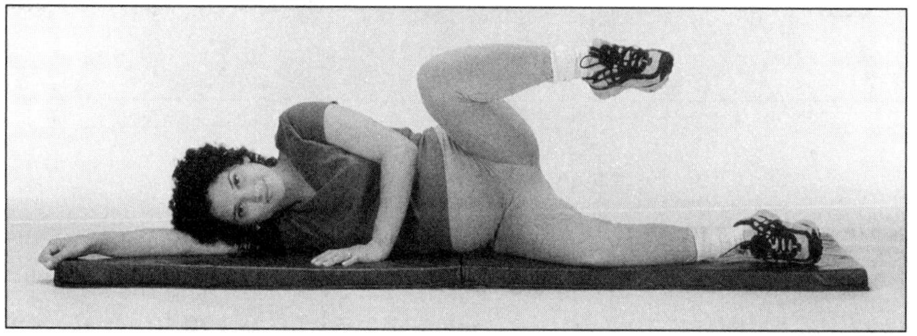
side-lying knee lift

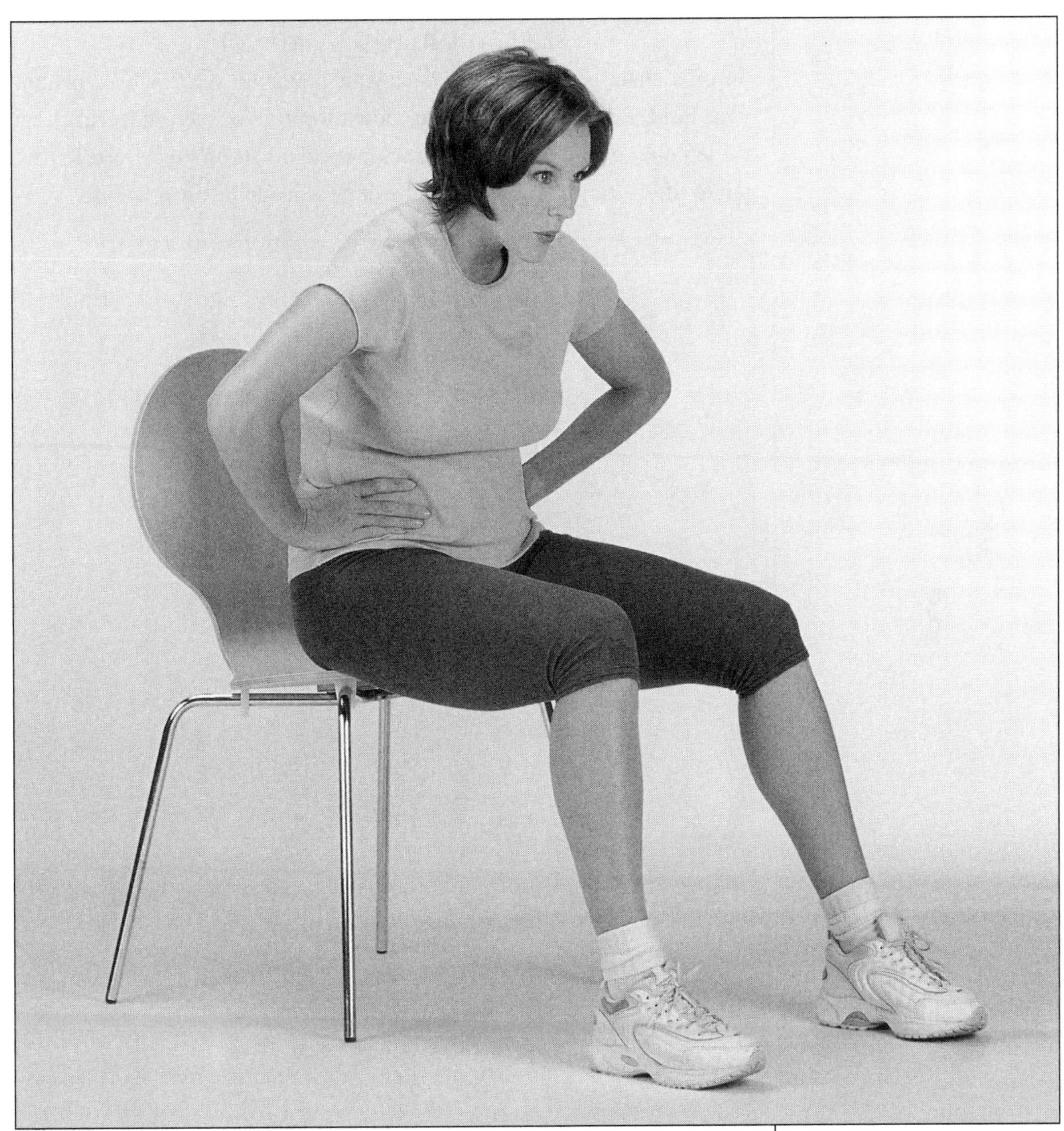

SEATED CRUNCH*

seated crunch

Sit on a chair, bench, or bed with your hands on your belly or behind your head. Contract the abdominals from the top, downward. Exhale as you crunch, inhale on the release. Repeat for two to three sets of ten to fifteen repetitions. Of course, the bigger your belly gets, the more difficult this exercise will become.

SEATED OBLIQUE CRUNCH*

Sit on a chair, bench, or bed. Place your hands on your belly or behind your head. Pull your left shoulder down toward your left hip, crunching the left obliques. Exhale while crunching and inhale on the release. Repeat ten to fifteen times. This can also be done while lying on your side.

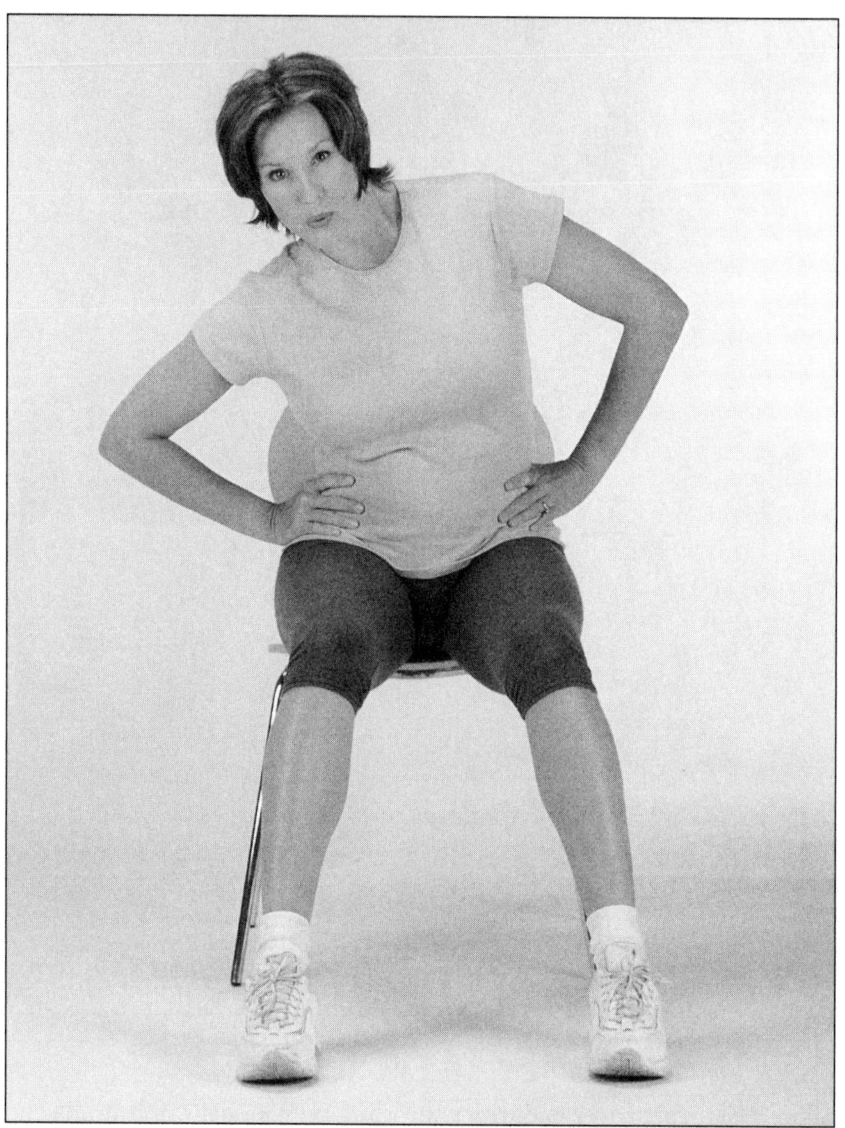

seated oblique crunch

SIDE-LYING ABDOMINAL CONTRACTION*

Lie on your side with your knees bent in front of you and your hands on your belly or behind your head. Contract and pull in your abdominals as

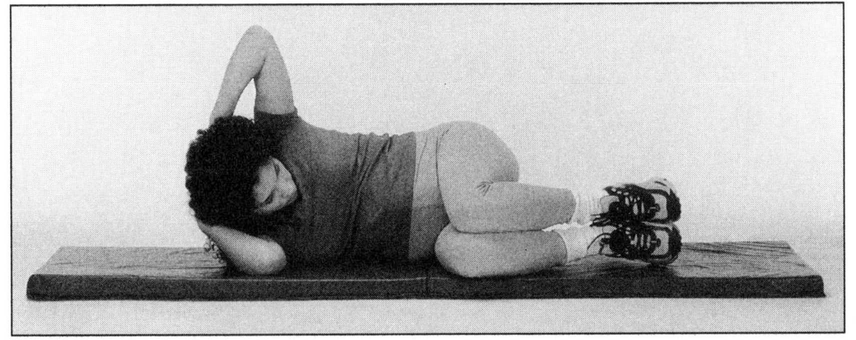

side-lying abdominal contraction

much as you can and exhale. Release and inhale. Repeat ten to fifteen times for two sets. Of course, the bigger your belly gets, the more difficult this exercise will become.

PELVIC TILT

This exercise can be done supine**, standing**, seated*, side lying*, on all fours**, or on ball**. Sit on the ball and walk forward, rolling with it until your shoulders and head are resting on top of the ball. Pull the abdominals in and contract your glutes as you tilt your pelvis forward to round the lower back and exhale. Release and inhale. Repeat ten times for two sets.

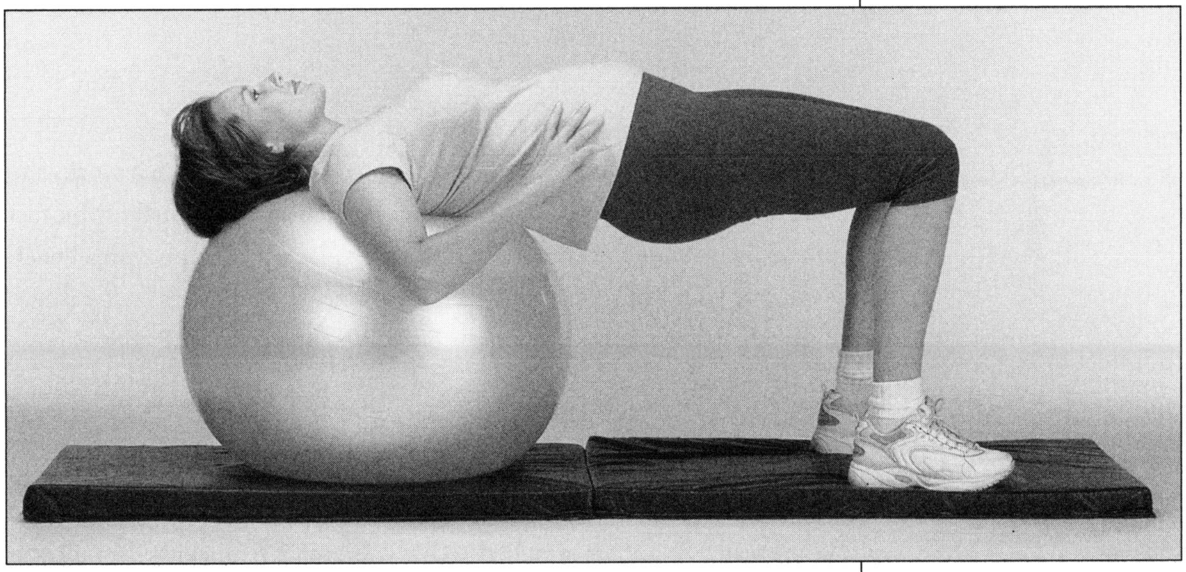

pelvic tilt on ball

PLANK POSE**

Position yourself on all fours, supported by your forearms and knees, or if you are very strong, on your forearms and toes. Your body should be in a

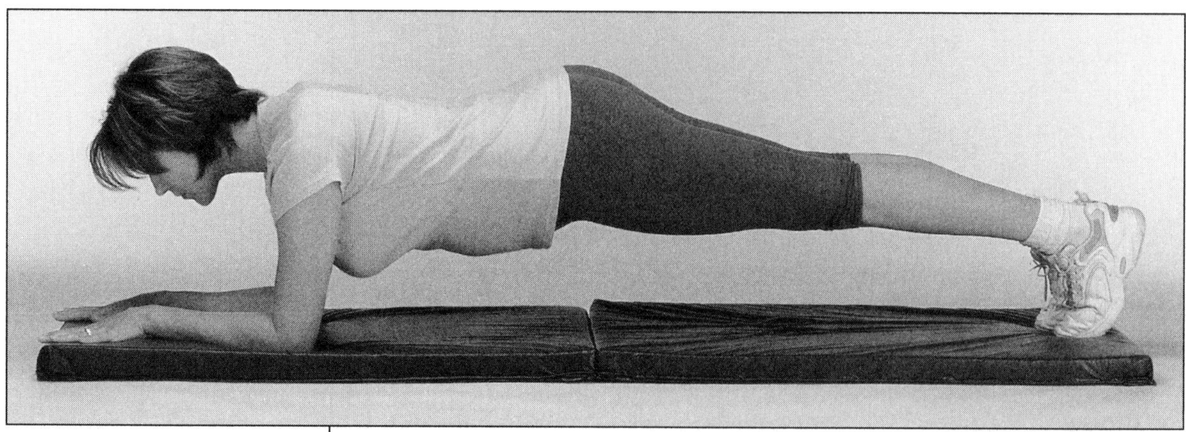

plank pose

straight line from your knees or heels to your shoulders. Pull your stomach in and up as much as you can. Hold the pose for five to fifteen seconds. Or, if you are very strong and there is no strain on your back, hold for up to one minute. If you are doing this exercise on your toes, add a pelvic tilt. Repeat two to three times.

As your pregnancy progresses, this yoga-type exercise may become too uncomfortable or make you dizzy. In that case, either discontinue or try elevating your elbows onto a low bench or chair. Postpartum, you will find that this exercise is great to flatten your stomach again.

lower back exercises

Many of these exercises require you to be on all fours (which works the transverse abs as well as the lower back). If that position makes you feel dizzy, discontinue the exercise or modify by placing your arms on a bench to elevate your head above the level of your heart. Because the latter stages of pregnancy will cause your lower back to be in a perpetually flexed position, the goal of most of these exercises is to stretch rather than strengthen the lower back.

PELVIC TILT*

While seated in a chair or in bed, rotate your pelvis by tucking the tailbone and hips in and under. Think of your pelvis as a salad bowl that is tipped forward and is about to spill its contents and you're tilting backward to prevent it. Contract and pull in your abdominals. You can also add a Kegel squeeze. Repeat for two to three sets of ten to fifteen repetitions. This exercise can also be done standing against a wall with your knees slightly bent**, or lying in bed on your side if you are on bed-rest*.

CAT STRETCH (PELVIC TILT ON ALL FOURS)**

If you've ever seen a cat arch its back, you'll understand how this exercise got its name. Position yourself on all fours, with your back straight but relaxed (don't let it sag). Take a deep breath in. Exhale as you pull in the abdominals, round the spine up, and tuck the hips and pelvis in and under. For maximum benefit, add a Kegel. Release and inhale. Repeat for two sets of ten to fifteen repetitions.

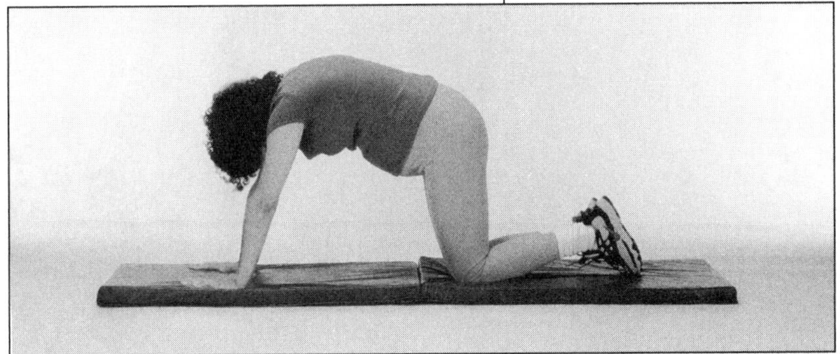

cat stretch

OPPOSITE ARM AND LEG RAISE**

Position yourself on all fours, with your back straight and abdominals pulled in. Slowly extend the left leg, then the right arm up in a straight line. Hold for a couple of seconds before lowering. Do ten to fifteen repetitions, then repeat using the opposite limbs. Do two sets. If it's difficult to maintain balance while doing this exercise, extend just one arm or leg at a time. (This is the only exercise you can do while pregnant to strengthen your back.)

opposite arm and leg raise

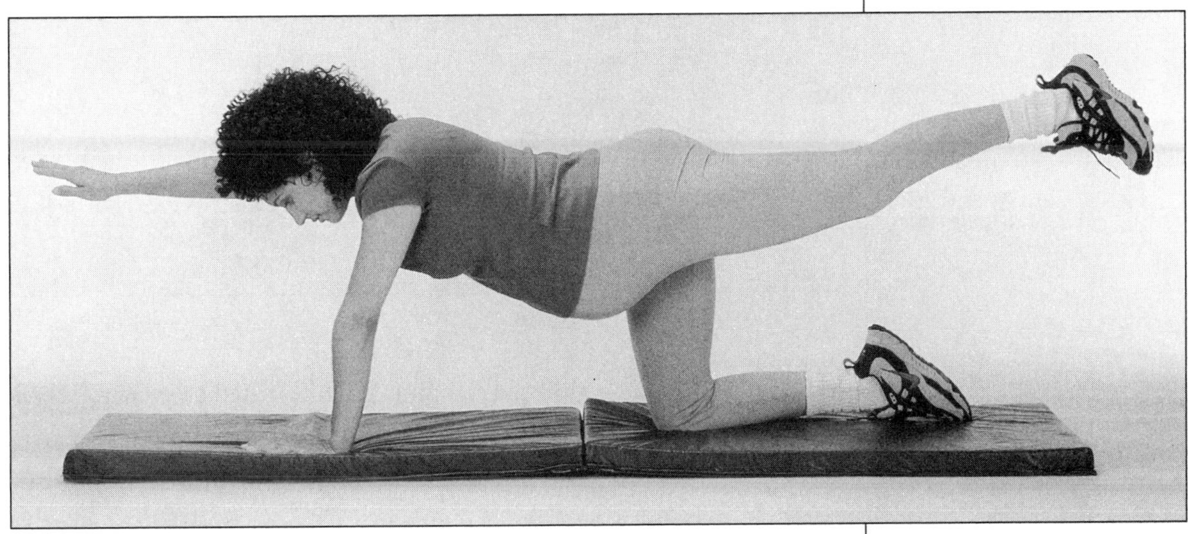

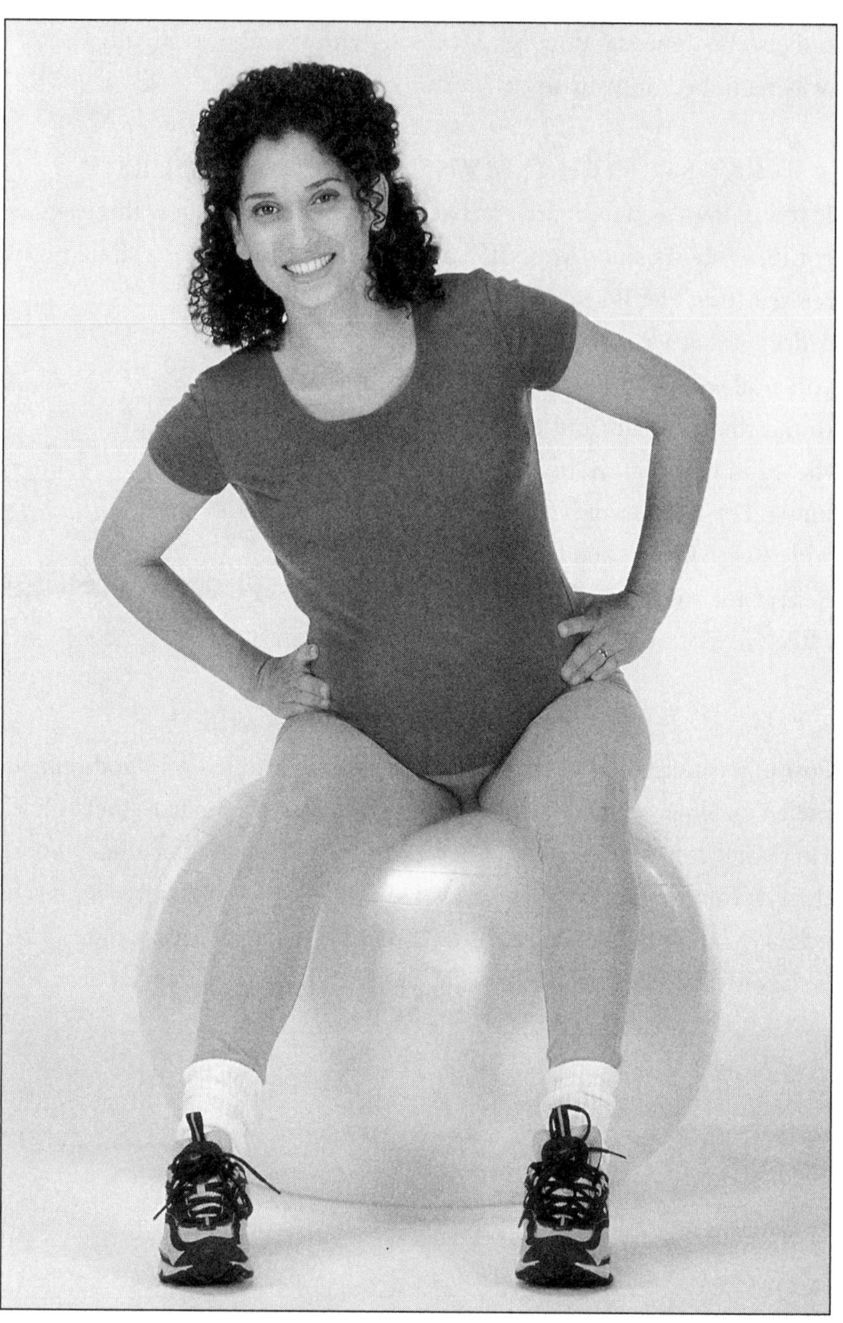

pelvic hip circles

PELVIC HIP CIRCLES**

This exercise can be performed standing or while seated on a Gymnic ball (a large, inflated ball found in most gyms and sporting goods stores). Move your hips and pelvis in a gentle circle. Do two sets of ten to fifteen circles in each direction.

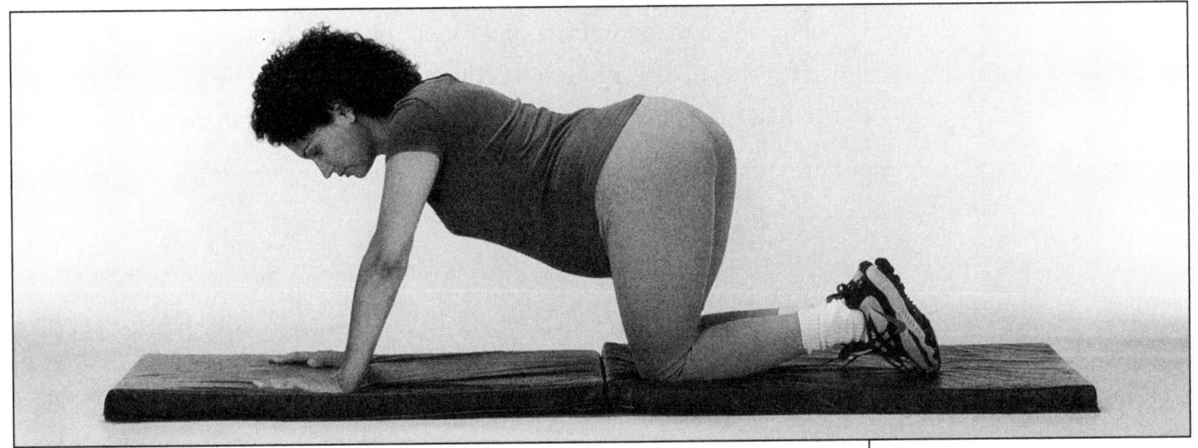

dog wag

DOG WAG**

Position yourself on all fours, with your back straight and abdominals pulled in. Gently wag your tailbone from side to side, contracting the obliques, to loosen the lower back and hip area. Do two sets of ten to fifteen repetitions.

SIDEWAYS HIP LIFT**

From a standing position, gently lift the left hip up toward the left shoulder, lifting the left heel off the floor. Relax and lower. Repeat on the right side. This can also be done while lying on your side*. Do two sets of ten to fifteen repetitions.

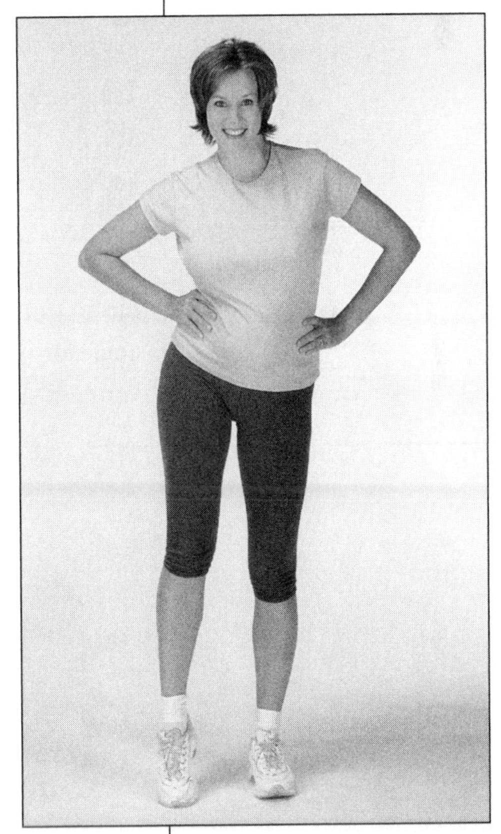

sideways hip lift

childbirth preparation exercises

To further prepare yourself for labor and delivery, it is helpful to do exercises that mimic your childbirth position and stretch the inner thighs (opening the hips) and lower back.

THE C-CURVE

This exercise almost perfectly mimics labor—without the pain. Sit on the floor with knees bent and hold on to your legs behind your knees. Take a deep breath and try to straighten your back by lifting your chest up high. Forcefully exhale, pulling in your abdominals, and round the lower back as much as possible. Do two sets of ten to fifteen repetitions. You can add a Kegel squeeze during the inhalation phase and let go on the C-curve stretch, but do not bear down.

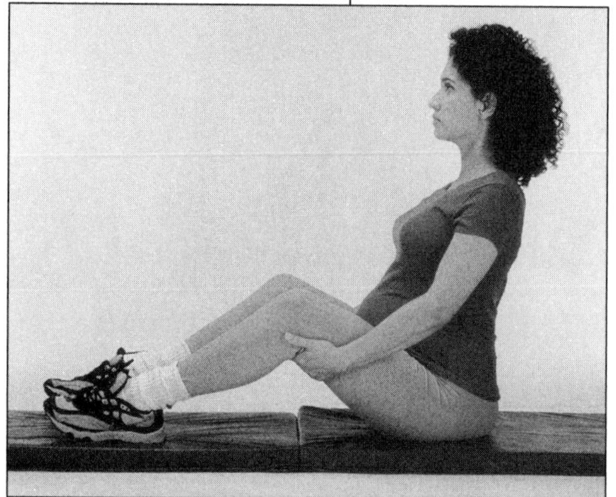

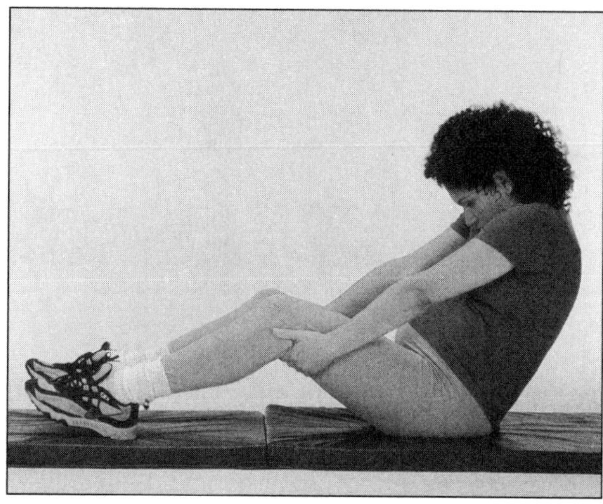

C-curve beginning (left) and end (right)

ABDOMINAL PULSE*

Tailor-sit against a wall, in bed, or sit on a chair with your hands on your stomach. Inhale and let your lungs expand with air. Relax your abdominals. Exhale and contract the abdominals tightly. Repeat ten to fifteen times for two sets.

SIDE-LYING KNEE TUCK*

Lie on your right side with the right leg bent in front of you at a 90-degree angle for support. Grab your left knee with your left hand and pull toward your left shoulder (to open the hip) for ten seconds. Repeat on each side.

side-lying knee tuck

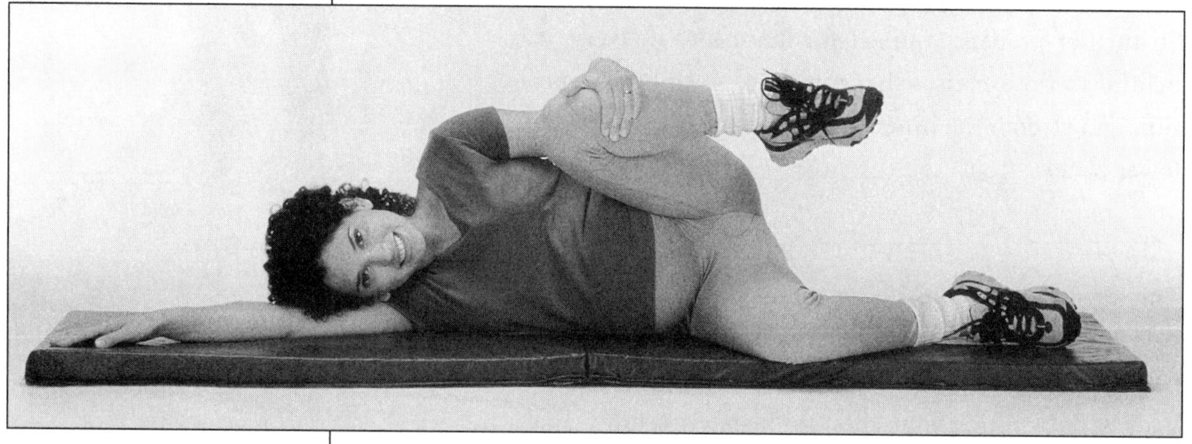

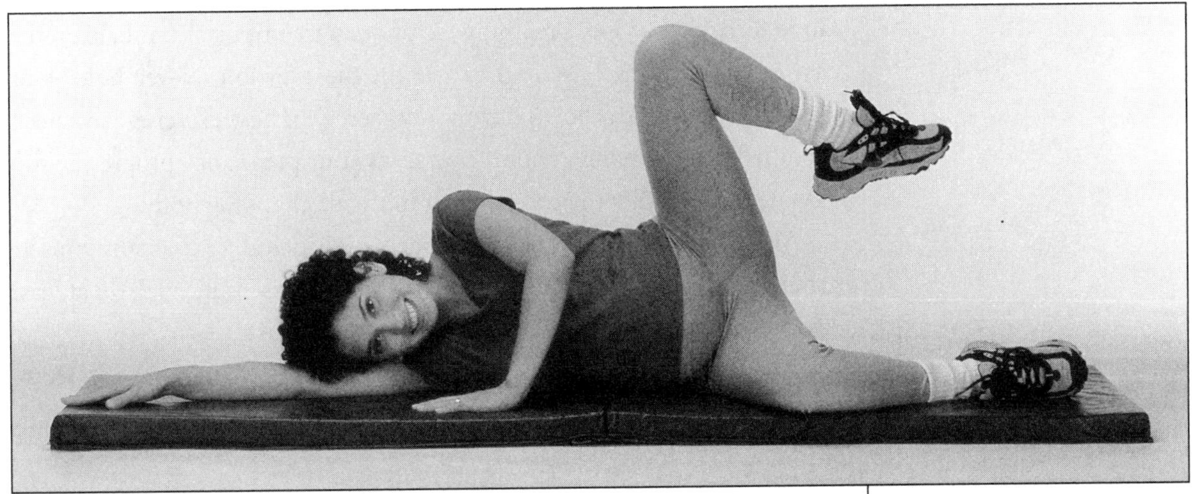

side-lying hip opener (clam)

SIDE-LYING HIP OPENER*

Lie on your right side with both legs bent in front of you at a 90-degree angle. Open your hips by lifting the left leg until it is perpendicular to the floor. Repeat for ten to fifteen repetitions on each side.

SUPPORTED SQUAT**

This exercise mimics the labor position very well. Hold on to something sturdy for support, such as a desk or table. Stand with your feet about a foot apart. Squat down as far as you feel comfortable. Keep your back straight, your chest up, your abdominals in, and your knees behind your toes. Inhale while squatting, and exhale as you rise. Use your thighs to push up, pressing through your heels. Do two sets of ten to fifteen repetitions (see page 141 for photo).

additional strength, toning, and flexibility exercises

During pregnancy, your muscles, joints, tissues, and organs go through some drastic changes and are put under a lot of stress. To get through pregnancy as easily as possible, and to prevent any future health problems, it is very important to prepare your body properly. The exercises in this section will help you maintain good posture, prevent back problems, and increase strength and flexibility.

As with everything else, of course, moderation is the key. Do not overwork, strain, or be careless. Execute each exercise slowly and smoothly.

Good form and proper breathing techniques are important. Inhale on the easy part of the exercise and exhale on the exertion. Never hold your breath, strain, or bear down during any exercise. These exercises have been modified for pregnancy, and of course, as your pregnancy progresses you may need to modify them further to suit your changing body.

Work out at least three times per week, including as many muscle groups as possible in your routine. Unless otherwise indicated, do at least two sets of ten to fifteen repetitions for each exercise.

You should try to exercise all areas of the body when pregnant. However, if you want an order of importance to guide you in planning your workout, here it is:

1. pelvic floor muscles (strengthening)
2. abdominals (strengthening)
3. lower back (stretching)
4. upper back (strengthening)
5. heart and lungs (cardiovascular exercise)
6. thighs and buttocks (strengthening)
7. hips (stretching)
8. chest (stretching)
9. shoulders and arms (strengthening)

leg, hip, and buttock exercises

SUPPORTED SQUAT

Unless you are a bodybuilder or professional athlete, avoid doing any unsupported squats after the first trimester. Hold on to something sturdy for support, such as a desk or table. Stand with your feet shoulder-width apart. Squat down as far as you feel comfortable. Keep your back straight, chest up, abdominals in, and knees behind your toes. Inhale while squatting, and exhale as you rise. Use your thighs to push up, pressing up through your heels. Do two to three sets of ten to fifteen repetitions.

There is no need to add any additional weight for resistance. After all, as you gradually gain weight, you are naturally increasing your own workload.

If your knees or back are weak, do only half-squats. If you still experience discomfort, the squat is not an appropriate exercise for you. If at

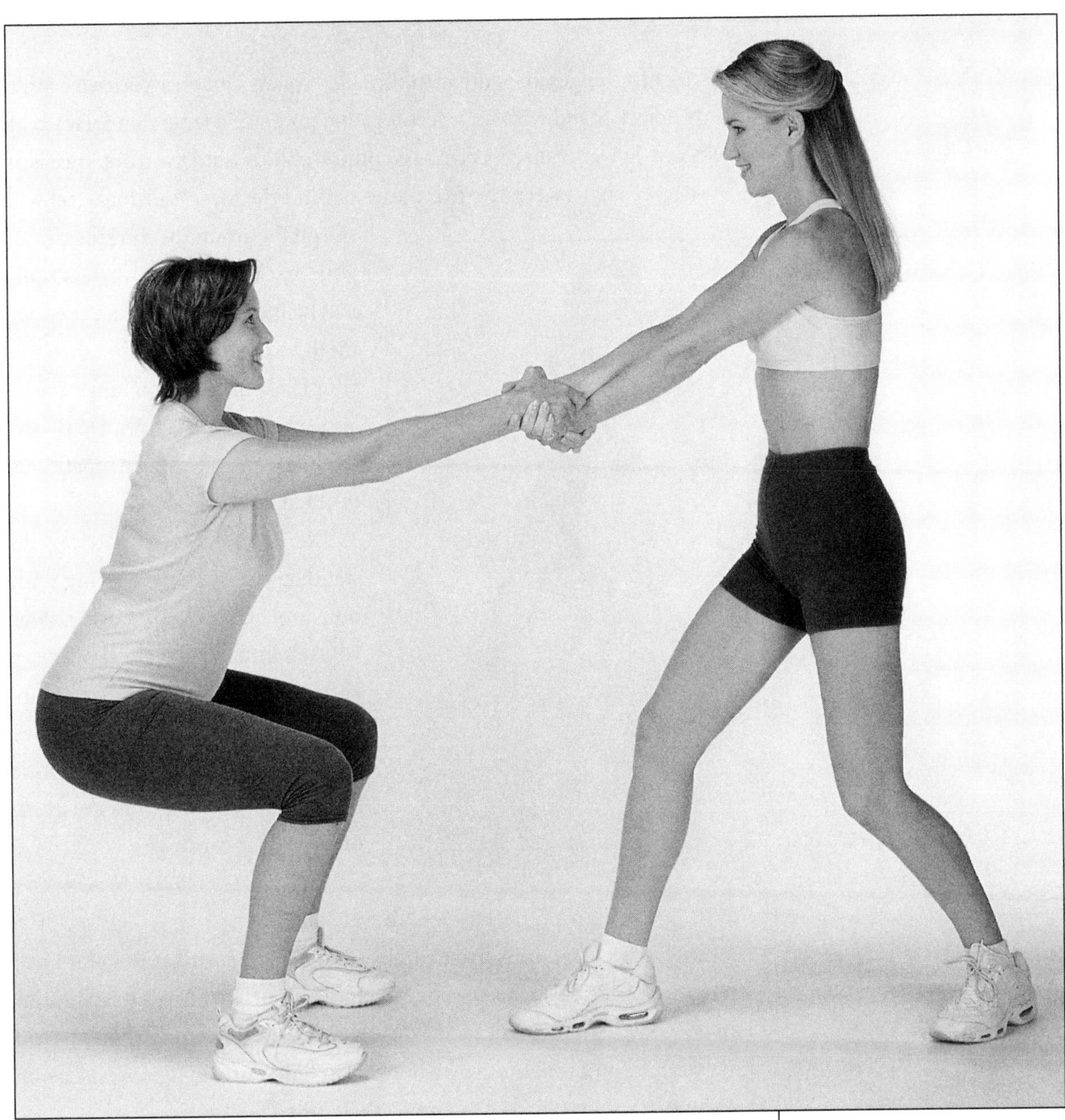

supported squat

any time during your pregnancy you are no longer able to do squats, find another leg exercise that better suits your needs, such as the elastic single leg press.

You can vary this exercise by adding a Kegel or a pelvic tilt at the bottom of the squat, or lean up against a wall with a big ball between your back and the wall. Press your back into the ball as you roll up and down to perform your squats.

SUPPORTED LUNGE

The rules for lunges are similar to those for squats. Support yourself with a sturdy object. Stand with your feet together and take a large step forward or backward. Lower yourself as far as is comfortable or until the front knee is at a 90-degree angle. Keep the front knee behind the toes. Your rear heel will rise off the ground as you lunge. Keep your back straight, your abdominals tight, and your chest up. Use your thigh to push up, pressing through your heel. Inhale as you lunge down, and exhale as you return. Do two to three sets of ten to fifteen repetitions on each leg.

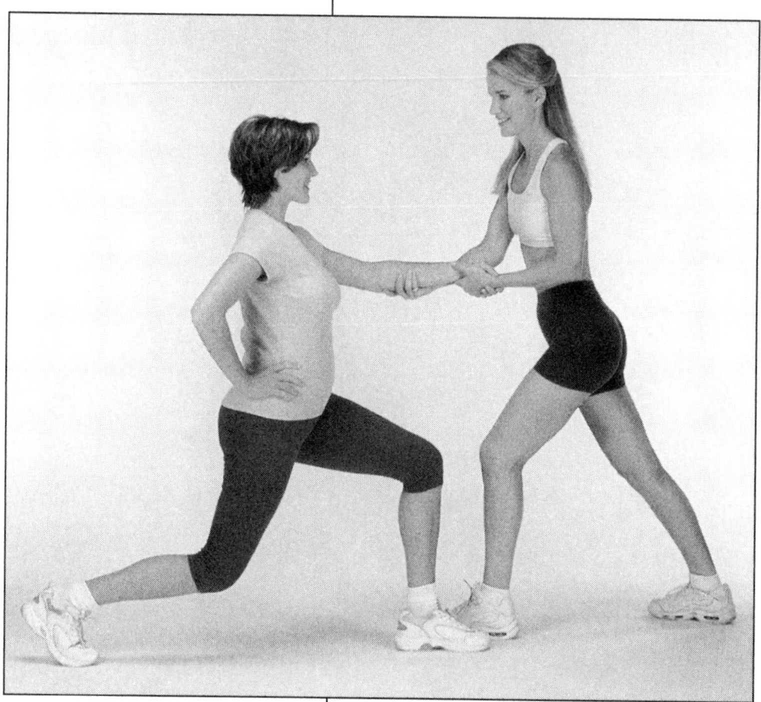

supported lunge

As an alternative, you can do stationary lunges, by starting with one foot already forward. Lower yourself into the lunge and push up, keeping your back straight, chest up, abdominals tight, and the front knee behind the toes. Lunges give your legs a nice shape and work the front, outer, and inner thighs.

LEG EXTENSION

Leg extensions work your front thighs or quadriceps, and are a great knee strengthener. Sit on a chair or bench that supports your leg to the knee. Extend your leg out straight by flexing your quadriceps. Exhale as you raise your leg and inhale as you lower it. Do ten to fifteen repetitions using the same leg, then switch. Do two to three sets.

You can do leg extensions while wearing ankle weights or working on a leg extension machine. The use of Dyna-Bands, wide stretchy rubber bands used for resistance exercises, is another option. If your knees are weak, do not add ankle weights or any other form of resistance. If your knees are very weak from an injury or surgery, have someone lift your leg out straight as you flex your thigh and hold the contraction for a few seconds.

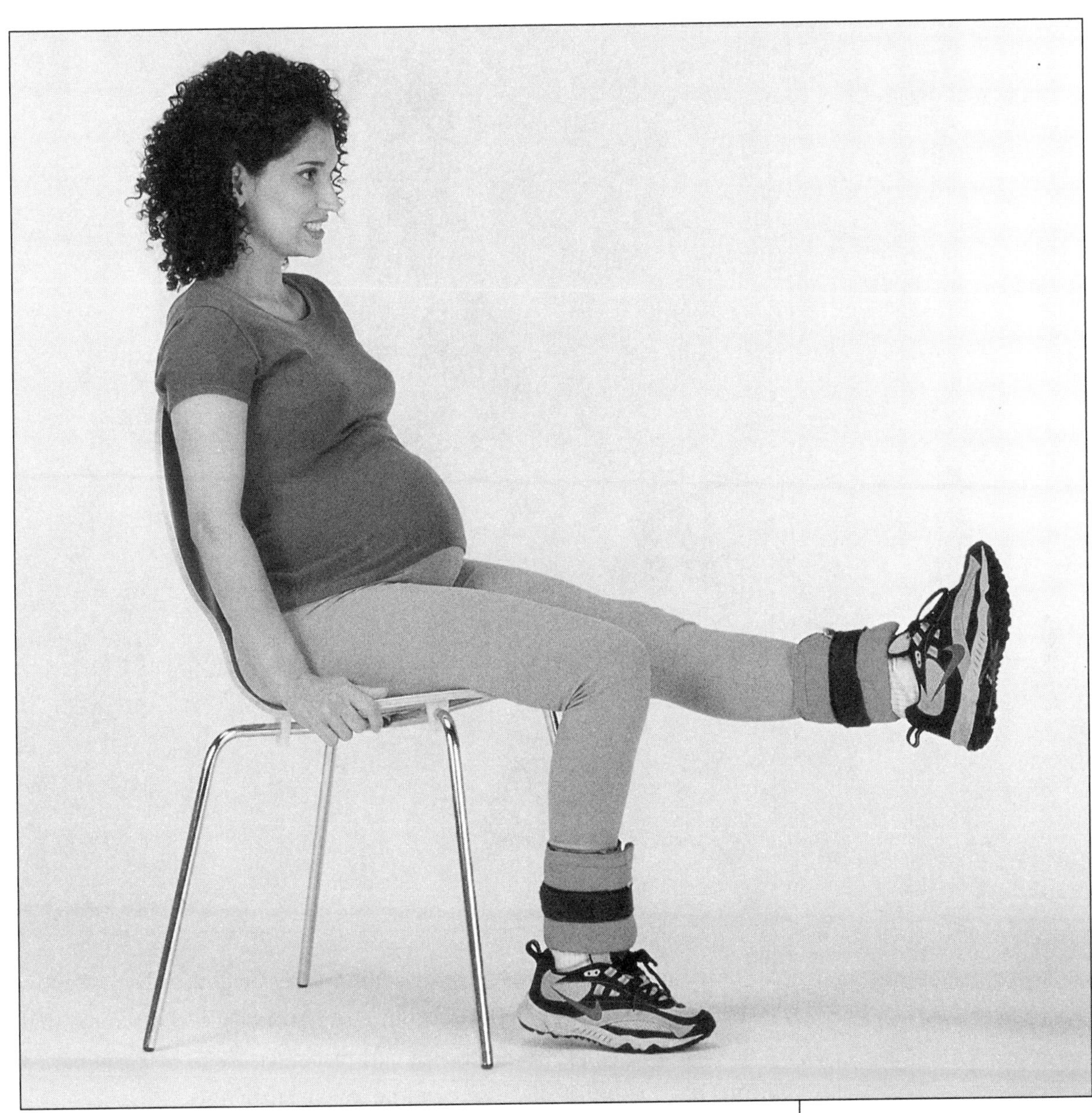

leg extension

LEG CURL

Stand with your legs together, holding on to a sturdy object such as a chair for support. Bending at the knee, raise one foot up toward your buttocks by flexing your hamstring. Your knees should stay together, and your foot should be flexed to prevent cramps. Return to your starting position. Exhale as you curl, inhale on the return. Do ten to fifteen repetitions using the same leg, then switch for two to three sets.

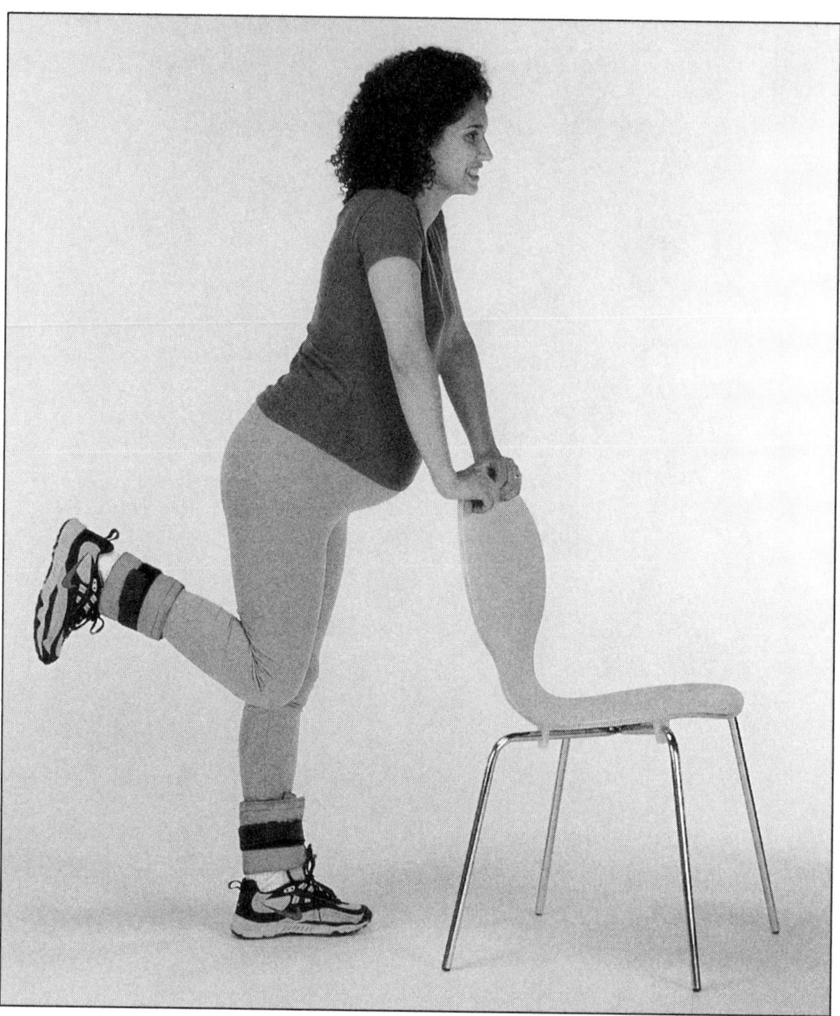

leg curl

You can modify this exercise by adding ankle weights or Dyna-Bands, or by squeezing a soft ball behind your knee. Avoid leg curl machines that require you to lie prone. Seated leg curl machines are fine. If you have a strong back, you may also use standing leg curl machines.

Leg curls strengthen your hamstrings, which helps straighten your posture by reducing lumbar lordosis (sway back).

LEG PRESS—MACHINE AND ELASTIC SINGLE

Leg presses are like squats, but they are usually performed using a machine. Avoid leg presses that require you to lie flat on your back. Also, be careful with seated and angled-seat leg presses after your fourth month of pregnancy—they may crowd your uterus. You may have to do partial presses. Place feet shoulder-width apart on the platform, with your toes pointing slightly out. Lower your knees toward your shoulders and inhale. Exhale as you press up. Repeat for two sets of ten to fifteen repetitions. If this exercise bothers you, try increasing your knee angle by moving your feet up.

Another option is the elastic single leg press, which is performed using a Dyna-Band. Sit on a chair, place one foot in the center of the Dyna-Band, and hold on to both ends. Flex your thigh, pressing the Dyna-Band with your heels, not your toes, as you extend the leg. If you have knee problems, or experience any discomfort doing this exercise, switch to something else.

LYING ADDUCTOR LIFT (INNER THIGH LEG LIFT)

Lie on your side with your head resting on your arm to keep your spine aligned. Do not prop your head up with your hand. Place your top leg on a ball or bench-step to ensure that your hips are straight. Make sure your top hip does not lean forward or backward. Keep your bottom leg straight. Lift the bottom leg up and down, using your inner thigh muscles. This requires only a small movement to be effective. If you need more resistance, strap on some ankle weights. Repeat for two sets of fifteen repetitions on each side.

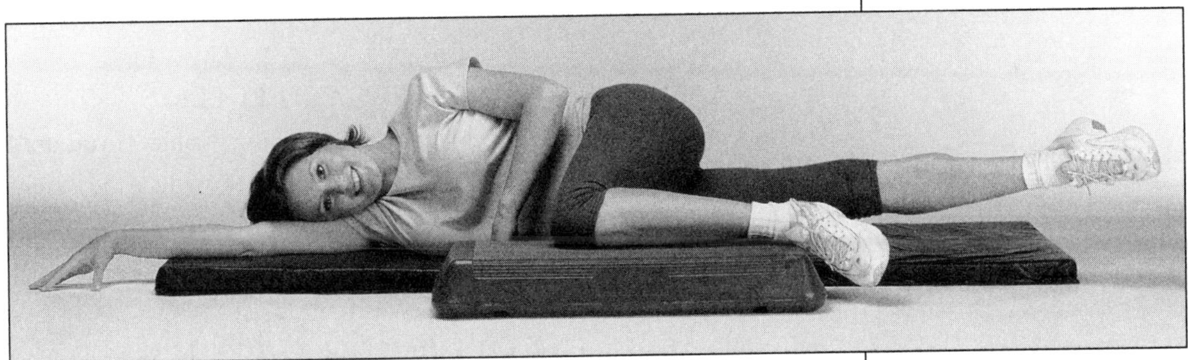

lying adductor lift

ADDUCTOR SQUEEZE

You can work your inner thigh muscles by sitting on a chair and squeezing a soft ball between your knees. Or you can sit on the floor, place the soles of your feet together, and press the inside of your legs gently up against the resistance of your elbows. Do two sets of fifteen repetitions.

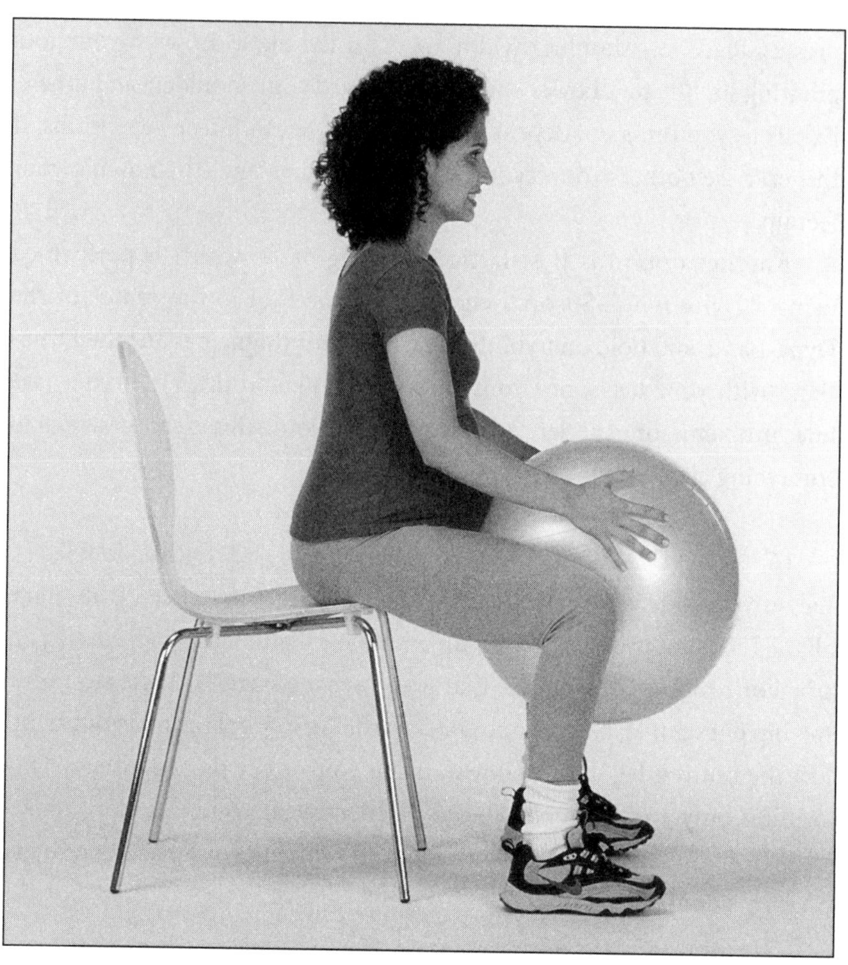

adductor squeeze

ADDUCTOR MACHINES AND PULLEYS

You can continue using inner thigh machines or pulley cables if you used them prior to conceiving. However, you should probably reduce the weight load. If your inner thighs are not conditioned to this type of apparatus, you should avoid it, as it may put undue strain on the pubic bone.

LYING ABDUCTOR LIFT (OUTER THIGH LEG LIFT)

Lie on your side with your head resting on your arm. Your spine and neck should be aligned straight. Bend your lower leg in front of you for balance and keep your hips stacked straight. Keeping your top leg straight and your foot flexed, lift the leg slowly as far as it will go, which should not be very far if you are doing it right. Lower your leg slowly and repeat ten to fifteen times before switching to the other side. Do two to three sets on each side.

You can use ankle weights or lower body Dyna-Bands to add resistance. Place the Dyna-Band around both ankles. You'll have to keep both legs straight, unless the band is placed above your knees.

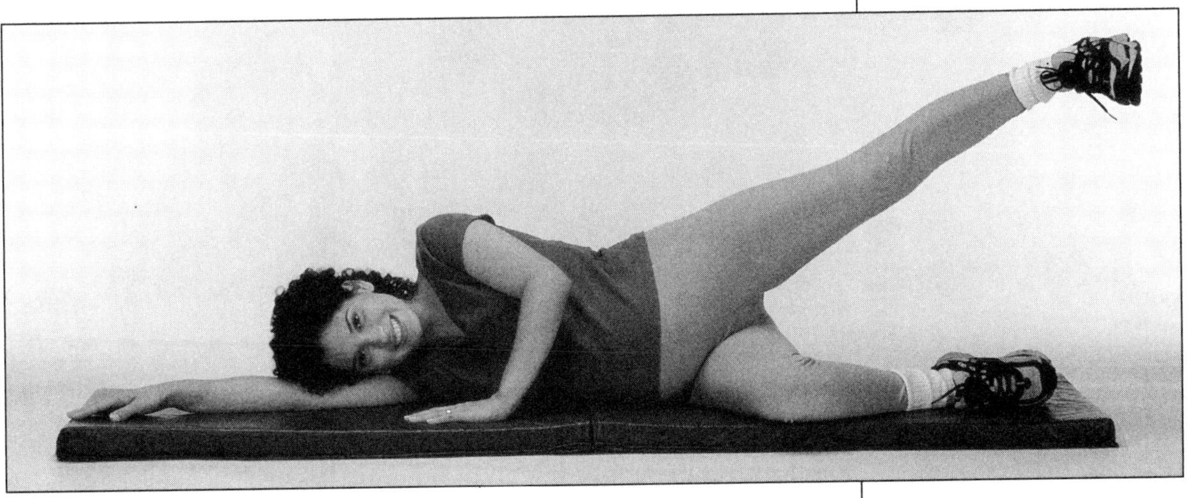

lying abductor lift

ABDUCTOR MACHINES AND PULLEYS

If you used them before becoming pregnant, you may use outer thigh machines or pulley cables to work the abductors. You may need to reduce the weight to avoid abdominal strain. You can also simulate the abductor machine by sitting at the edge of a chair, with a Dyna-Band wrapped around your legs, above the knees, and move your knees apart against the resistance.

TRAVELING LEG ABDUCTION

Stand with a Lower Body Dyna-Band wrapped around your ankles (or a regular Dyna-Band tied around them). Keep your feet far enough apart to keep tension in the band. Walk sideways, four steps to the right, then four steps to the left. Repeat five to ten times in each direction for two sets. If your balance is off, find a partner to do this exercise with.

BUTTOCK LEG LIFT

Get on your knees and elbows. Hold your abdominals and lower back tight and straight for support. Extend one leg behind you. Lift the leg up slowly by squeezing the buttocks until there is a straight line from your foot to your shoulder. Ankle weights will add resistance. Do two sets of twenty repetitions. If this position makes you dizzy, try placing your arms

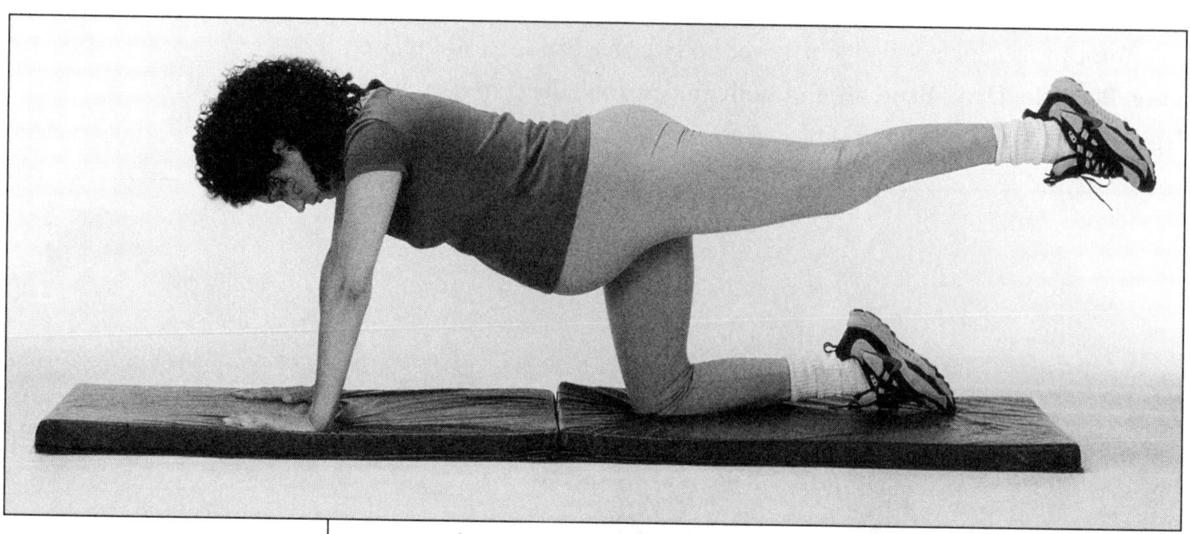

buttock leg lift

higher up on a chair. If that is still uncomfortable, do it while standing. Hold on to a chair or table and extend one leg behind you by squeezing the buttocks. Lean forward slightly so that your back will not arch as your leg rises. You can use ankle weights, Dyna-Bands, or pulleys as well.

Most weight machines that claim to isolate the buttocks are rather ineffective and uncomfortable. Furthermore, many of these machines are too difficult for a pregnant woman to get in and out of.

CALF RAISE

Full-range calf raises, those requiring you to lift your heels high off the ground, may cause leg cramps. If you really want to work your calves, do partial raises. Stand near an object you can hold for support and place the balls of your feet on a big book or plank. Lower your heels to the ground, stretching out the calf muscles, and inhale. Flex your calves, lifting your heels up to a horizontal position, and exhale. Do two sets of ten to fifteen repetitions.

upper back exercises

LAT PULLDOWN

The latissimus dorsi muscles work by squeezing your shoulder blades together and moving your elbows down and back. Pulldowns work these muscles and will help you maintain good posture during and after your pregnancy. You can use a lat pulldown machine or Dyna-Bands to work these muscles.

Stand or sit up straight with your abdominal muscles pulled in tightly. Make sure to wrap the Dyna-Band around your fingers, and not your wrists. Start with your arms over your head at an outward angle, in the shape of a "V". Next, slowly, pull the band down behind your neck, bending your elbows and squeezing your shoulder blades together to increase tension in the band. Do not attempt to push the band beyond the point of comfort. Return to the starting position and repeat the exercise ten to fifteen times for two sets. If you're using a lat pulldown machine, remember to pull the bar down in front of your chest.

If stretching your arms over your head is not a comfortable position for you, causes dizziness or places too much pressure on your sides, try substituting a rowing exercise instead.

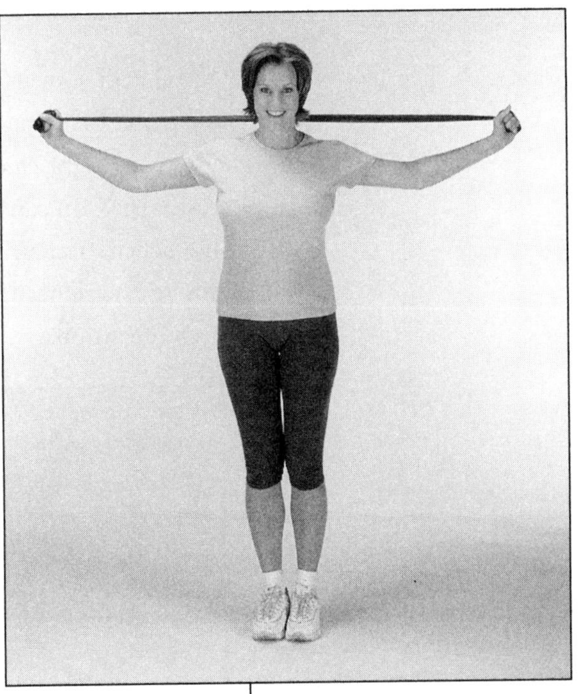

lat pulldown

SEATED ROWING

Rowing machines can cause problems for pregnant women if not used properly. You may develop back strain from leaning forward to grasp the handles on a rowing machine. Also, your belly will soon grow so big that you may not be able to pull your elbows back far enough to do the exercise properly.

Dyna-Bands may be a better option for you. Sit very straight in a chair or on the floor. Place your feet together on the center of the band and hold on to either end with your hands. Keep your knees slightly bent, and use your upper back muscles to pull your elbows behind you, squeezing your shoulder blades together. Exhale on the exertion. Inhale as you bring your arms slowly forward, and stay as upright as possible. Repeat for two sets of ten to fifteen repetitions.

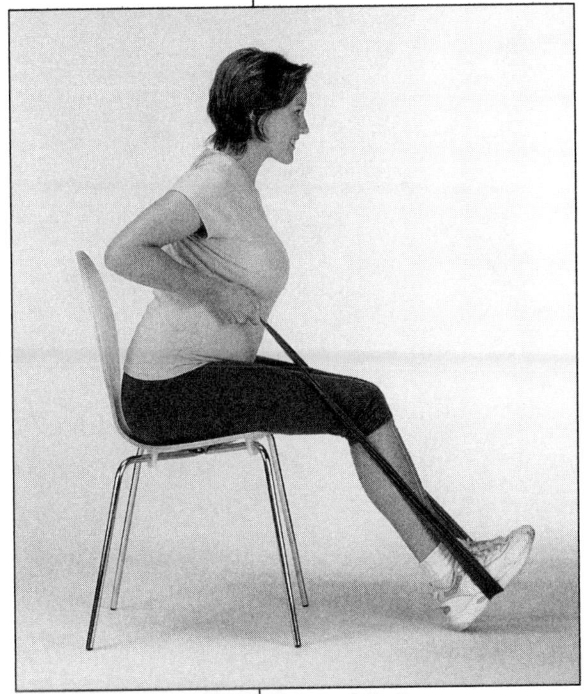

seated rowing

SINGLE ARM ROW

Kneel with your left knee on a bench or chair. Support yourself with your left hand. Make sure to keep your back straight and abdominals tight, and pull your right elbow up behind you, using the right back muscles. For resistance, you can use a dumbbell, or you can secure a Dyna-Band under the bench or chair leg. If you're a beginner, use five-pound dumbbells. If you're experienced, use a weight you are accustomed to. Do two sets of fifteen repetitions.

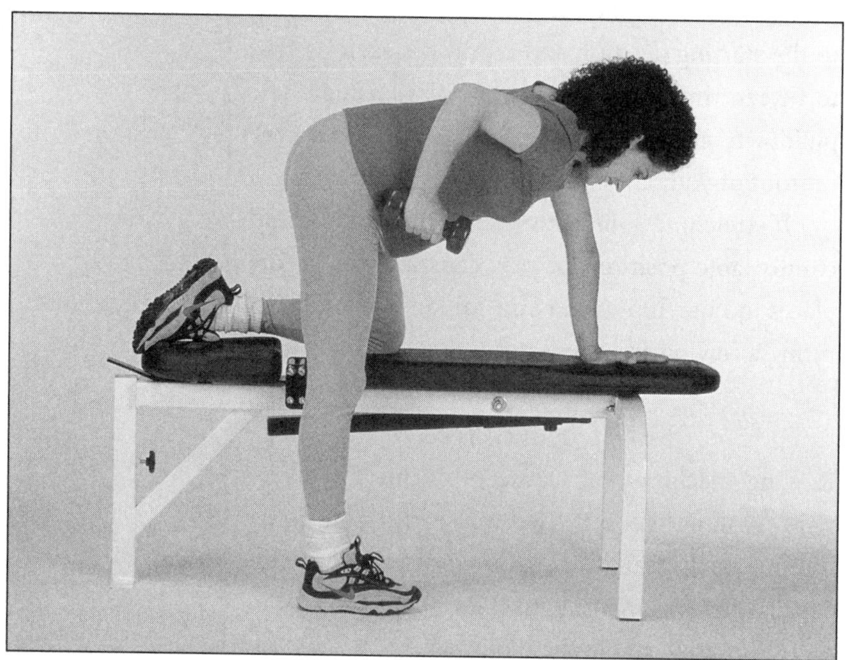

single arm row

chest exercises

INCLINE CHEST PRESS

Lie on an incline bench set on at least a 45-degree incline. Keep your back flat against the bench; do not arch. Hold a BodyBar or barbell out at shoulder level. Squeeze your shoulder blades together and lower the weight toward your chest while inhaling. Press the weight back up, using your chest muscles to push your arms up, and exhale. Do two sets of fifteen repetitions.

This exercise can also be done while standing or using a Dyna-Band. Wrap the band behind your back, grasp the ends, and press your hands forward, flexing your pectoral muscles.

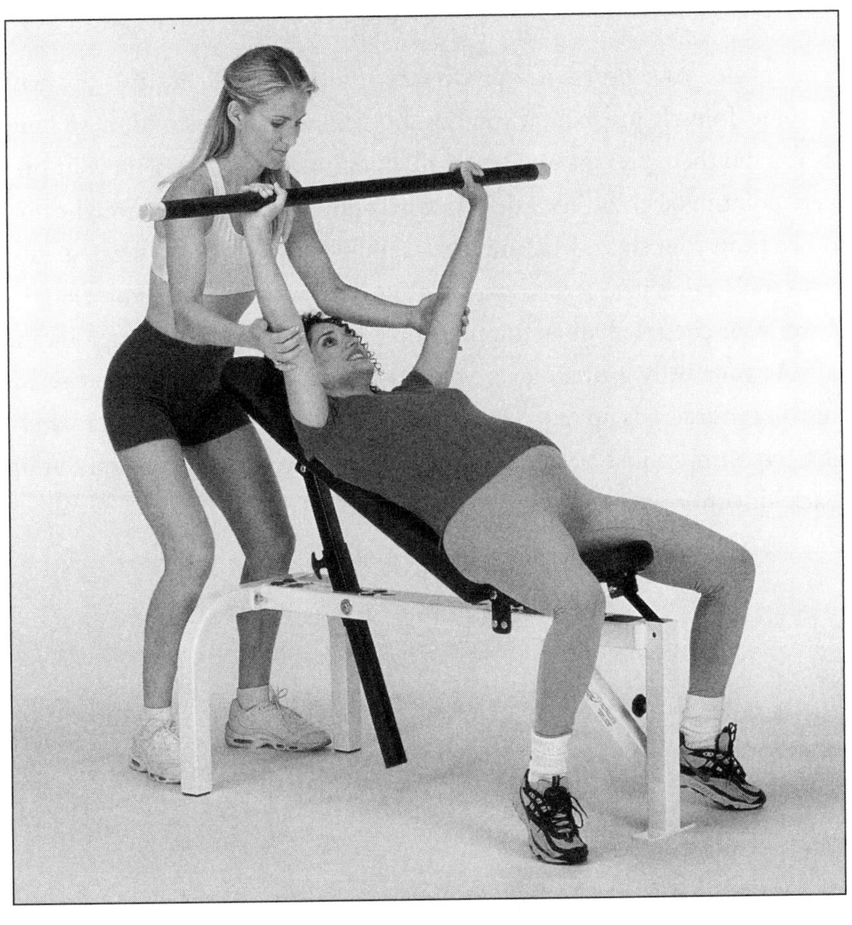

incline chest press

INCLINE CHEST FLY

Lie on an incline bench set on at least a 45-degree incline. Keep your back flat against the bench; do not arch. Hold a dumbbell in each hand. Extend your arms, slightly bent, in front of you at shoulder level, with your palms facing each other. Lower your arms out to the side, elbows first, while stretching your pectorals and inhaling. Exhale and use your chest to bring the weights back to the starting position. Do two sets of fifteen repetitions. Due to the instability of your joints and the possibility of elbow or shoulder injuries, avoid using dumbbells after twelve weeks of pregnancy. You can still do this move, working against an imaginary resistance, or do another chest exercise.

PEC DEC AND CHEST MACHINES

So long as you are sitting up and your back is supported, the various chest exercise machines are fine to use during pregnancy.

PUSH-UP

The further your pregnancy progresses, the more difficult push-ups will become. In early pregnancy, you can do them without restriction, so long as you did them previously. Get on all fours (knees or toes), with your fingers pointing slightly inward. You arms should extend in a straight line down from your shoulders. Your back should be straight—no sagging. Pull your midsection in as tight as you can and keep your hips up. Inhale as you lower your chest. Exhale as you press up. Do as many push-ups as you can.

As your belly grows bigger you may have to modify this exercise by moving your hands up onto a bench-step or table. You can also do a standing push-up against a wall. If push-ups make you dizzy or strain your back, discontinue.

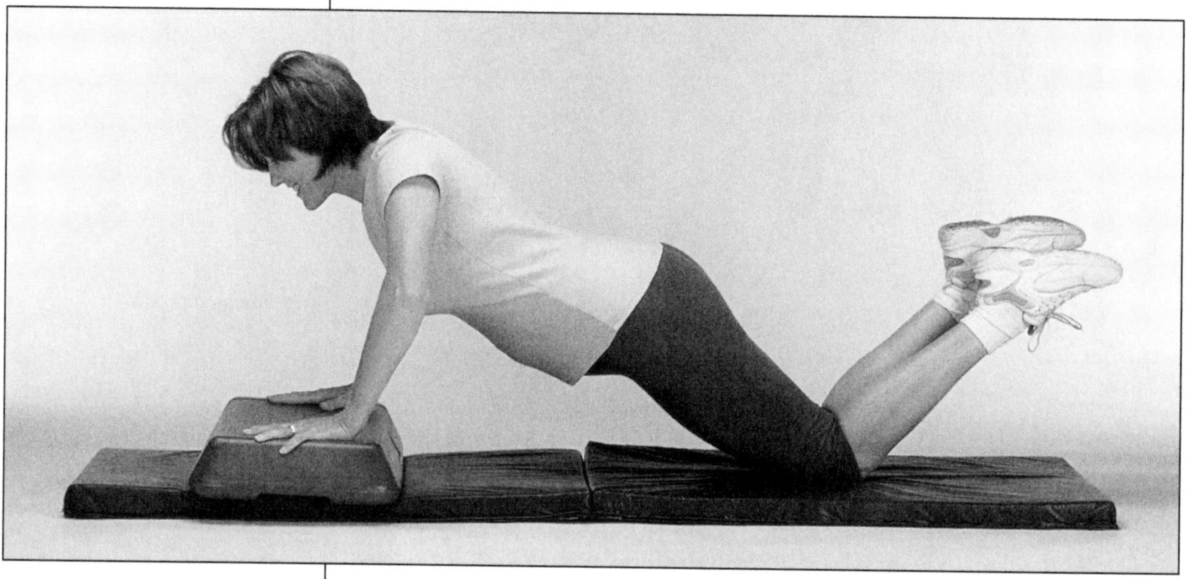

modified push-up

shoulder exercises

REAR SHOULDER PULL

Strengthening the rear shoulder muscles will prevent rounded shoulders. Stand up straight. Hold a Dyna-Band in front of you, with your hands about shoulder-width apart. Make sure to wrap the Dyna-Band around your fingers and not your wrists. Use your rear shoulder muscles to press your arms apart and backward while exhaling. Resist as you slowly move your arms forward again and inhale. Do two sets of fifteen repetitions.

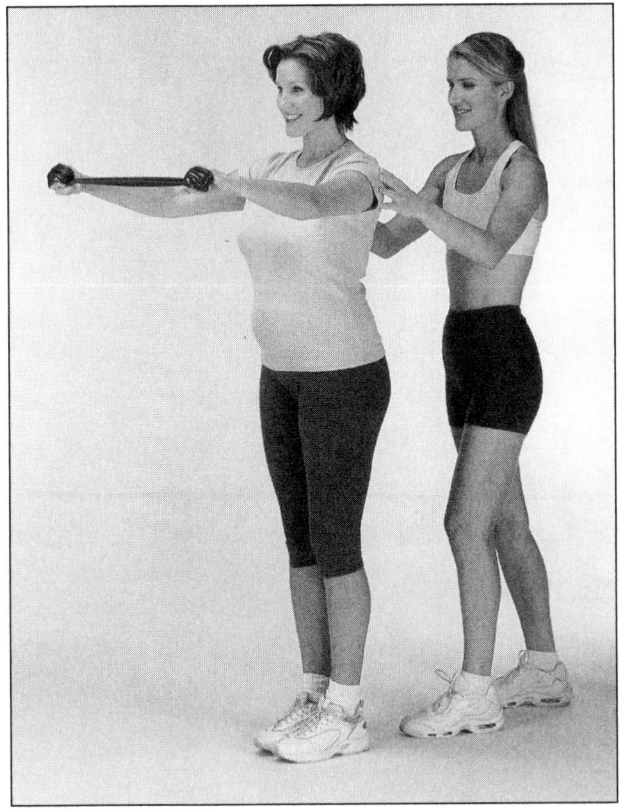

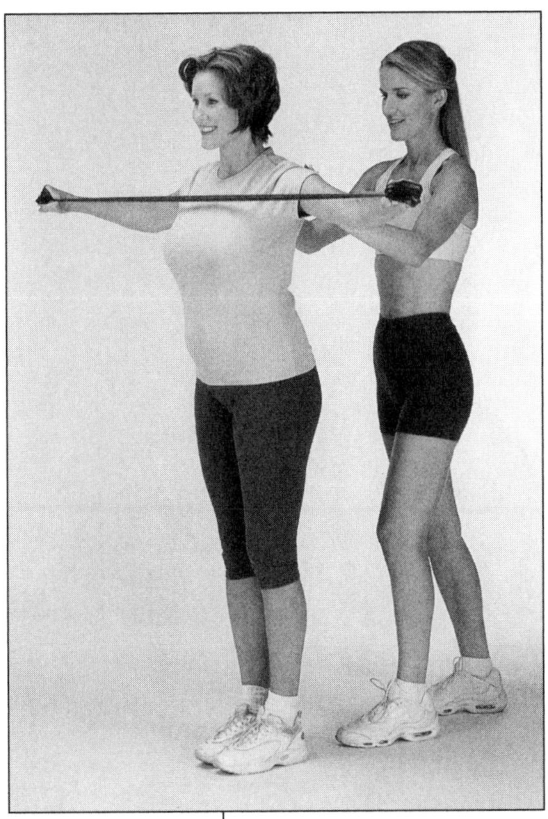

rear shoulder pull beginning (left) and end (right)

SHRUGS

This exercise feels wonderful on tired shoulders. Stand up straight with pelvis tucked in. Lift and squeeze your shoulders up toward your ears, then move them back down in a circular motion. Do two sets of fifteen repetitions.

SCAPULAR RETRACTION

This exercise is easy to perform, even while sitting in bed. Sit or stand with a straight back and your arms either lifted in front of you or relaxed at your sides. Retract and squeeze your shoulder blades together. While still contracted, rotate your shoulder blades down while exhaling. Release and inhale. Repeat fifteen times for two sets. You can add resistance by using dumbbells or a Dyna-Band secured around a door handle.

TRICEPS KICKBACK

Kneel with your left knee on a bench or chair, and lean forward, supporting yourself with your left hand. Hold a dumbbell in your right hand.

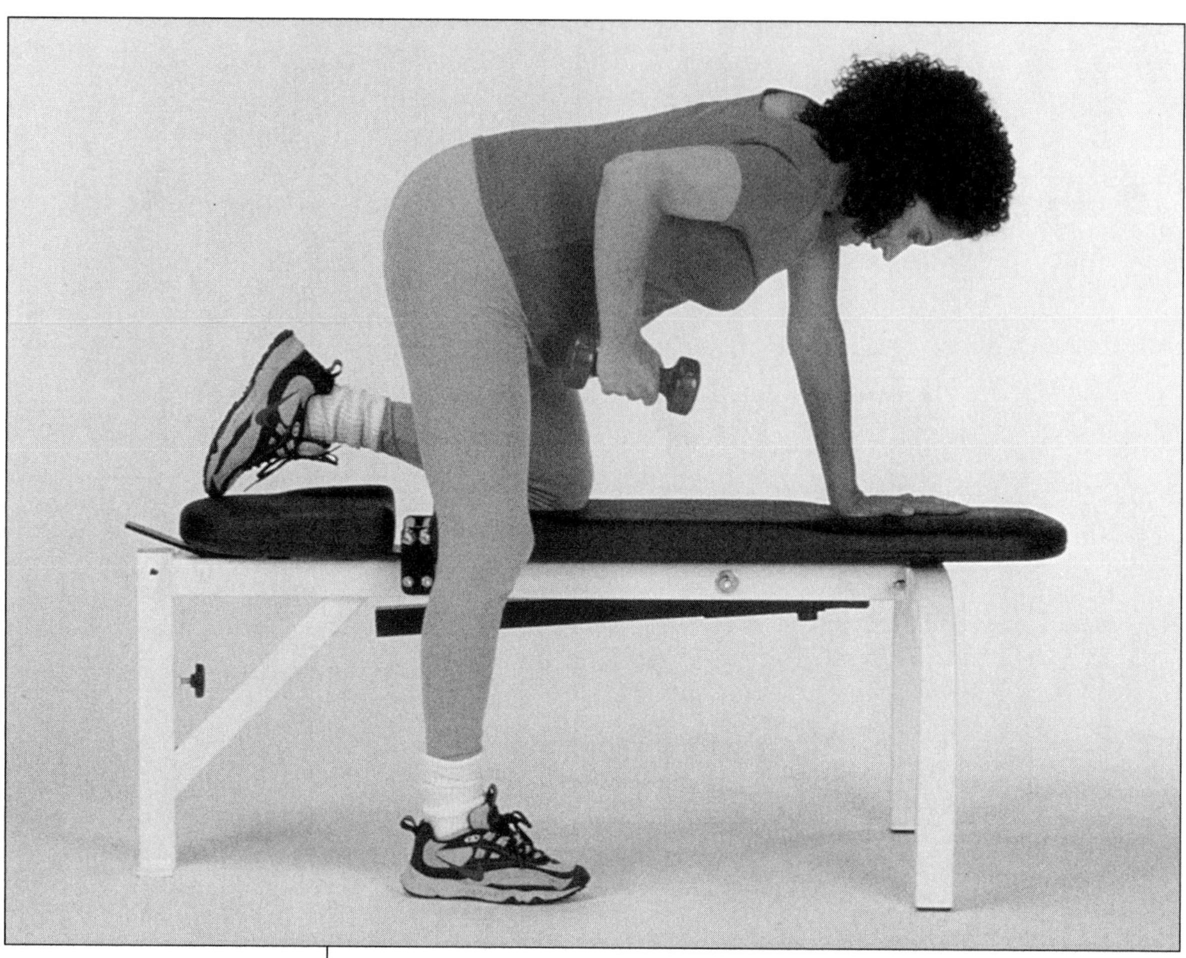

triceps kickback

Keep your back straight and hold your right elbow high and close behind you. Press your right forearm straight back, flexing the back of your arm as you exhale. Resist as you bend the elbow and return to starting position, and inhale. In this movement, the upper arm should remain stationary, while the forearm moves back and forth. Do two sets of ten to fifteen repetitions with each arm.

STRAIGHT TRICEPS ARM PRESS

Stand with your pelvis tucked in. With your arms hanging down straight, hold a Dyna-Band at shoulder-width in front of your hips. Press both arms straight back as far as you can, flexing the triceps. Your arms will not go very far. Exhale on the exertion. Return your arms slowly and inhale. Repeat ten to fifteen times for two sets. You may also do this exercise with dumbbells instead of the Dyna-Band.

TRICEPS MACHINE

Any triceps machine or cable exercise machine should be okay so long as your belly does not get in the way. Avoid machines with chest pads in front.

BICEPS CURL

Stand with your pelvis tucked in. Hold dumbbells, a BodyBar, or use rubber tubing or a Dyna-Band placed under your feet. Flex your biceps to slowly lift the weight toward your shoulders, exhaling as you do. Resist as you slowly lower the weight and inhale. Walk around in between sets to keep your blood circulating. Repeat for two sets of fifteen repetitions.

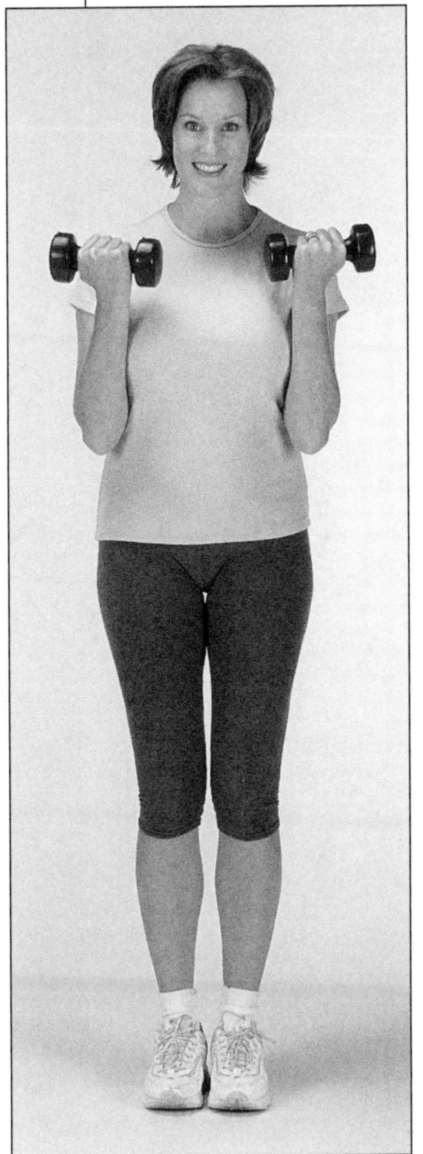

biceps curl

BICEPS CURL MACHINE

You can safely use any biceps curl or cable machine, unless there is a support pad in front of your belly.

WRIST CURL

Working your forearms and strengthening your wrists is optional; it is not vital to your fitness. However, it may help your circulation and prevent edema or carpal tunnel syndrome. Sit with your forearms on your thighs and your wrists on top of your knees. Hold on to dumbbells or a BodyBar. Bend your wrists up and down slowly. Do one set with the palms facing down and one set with the palms up.

Chapter Six

exercises for high-risk and bed-rest pregnancies

IN THIS CHAPTER

- *High-risk categories and special concerns*
- *"In bed" doesn't mean out of commission*
- *Simple but crucial exercises you can perform in bed*

Being categorized as a high-risk pregnancy does not mean that you have been rendered disabled—even if you've been ordered on bed rest. Too often, high-risk pregnant women—especially those on bed rest—are instructed not to do anything in order to protect the fetus. However, so long as a pregnant woman is well monitored, and performs only special bed-rest exercises, she *can* exercise safely, without jeopardizing her baby. Being pregnant can be quite an ordeal in itself. Immobility or inactivity will only make you feel worse, and also fare worse during labor. If you are in a high-risk category, it is even more important that you do some kind of exercise, however limited, to help your strength, endurance, flexibility, and self-esteem.

Inactivity contributes to heart disease, aches and pains, fatigue, osteoporosis, and unnecessary weight gain. Though the effects of bed-rest on pregnant women have yet to be studied specifically, research on the immobilization of bed-rest has shown that inactive muscles deteriorate very quickly, decreasing strength and endurance, while the bones lose calcium, reducing skeletal strength. After only twenty-one days of total bed-rest, the body deconditions by 25 percent, which is equivalent to the effects of thirty years of aging! To cope with the nine-month marathon of pregnancy and a possibly difficult labor, you need and deserve all the strength and endurance possible.

what is a high-risk pregnancy?

The category "high-risk" is a broad one, and difficult to define. It includes just about anything that is not perfectly healthy and normal, that may or will complicate or jeopardize the pregnancy or delivery. It ranges from mild to severe problems requiring bed-rest.

You should go straight to the hospital if:

- your water has broken
- you are suffering from preeclampsia
- you are having uterine contractions

You will most likely be ordered on bed-rest at some time during the pregnancy if:

- you have placenta previa (placenta covering the cervix) or placenta abruption (placenta has broken away from the uterus)
- you have gone into labor prematurely before
- you have been diagnosed with a weak or incompetent cervix

You may be ordered on bed-rest if:

- you have had three or more miscarriages
- you are carrying two or more babies
- you are bleeding
- there are signs of growth retardation

You may not be ordered on bed-rest, but are still considered high risk and will need extra monitoring if:

- you suffer from chronic hypertension
- you suffer from thyroid, cardiac, vascular, or lung disease
- your baby is in breech position
- you are anemic
- you are a very fit mother carrying twins

You should not require bed-rest, but will require monitoring, if:

- you have gestational diabetes
- you have any joint or muscle pain or problems
- you have a back problem
- you have a seizure disorder
- you have been very sedentary, or are very overweight (200 pounds or more)
- you are very underweight
- you are older than thirty-five years of age
- you are a disabled person

If there is any risk of premature delivery, you should not participate in a regular exercise program, but there is still quite a bit that you can do.

Only 50 percent of premature deliveries have known causes. However, research has found a correlation between risk level and factors such as socioeconomic status, medical history, and lifestyle. Statistically, the following socioeconomic factors *may* place you in a higher risk category: low income, single-parent household, more than two children, poor or no prenatal care, poor nutrition, younger than age eighteen or older than thirty-five. Medical factors that tend to increase risk include: less than a year between pregnancies, serious maternal diseases, an incompetent cervix, or previous preterm labor. Lifestyle factors that can increase your risk include: alcohol, cigarette, and/or drug use, excessive stress, performing very heavy physical work, and physical abuse.

high-risk exercise guidelines

If there is any risk of premature delivery, you should not participate in a regular exercise program, but there is still quite a bit that you can do. Even on bed-rest, you can safely work and stretch your entire body with light exercises, concentric and isotonic contractions (muscle shortening against resistance), and static stretches. These exercises can be performed seated or lying on your side in bed. If you are strong enough, you may add Dyna-Bands, light dumbbells, or ankle weights for resistance. If you have been ordered to move around as little as possible in bed, do every seated exercise first, then do every side-lying exercise on one side before turning over and doing them on the other side. Switching positions between every exercise can be a workout in itself!

If you have an incompetent cervix, you may not even be allowed to sit up. If so, all exercises should be done lying on your side and briefly on your back.

If you are not on bed-rest, you can probably enjoy walking or swimming for cardiovascular exercise as a supplement to your toning and stretching routine. Of course, you should *consult with your doctor and instructor before doing any form of exercise.*

toning exercises

These exercises can all be performed in bed. Prop yourself up with pillows for support as needed. For a description of the major muscle groups of the body and how they function, refer to chapter 5.

KEGELS

Kegel exercises are essential for every pregnant woman. Even if you are confined to bed, you still can and must perform your Kegels. Squeeze your pelvic floor muscles, pulling up through the pelvic cavity. Visualize the muscles as if they were on a drawstring and you could pull them closed. Do not hold your breath. Exhale as you squeeze and pull up, and inhale as you release. Do five Kegels at a time. Repeat at least three to four times a day. For more detailed information on this exercise and its benefits, see pages 124–125.

upper body exercises

LAT PULL

The latissimus dorsi muscles work by squeezing your shoulder blades together and moving your elbows down and back. Lat pulls work these muscles, along with the rhomboids, rear shoulders, and biceps.

Sit up straight in bed, propped up on pillows. Hold a Dyna-Band in front of you or over your head. Pull your arms apart and back, squeezing the shoulder blades together. Exhale. Inhale as you slowly return to your starting position. Repeat ten to twenty times.

ROWING

Lie on your right side with both knees bent and your head down to keep the neck straight. Stretch your left arm forward and inhale. Pull your

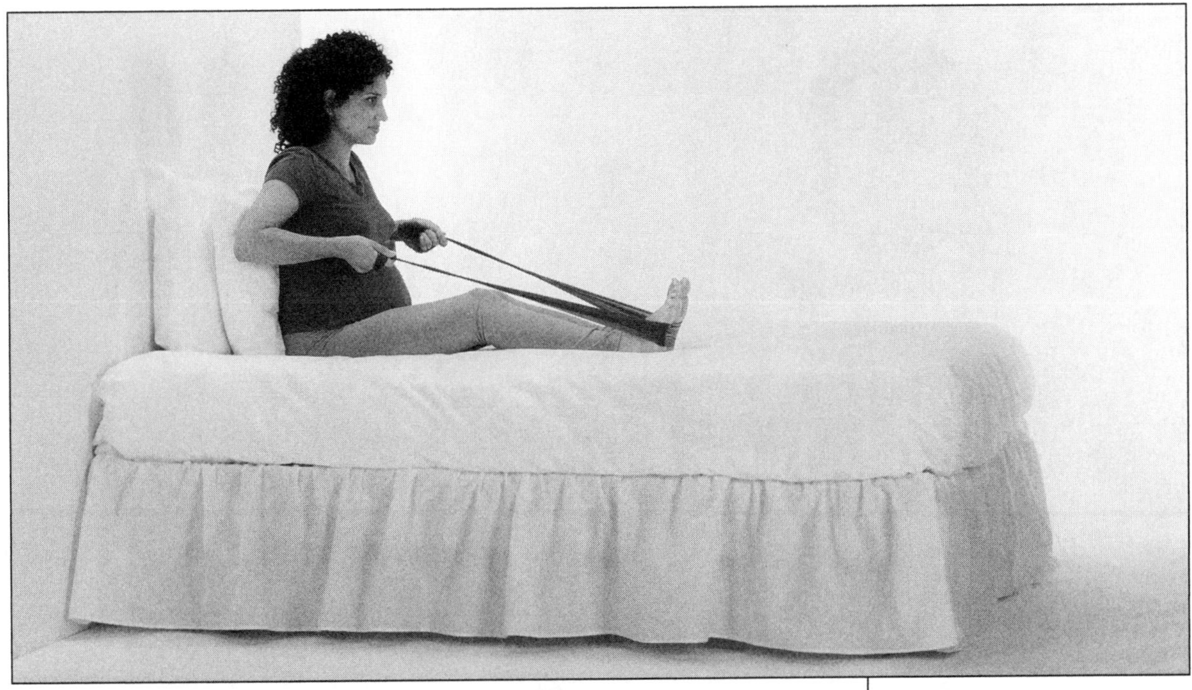

rowing

elbow back, squeezing the left shoulder blade toward the middle of the back and exhale.

Hold the squeeze for a few seconds without holding your breath. Repeat ten to twenty times on each side. This exercise works the latissimus dorsi muscles, rhomboids, and biceps. It can also be performed seated upright holding a Dyna-Band secured around your feet.

SHRUG

Sit up straight in bed. Shrug your shoulders up to your ears and rotate backward, squeezing the shoulder blades together, while exhaling. Hold the squeeze for a couple of seconds. Release and inhale. Repeat ten to twenty times. Shoulder shrugs work the trapezius, rhomboids, neck, and shoulder muscles.

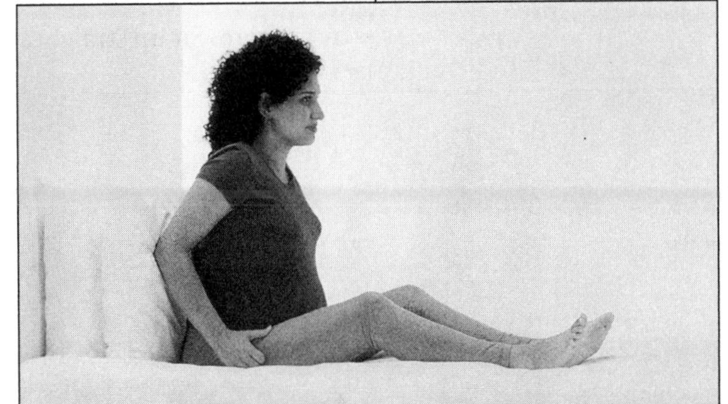

shrug

CHEST PRESS

Sit up straight in bed. Place a Dyna-Band behind your back and hold the ends at the sides of your chest. Press your hands forward, flexing your

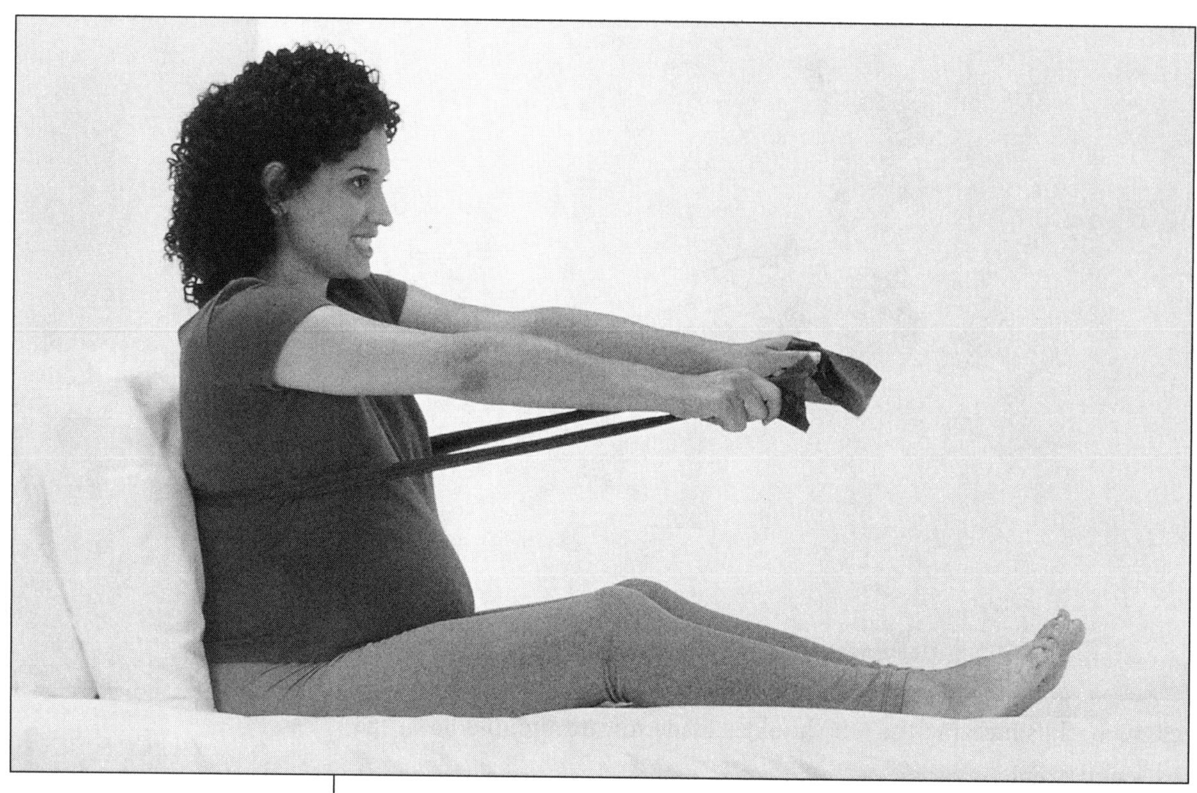

chest press

chest muscles (pectorals), and exhale. Release slowly and inhale. Repeat ten to twenty times.

PEC SQUEEZE

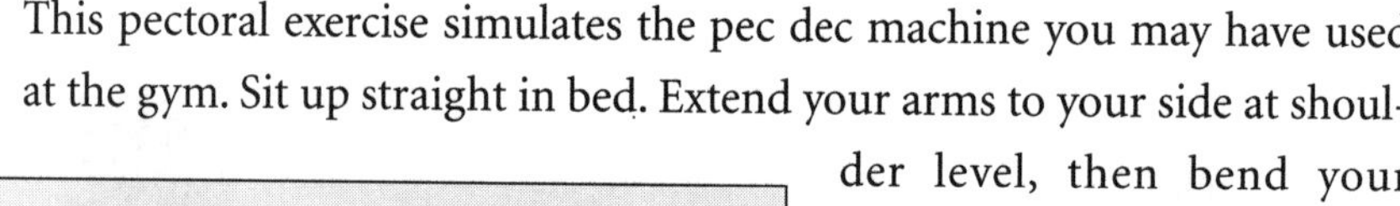

This pectoral exercise simulates the pec dec machine you may have used at the gym. Sit up straight in bed. Extend your arms to your side at shoulder level, then bend your elbows to a 90-degree angle. Flex your pectorals as you bring the elbows together as close as possible and exhale. Your growing chest may be too big to allow the elbows to actually touch. Hold the contraction for a second, release, return to your starting position, and inhale. Repeat ten to twenty times.

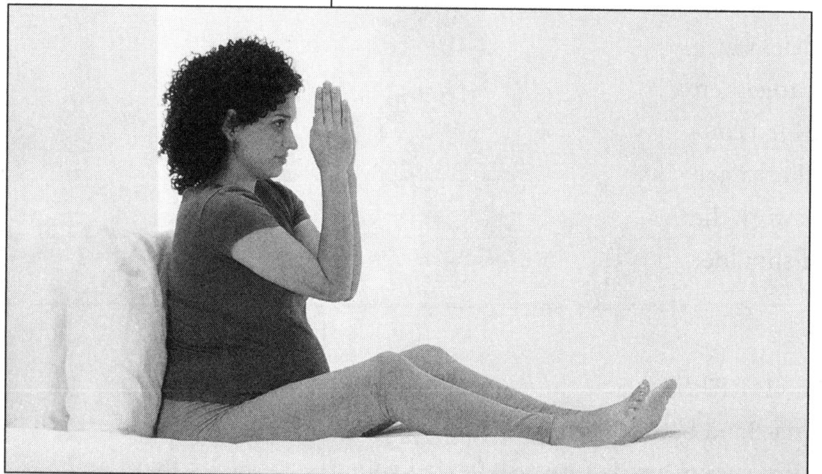

pec squeeze

BICEPS CURL

Sit up straight in bed with your arms down by your sides. Keeping your elbows tight at your sides, curl your forearms up to your shoulders and flex the biceps while exhaling. Hold the contraction for a couple of seconds. Release down and inhale. Repeat ten to twenty times. If you're strong enough, you can add resistance by using dumbbells or a Dyna-Band. Sit on the band and pull the ends up as you curl. This exercise can also be done lying on your side, exercising one arm at a time.

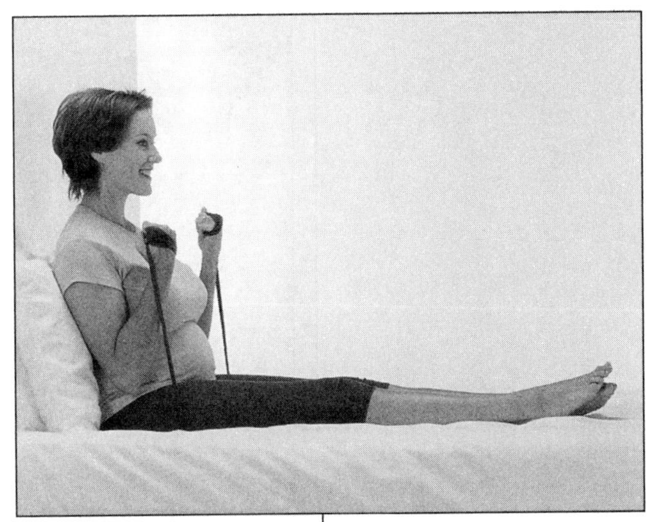

biceps curl

TRICEPS EXTENSION

Sit up straight in bed with your arms extended straight forward. Flex the triceps muscle hard and exhale; hold for a few seconds without holding your breath. Release and inhale. Repeat ten to twenty times. This can also be performed one arm at a time, lying on your side.

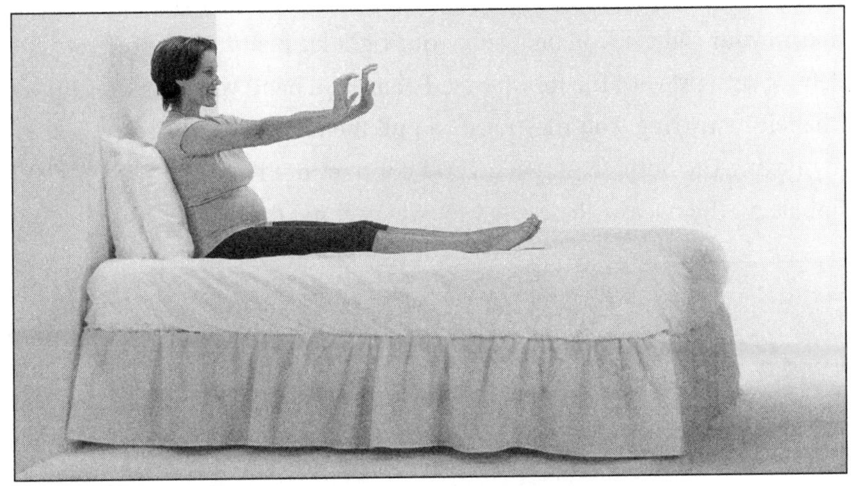

triceps extension

lower body exercises

LEG EXTENSION

Sit up straight in bed with your knees bent and pillows under your knees. Keeping your knees together, extend the right leg out straight. As you flex

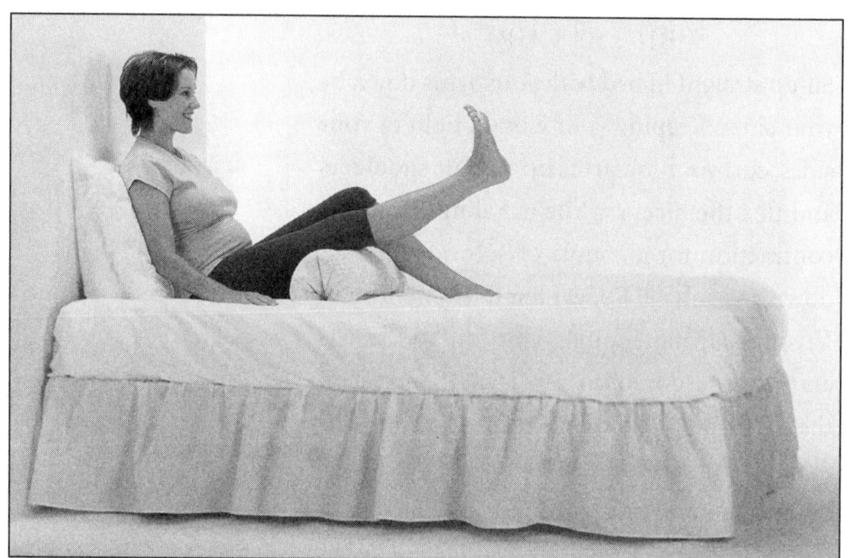

leg extension

the thigh muscles, exhale and hold it for a second. Release as you inhale. Repeat ten to twenty times on each leg. This exercise can also be done lying on your side. This exercise works the quadriceps, hip flexors, and abdominal muscles.

LEG CURL AND BUTTOCK SQUEEZE

Lie on your right side in bed, with your right leg bent for support, and the left leg straight with the foot flexed. Exhale and bend your left knee to flex the left hamstring. You may need to pull the knee back just a few inches, by flexing the buttock, to get a good contraction. Hold for a second and inhale on the release. Repeat ten to twenty times on each leg.

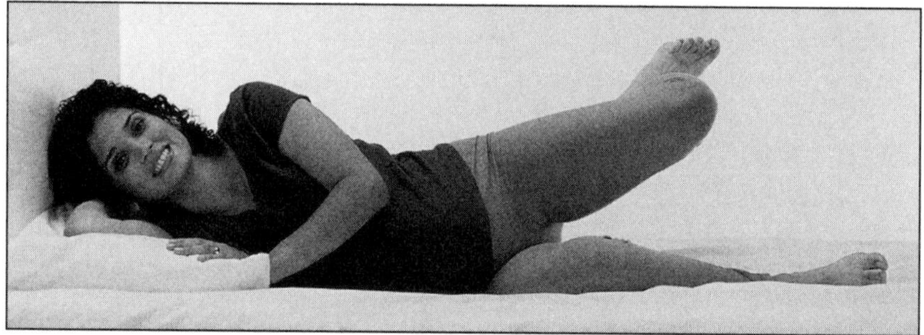

leg curl and buttock squeeze

ABDUCTOR LIFT

Lie on your right side in bed, with the right leg bent for support, and the left leg straight with a flexed foot. Slowly raise the left leg up as far as comfortable

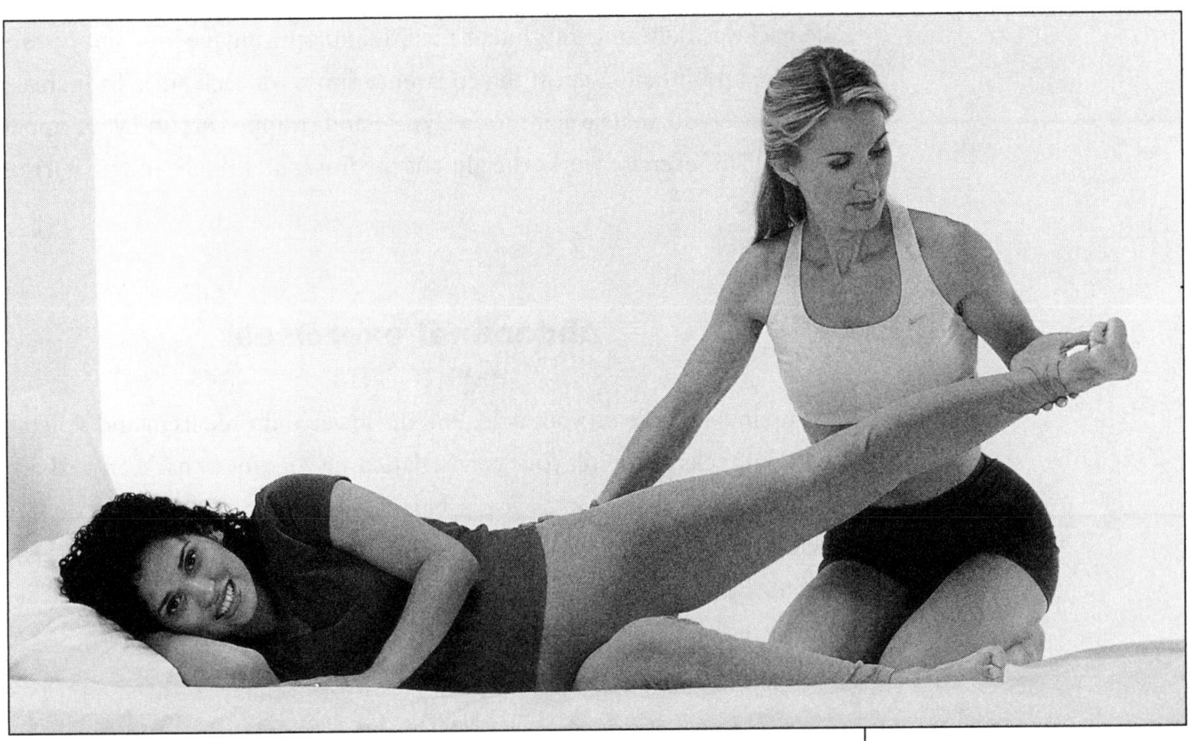

abductor lift

(about twelve inches) and exhale. Lower the leg and inhale. Repeat ten to twenty times on each leg. A light ankle weight may be used for added resistance. This exercise works the outer thigh and gluteus medius muscles.

HIP OPENER

Lie on your right side, with both legs bent in front of you at a 90-degree angle. Slowly lift the left knee up until it is perpendicular to the bed (don't

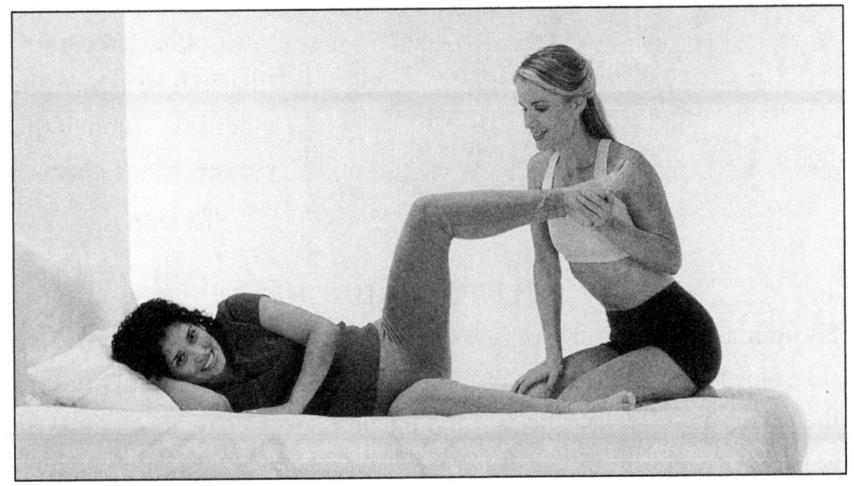

hip opener (clam)

go backward), flexing the gluteus medius and opening the hip joint. Slowly release and inhale. Repeat ten to twenty times on each side. To increase resistance, add ankle weights or a Dyna-Band strapped around your upper calves. This exercise works the gluteus medius, outer thigh, and piriformis muscles.

abdominal exercises

PELVIC TILT

Sit up in bed or lie on your side. Pull the lower abdominals in and squeeze your buttocks as you tilt your pelvis, flattening your lower back, and exhale. Release the contraction as you inhale. You can also add a Kegel squeeze before you release. Repeat ten to twenty times. In addition to strengthening the pelvic floor, glutes, and abdominal muscles, this exercise also stretches the lower back.

ABDOMINAL CRUNCH

Sit up in bed or lie on your side. Place your hands on your belly. Contract the abdominal muscles as tight as you can, rounding your back, as you would for a C-curve, and exhale. Release the contraction as you inhale, straightening your back. Repeat ten to twenty times. If your abdominal muscles have separated (diastasis recti), do the modified version of this exercise, which is shown on page 127.

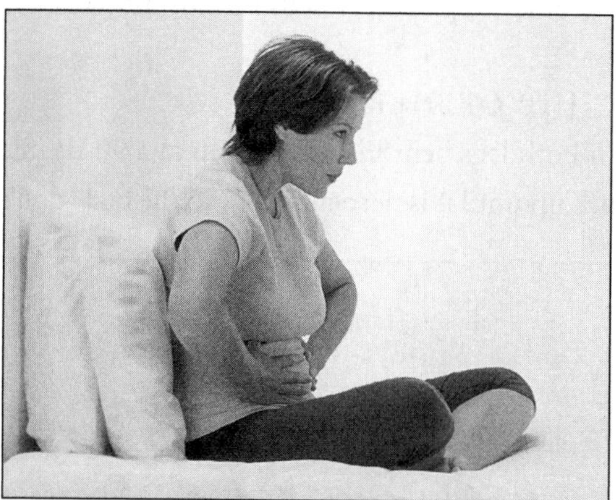

abdominal crunch

OBLIQUE CRUNCH

Sit up in bed with your hands resting by your sides or lie on your right side. Slowly contract the left obliques, bringing the left shoulder toward the left hip as you exhale. Release and inhale. Repeat ten to fifteen times on each side.

KNEE LIFT

Lie on your right side with your knees bent in front of you for support. Bring your left knee toward your left shoulder by contracting the obliques. Exhale on the contraction; inhale as you release. Repeat ten to fifteen times on each side.

ABDOMINAL PULSE

Sit up in bed or lie on your side with your hands on your belly. Inhale and relax your abdominals. If your belly is really big, you may need to lift your arms out to the side to expand your lung capacity. Exhale, pull in and contract the abdominals as best you can. Inhale and release. This can be tricky until you get used to it, but practice makes perfect. When you get better at it, speed up the repetitions. Repeat at least fifteen times.

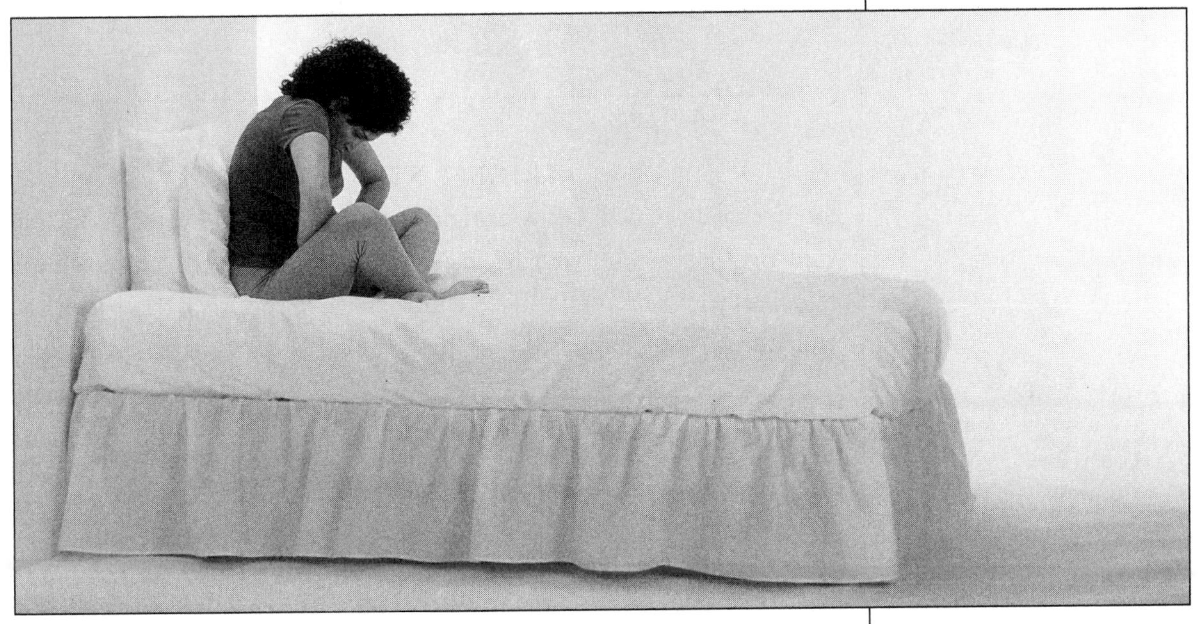

abdominal pulse

stretches

As with the other exercises, prop yourself up with pillows for support.

ELBOW CHEST STRETCH

Sit up in bed and place both hands behind your head. Gently press your elbows backward to stretch the shoulders and pectorals. Hold the stretch for at least ten to thirty seconds. Don't forget to breathe. This is more effective if someone else presses your elbows backward.

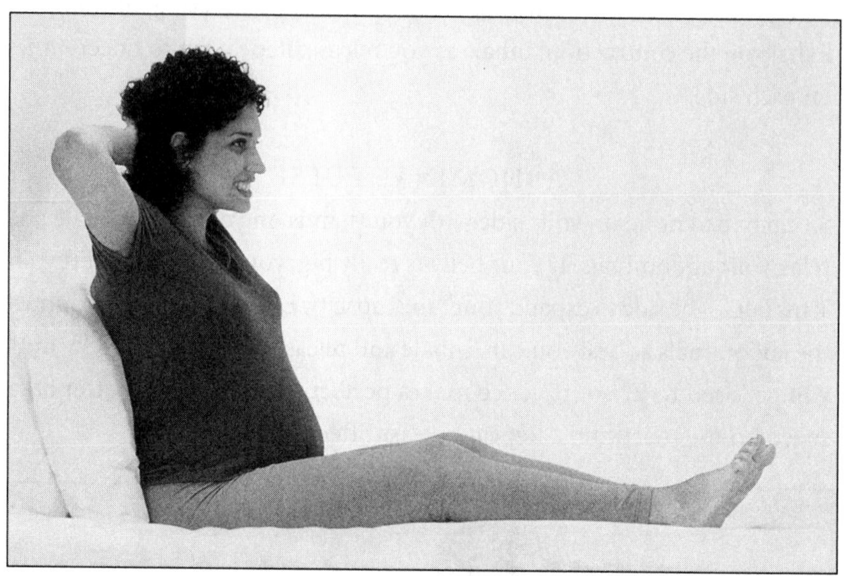

elbow chest stretch

TRICEPS STRETCH

Sit up straight in bed. Lift your right arm up and behind your head. Grab your right elbow with your left hand, and press the right hand down the middle of your back until you feel a nice stretch in your right triceps muscle. Hold the stretch for at least ten to thirty seconds. Repeat on the other side.

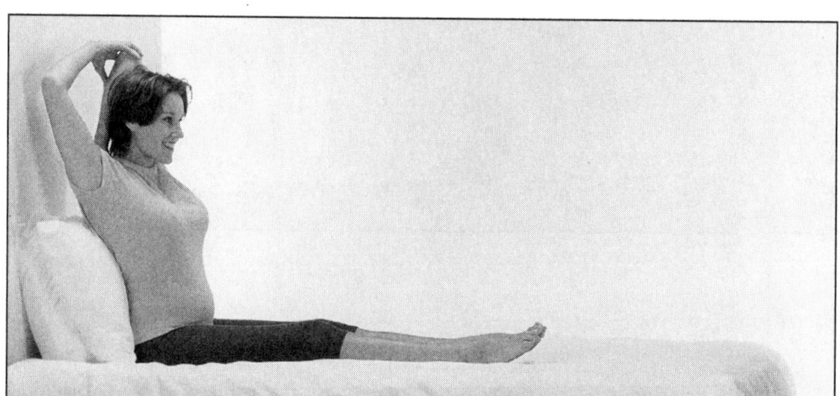

triceps stretch

SHOULDER STRETCH

Sit up straight in bed. Draw your left arm across your chest, using your right hand to press the elbow toward you until you can feel a stretch in your shoulder. Hold the stretch for ten to thirty seconds. Repeat on the other side.

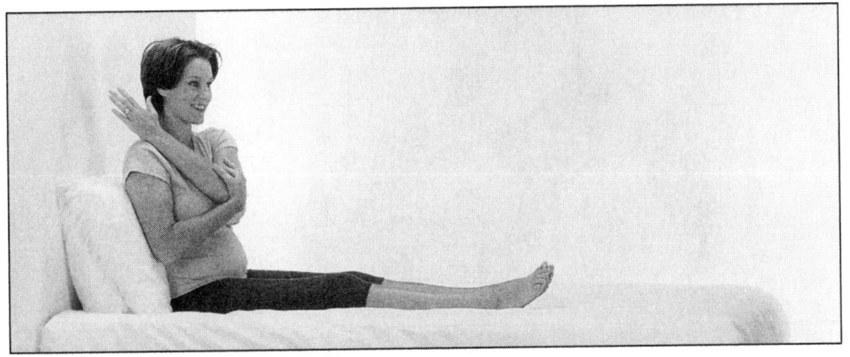

shoulder stretch

QUADRICEPS STRETCH

Lie on your right side with both legs bent. With your left hand, grab your left foot and pull it close to your buttocks. Gently move the left knee down toward the other knee until you feel a stretch in the front thigh. Hold the stretch for ten to thirty seconds. Repeat on the other side.

quadriceps stretch

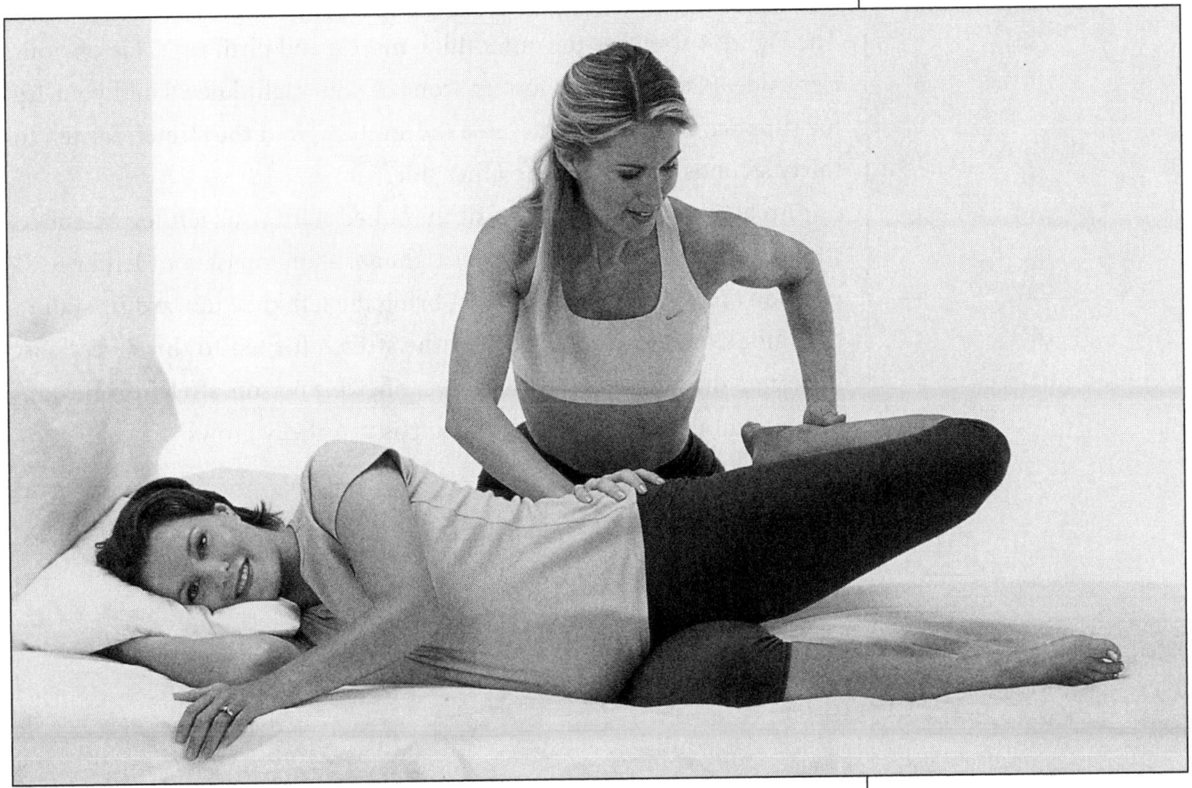

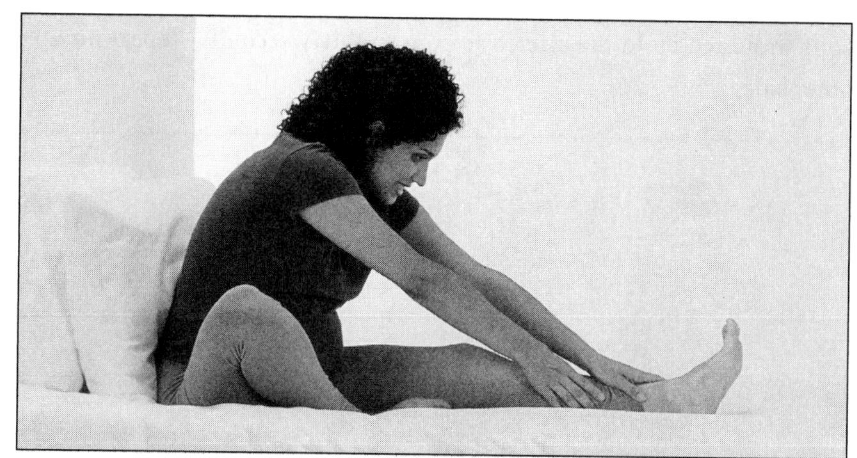

hamstring stretch

HAMSTRING STRETCH

Sit up or lie on your right side with the right knee bent for support. Grab your left ankle or calf with your left hand, and keep your leg as straight as you can. If you are very flexible, you can hold on to your foot. Hold the stretch for ten to thirty seconds. Repeat on the other side.

FIGURE 4

The Figure 4 stretches the outer thigh muscle and piriformis. Lie on your right side. Place your left foot in front of your right knee. Hold your leg for support, or to gently increase the stretch. Hold the stretch for ten to thirty seconds. Repeat on the other side.

An alternate method is to sit up in bed with your left leg extended straight in front of you. Place your right ankle on top of your left knee. If you don't feel enough of a stretch, bring the left knee upward by sliding that foot closer toward you. Hold the stretch for ten to thirty seconds. Repeat on the other side. If you're a very flexible person, stretching the piriformis "enough" will become difficult as your belly grows.

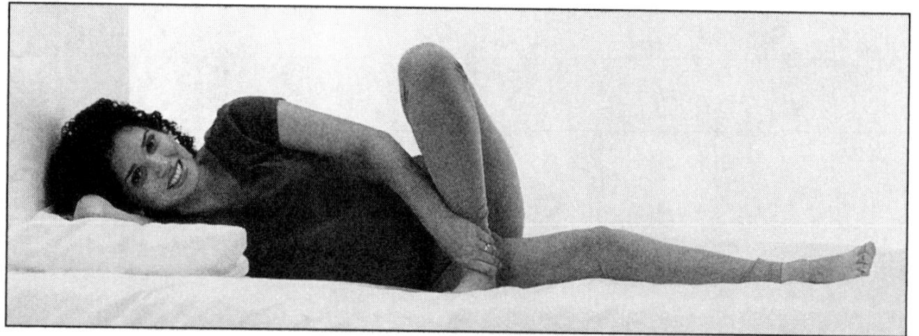

figure 4

KNEE TUCK

Lie on your right side with the right leg bent for support. With your left hand, pull your left knee up as close to the left shoulder as possible. Hold the stretch for ten to thirty seconds. Repeat on the other side. This exercise stretches the inner thigh, buttocks, and lower back.

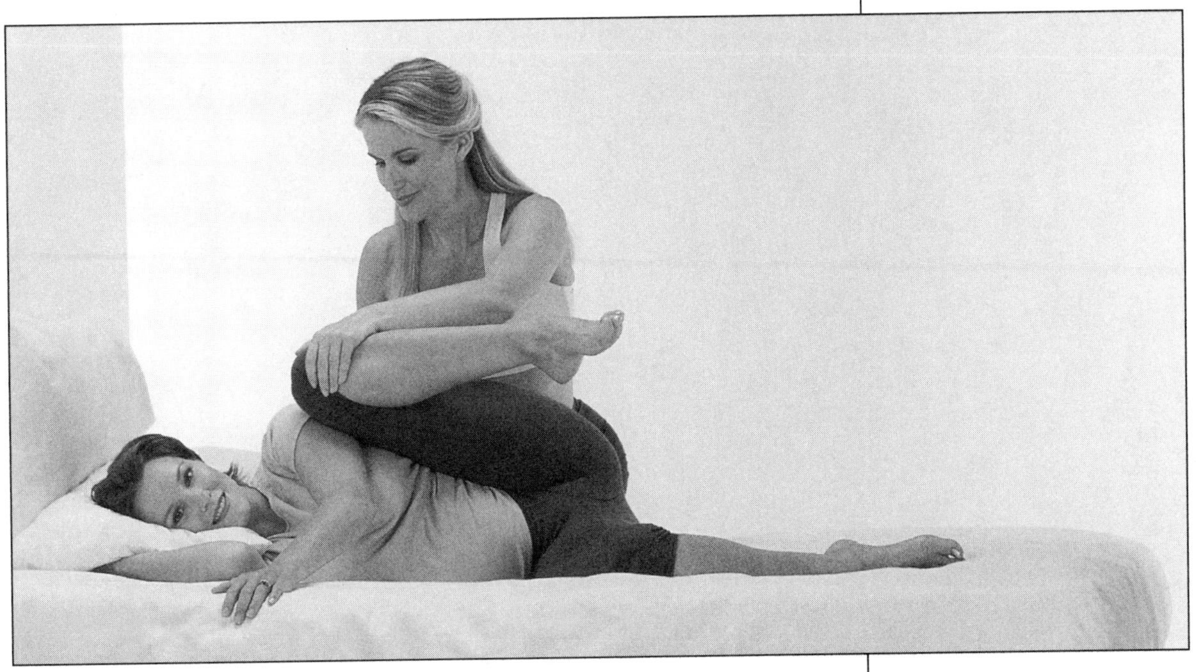

knee tuck

C-CURVE

This exercise stretches the lower back and buttocks. Sit up straight in bed with your knees pulled up toward you. Hold on to your legs behind your knees for support, and pull your abdomen in and round your back. Hold the position for ten to thirty seconds. Release and repeat. You can also add a Kegel to this exercise.

C-curve beginning (left) and end (right)

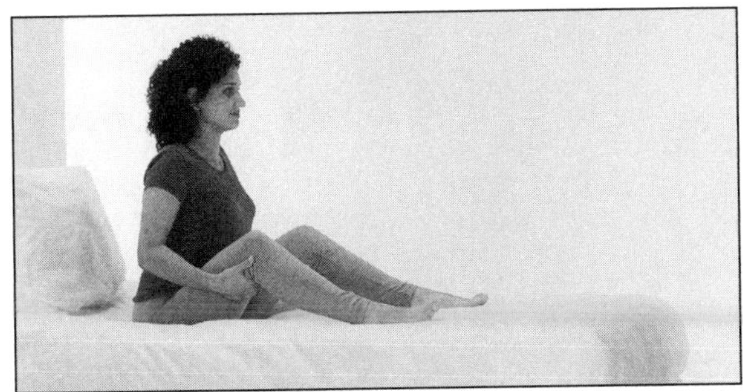

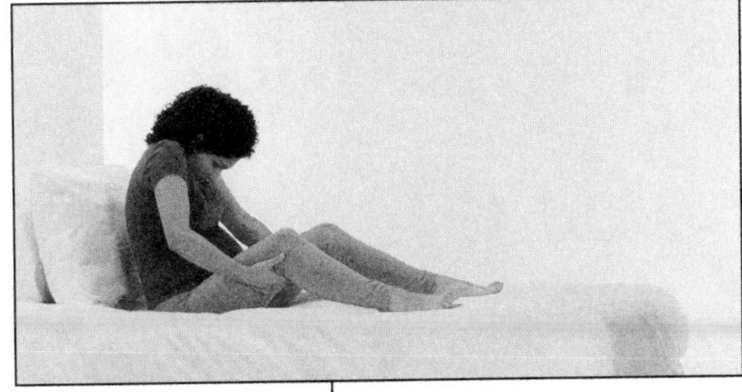

Chapter Seven

posture, stretching, yoga, relaxation, and correct breathing

IN THIS CHAPTER

- *Postural self-test and guidelines for good posture*
- *Stretches for every muscle group*
- *Stress-reduction techniques including: meditation, visualization, and breathing exercises*

Posture, stretching, relaxation, breathing, and yoga may seem like an awful lot to cover in one chapter. Indeed, I could write an entire chapter about each of these topics. But they are all interrelated, especially during pregnancy, so it seems fitting to combine them here. In previous chapters, you read about the effects that pregnancy has on your body. In addition to pushing your body to new limits, pregnancy causes a surge of new hormones. These changes affect your body, mind, and emotions, adding to whatever pressures you are already under in your daily life—from your job, mate, children, and other responsibilities—not to mention the anxiety you may be feeling about pregnancy and motherhood.

The techniques in this chapter can help alleviate both the physical and emotional challenges that pregnancy brings. Practicing good posture will minimize the strain on the musculoskeletal system. Yoga and stretching lengthen the muscles, improve posture, and aid in relaxation. Practicing breathing techniques can expand your lung capacity, which will offset the effect of your growing uterus on your lungs. Correct breathing also works in concert with the relaxation methods covered here, such as meditation and visualization. The techniques in this chapter, whether you practice

Your feet will thank you for investing in a pair of good, supportive sneakers.

them all or mix-and-match, can help bring your mind, body, and soul into balance—making the road to motherhood a more harmonious one.

posture

A person with good posture exudes confidence, vitality, and a fit, healthy image. Your posture affects your health, balance, comfort, and breathing. Proper posture means the spine is efficiently aligned in any position, whether working or resting, with minimal exertion. As your belly grows bigger and you are carrying more weight in front, you will need to readjust your center of gravity, which takes practice and effort. Pregnancy makes perfect alignment difficult, if not impossible. But it is vitally important that you try to maintain as close to perfect posture as you possibly can.

During pregnancy, you may be inclined to stand on the back of your heels, arching your back, with your belly, shoulders, and head shifting forward. This position tightens the lower back muscles, weakens the abdominals, and overstresses the bones and ligaments, leading to backaches, painful joints, and other discomforts. Some pregnant women lock their knees to stay straight, but instead end up leaning back quite uncomfortably.

Another common trait of pregnant women is the wider foot stance for better balance. This would be okay if it wasn't for the "waddle" that usually accompanies it. If the hip extensors (buttocks, hamstrings) and abductors (outer thigh muscles) are weak, the result is a haphazard, sloppy waddle-walk or "duck-walk." This is not only an unattractive look, it can also be dangerous for your back, hips, knees, ankles, and feet.

When you are walking, remember the old adage, "Think tall." Lift your head and chin up, hold in your stomach, tuck your buttocks in and under, shoulders back, and chest up. Even more important for injury prevention, be careful to keep good posture, alignment, and balance when you exercise.

Wearing high heels during pregnancy is a no-no, because they can accentuate all of these postural problems and probably set you up for further injuries. Wear flat or low-heeled shoes with good arch support. However, avoid shoes that are too flat, such as cheap tennis shoes, especially when you exercise. Your feet will thank you for investing in a pair of good, supportive sneakers.

You should wear a good supportive bra daily—and nightly when necessary. It will help prevent upper back strain and keep your bust from sagging as it becomes heavier. During exercise you may need not just one, but two good jog bras for adequate support.

The strength of your upper back muscles determines your shoulder position (upper spinal alignment), and the strength of your abdominals determines your degree of pelvic tilt. Other muscles that need strengthening for good posture are the glutes, hamstrings, abductor (outer thigh), trapezius, and rhomboids (upper back). The muscles that need to be stretched are the hip flexors, quadriceps, lower back, piriformis, pectorals, and calves. (For an illustrated guide to the location and function of these muscle groups, see chapter 5.) Keep these areas in mind when customizing your workout.

POSTURAL SELF-TEST

The best way to check your own posture when pregnant is from the side. Look at your body profile in a full-length mirror and answer these questions:

1. Is your chest up—or flat/concave?
2. Are your shoulders up and back—or rounded forward or leaning too far back?
3. Is your back curved naturally—or arched too much, or is it flat?
4. Are your knees soft—or hyperextended backward or bent forward?
5. Do you have regular foot arches—or are they high or flat?

The first segment of each question demonstrates proper posture. If any of your answers were in the latter part, you need to work on improving your posture. The following postural problems can be checked from the front. These problems are not usually related to pregnancy, but they are equally important to check and address. Stand facing a full-length mirror and answer these questions:

1. Is your head straight and in the middle—or slightly bending to one side?
2. Are your shoulders even—or is one higher than the other?
3. Are your hips even—or is one higher than the other?
4. Are your knees pointing forward, inward, or outward?
5. Is there less than two inches between your knees—or more?

A tilted head could be an indicator of tight neck muscles, a pinched nerve, or stress. These problems may be alleviated by massage, stretching, special exercises, or acupuncture. Avoid cradling the phone between your shoulder and ear. If your hips or shoulders are uneven you may have scoliosis (curvature of the spine). Consult your doctor for a diagnosis. Your doctor and/or a knowledgeable instructor should prescribe some special postural exercises for you that will help counteract the effects of scoliosis. If your knees are not straight or they are too far apart, consult your doctor. If you have no injury or medical causation, it may be possible to correct postural problems with special strengthening exercises.

postural exercises

Properly executing postural exercises may take a little practice. But if you want to carry your pregnancy as effortlessly as is pregnantly possible, don't give up until you master them. Once you begin to reap the benefits of proper body alignment, you'll never want to slouch again—during pregnancy or afterward.

BEGINNER

Stand with your back against a wall and your feet a foot away from the wall. Do a pelvic tilt, tucking the buttocks in and under, and pressing the lower back into the wall by pulling in the abdominals. Your head, shoulders, and the entire back of your torso should touch the wall at the same time. This can be very difficult, especially when you're pregnant.

ADVANCED

Once you've mastered the beginner version, advance to this one. Stand with your back against a wall and your feet a foot away. Tilt your pelvis and press the lower back into the wall. Maintaining this posture, slowly lift your arms in front of you—using your upper back muscles, not your shoulders—until they are straight up over your head, as close to the wall as possible. This is a difficult exercise to master—your lower back wants to leave the wall as your arms rise. Lift your arms only as high as they can go without arching your back away from the wall. If you master this exercise, the entire back of your torso and arms will touch the wall.

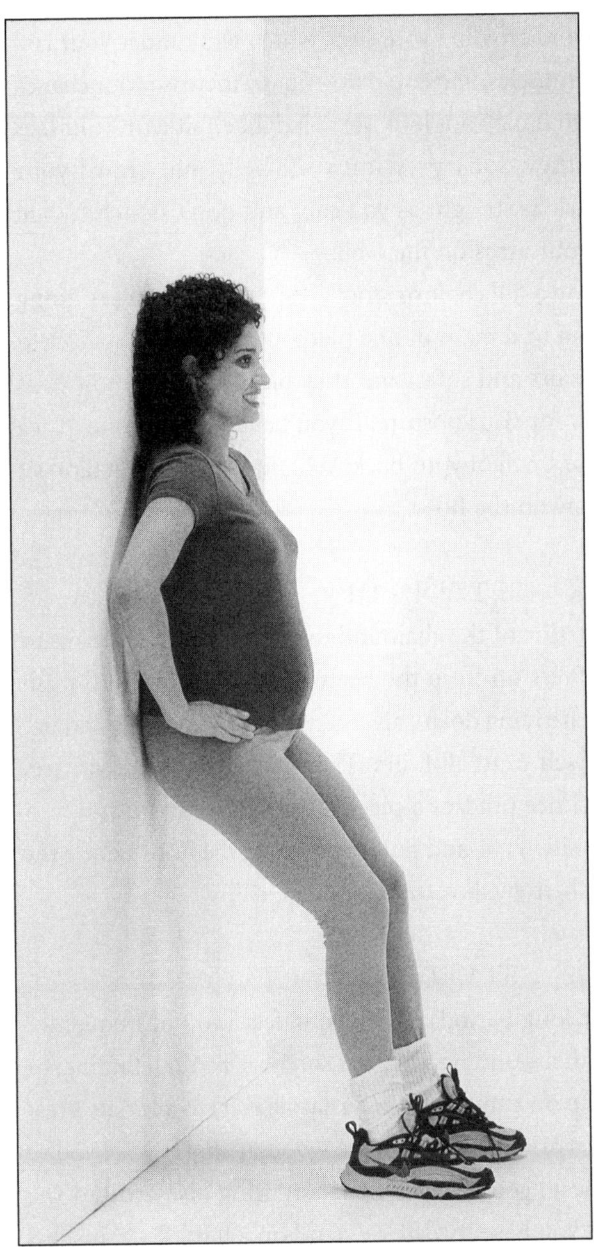

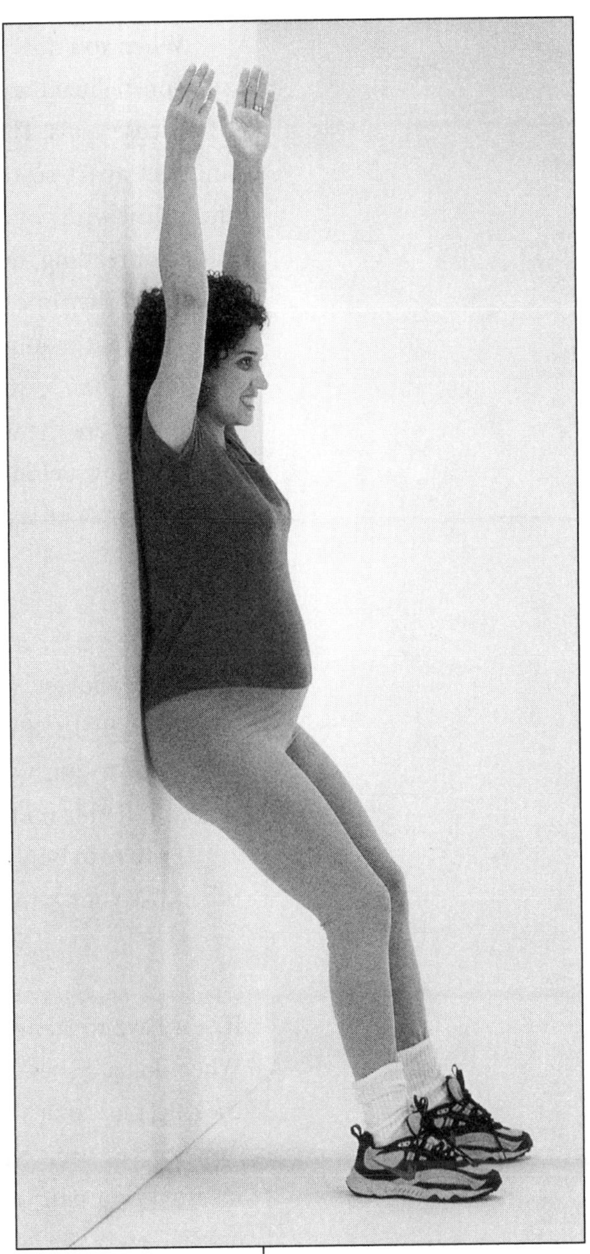

beginner (left) and advanced (right) postural exercise

good postural form

Stand up and walk around whenever you can; sitting for long periods while pregnant causes blood to pool in your legs. The more you sit, the more your hip flexors and piriformis flex, thereby shortening and tightening these muscles, resulting in hip and lower back stiffness. When you're standing or lying straight, the hip flexors get to relax.

When you do sit, avoid crossing your legs, which will hinder your circulation, tighten the hip muscles, and could potentially increase your chance of varicose veins. Though it may not look very "ladylike," sit with your legs and feet apart so that they don't press on your belly and crowd your uterus. Sit with your back as straight as you can, and don't slouch. When eating or reading, rest your arms on the table.

If you have one, sit on a tall chair or stool—especially if you are doing activities that require you to remain in one place—they're much easier to get out of than lower chairs and sofas, and they place less strain on your back. Sofas are the worst for your posture. If you have to sit on one, place a small pillow behind the small of your back. Whenever possible, tailor-sit (cross-legged) on a pillow on the floor.

GETTING UP

Grab on to a table or the side of the chair and use your hands and arms to help push yourself up. Press up from the heels—not the toes—and push with your thighs. If you are lying down, always roll onto your side, and use your arms to push yourself onto all fours. Then place one foot forward, and your hands on that knee (and/or a piece of furniture) to push up.

If you're in bed, roll sideways, and put one foot on the floor before the other. Use your arms to help push yourself up.

STANDING

If you have to stand for long periods, move your feet around frequently. When doing dishes or other standing activities, such as ironing, folding, or cooking, place one foot up on a small box (alternating feet) to alleviate pressure on your back. My favorite back-savers are wooden clogs. Once you've invested in a pair of these, you'll never wear anything else around the house—especially when you have to walk or stand on a hard floor. Instead of leaning over beds and bathtubs, bend your knees or kneel on the floor.

WALKING

Walk as upright as you can. Chin up, shoulders back, chest up, stomach in, buttocks in, pelvis tucked under, soft knees, and with straight controlled steps—no waddling. If you're vacuuming, or pushing a stroller or food cart, don't bend forward, keep the cart or vacuum close to you.

STAIR CLIMBING

Use a handrail if possible. Put your whole foot flat on every step, and press down with your heel. Use your thigh muscles to push yourself up. Keep the rest of your body as upright as possible.

While pregnant, try to avoid carrying another baby on your hip—it torques the spine.

LIFTING

With your torso upright, squat or lunge down, bending at the knees, not the hips. Grasp the desired object close to you. As your belly gets bigger, it won't be a good idea to lift something in front of you. Hold the object on the side, or divide it into two if possible, one object for each side. Keep your back straight and your abs and pelvis tight, and use your legs to lift up.

While pregnant, try to avoid carrying another baby on your hip—it torques the spine. Use other carrying tools and strollers.

If your belly has gotten very heavy, making exercise and other activities uncomfortable, try wearing a pregnancy belt or corset. Wear them only during such activity and do not become dependent on them. They could do more harm than good in that they weaken your abdominals by giving them a break.

KNEELING

At times when your body is really tired and you are home, get down on all fours. This position will help circulation, relieve aches, pains, cramps, and even hemorrhoids. I think if it was possible and practical, this is how all pregnant women would want to get around.

how to relieve posture-related aches and pains

Mild aches and pains are a fact of life during pregnancy. The following tips can help alleviate these pains when they occur. Worsening or chronic back, hip, neck, or shoulder pain should be brought to your caregiver's attention.

BACK PAIN

- Strengthen the upper back, abdominals, glutes, and hamstrings.
- Stretch the lower back, chest, hip flexors, and piriformis.
- Practice the postural exercises on page 176.

- Modify your workout and certain exercises to minimize back strain.
- Use a firm mattress or a bed board.
- Use a maternal back belt only when necessary (don't become reliant on it).
- For chronic pain, consider massage and physical therapy.

NECK AND SHOULDER PAIN

- Strengthen the upper back and neck.
- Stretch the chest.
- Stretch the neck forward, to the sides, and in half-circles from one shoulder to the other. (Bending your head backward could strain your cervical spine.)
- Use a firm mattress.
- Use pillows to rest your top arm and leg on when lying on your side.
- Wear a bra at night.
- Get neck and shoulder massages.

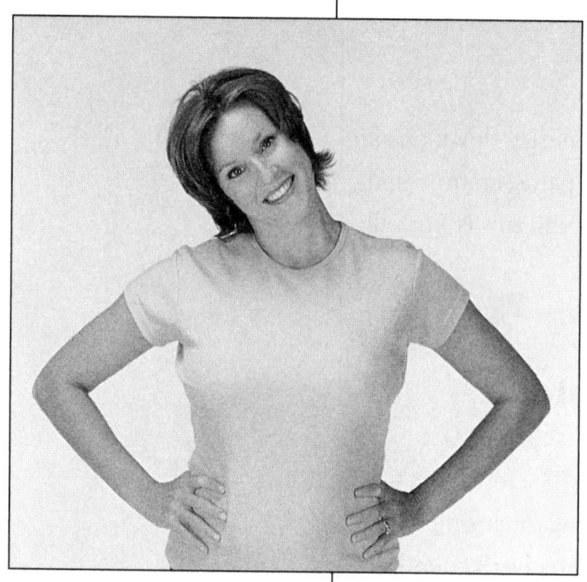

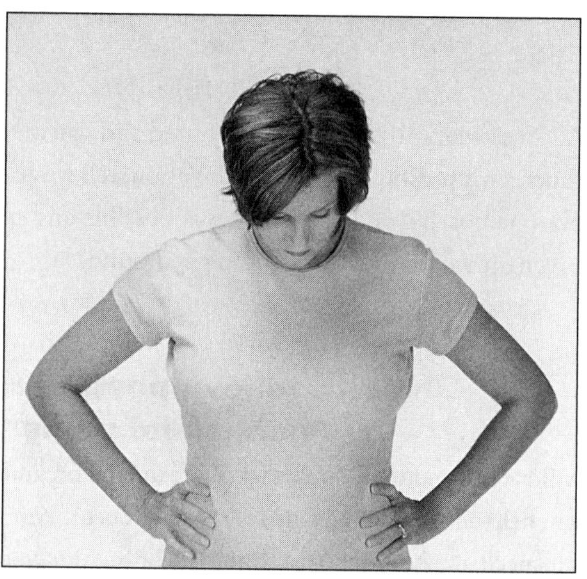

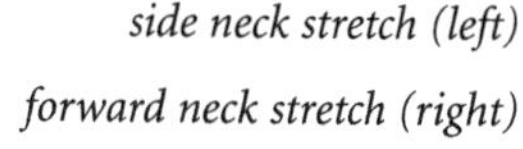

side neck stretch (left)
forward neck stretch (right)

HIP PAIN

- Wear low-heeled shoes.
- Spend less time sitting down (it tightens the hip flexors and piriformis).
- Stretch the hip flexors and piriformis.

- Try some hip mobility exercises, such as the pelvic tilt (see page 133), dog wag (page 137), and side-lying hip opener (page 139).
- If the pain is severe, you may need to walk with crutches until after your pregnancy.

SCIATIC PAIN

The best course for relieving sciatica depends upon its severity. If you experience temporary sciatic pain, such as when the baby moves into a position that pinches on a nerve, stretching the piriformis may help (see page 196 for a good piriformis stretch). If you experience chronic sciatic pain throughout your pregnancy, massage, rest, and relaxation may be your only relief.

Stretching itself is not a good way to warmup for a workout.

stretching

Stretching lengthens and makes your muscles more supple, which makes you more flexible. Flexibility is defined as joint mobility and range of motion (ROM), and the ability of a muscle to relax and lengthen. In essence, the greater your flexibility, the further your limbs can move in any direction, without discomfort and with less effort. Stretching should complement strength training and cardiovascular exercise, not replace it. If you have incredible ROM, but lack the stabilizing support of strong muscles, your risk of injuries is increased. Your natural ROM will decrease with age, inactivity, bad postural habits, and injuries, unless you stretch. Stretching helps you move more easily, decreases tension, and reduces the chance of aches, pains, and injury. Stretching after a workout prevents muscle soreness.

Stretching your muscles during pregnancy will not only *feel* great, it will also improve your posture, reduce many discomforts, and help make labor easier. But you need to be more careful than usual. Stretching too far or too fast, particularly when your muscles are not warm, could result in a pulled or strained muscle. Stretching itself is not a good way to warmup for a workout. Always warmup before you stretch, or stretch *after* a workout when your muscles are warm and pliable.

The best way to warmup and get your circulation going before working out or stretching is to either take a light ten-minute walk or bicycle

If it feels good, it probably is—and if it doesn't . . . well, you know the answer.

ride, or to use any other cardiovascular exercise or machine. Another great way to warmup is to do lighter and easier versions of the exercises you'll be doing in your workout. For example, if you plan to do squats with weights in your workout, do supported non-weighted squats to warmup. If you plan to run, warmup by walking.

If your intention in stretching is to lengthen the muscle permanently, increasing your flexibility rather than just maintaining it, the muscles being stretched need to be at least 100° to 102° Fahrenheit warm. Your muscles will be this warm only after a hard workout. You can't actually measure your muscle temperature, but when you're all hot and sweaty from working out, you'll know that you're there. However, there is no need at this time for you to permanently lengthen your muscles. Stretching during pregnancy should be about releasing and relaxing, not pushing your muscles and joints to their limits.

Whether you're a novice or an Olympic gymnast, when you are pregnant you should never take a stretch to the point of pain. Your joints and ligaments are softer and you could pull a muscle, or worse—severely injure a joint. Ease gently into a stretch until you can feel the muscle stretch (not hurt or burn), and hold for at least ten to thirty seconds. You may hold it longer if you want, your muscles will only relax more. Listen to your body. If it feels good, it probably is—and if it doesn't . . . well, you know the answer.

upper body stretches (chest, shoulders, and arms)

Remember to breathe during a stretch; do not hold your breath. Always elongate your muscles gently; do not bounce. Be careful not to take a stretch too far.

BODY STRETCH

Stand with your feet comfortably apart or sit on the floor. Reach with both arms up over your head as high as you can, stretching your whole body. When pregnant, avoid rising up on your toes, to prevent leg cramps and loss of balance. Hold the stretch for ten to thirty seconds. If this stretch strains your sides, discontinue.

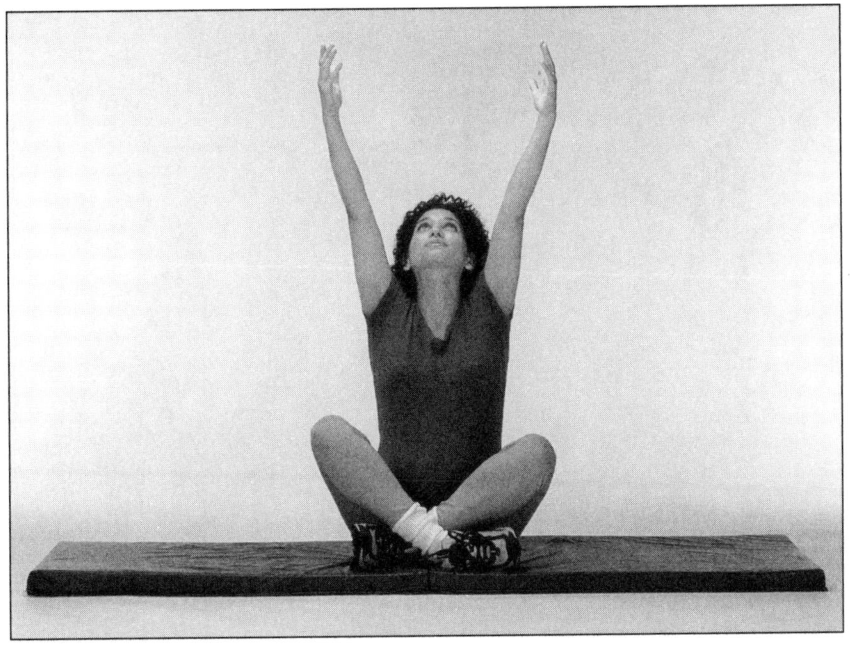

body stretch

SIDE STRETCH

Stand with your feet apart or sit on the floor. Raise one arm up as high as you can. You should feel the stretch on that side. If necessary, use the other arm for support. Hold the stretch for ten to thirty seconds. Repeat on the other side.

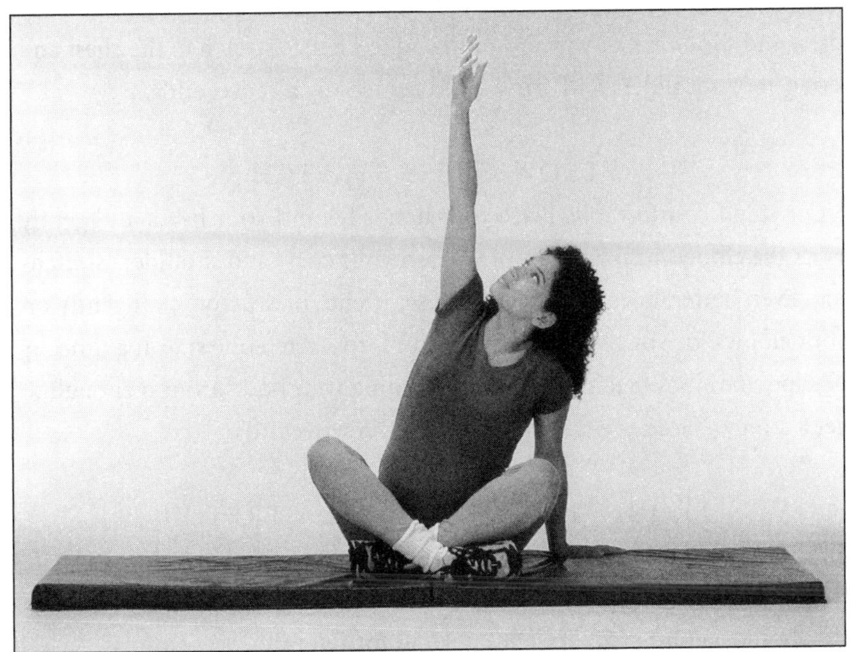

side stretch

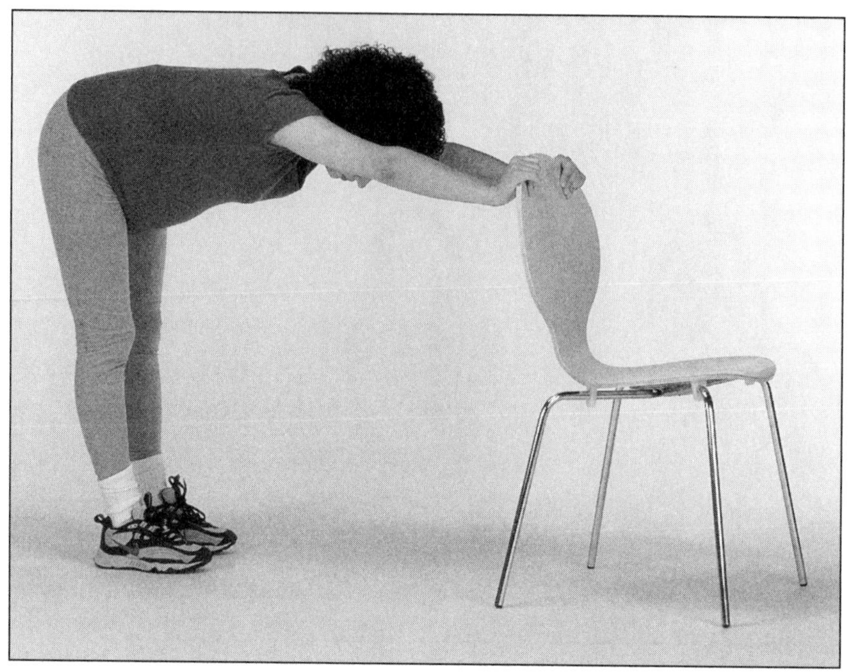
bent over chest stretch

BENT OVER CHEST STRETCH (MODIFIED DOWN DOG)

Place your hands or arms on the back of a chair or bench. Stand far enough away so that you can bend forward at the hips, creating a straight line from your arms to the buttocks. Your knees should be soft. Gently press your chest and shoulders downward until you feel a nice stretch in the chest and along your shoulders and arms. Hold for ten to thirty seconds.

ELBOW CHEST STRETCH

Sit or stand comfortably. Place your hands behind your head, and gently press the elbows backward until you feel your chest and shoulders stretching. Even better, have someone (spouse, friend, instructor) pull gently on your elbows for you. Another alternative is to stretch one side at a time, by placing one elbow against a wall and turning your body around enough to get a stretch. Hold the stretch for ten to thirty seconds.

FRONT SHOULDER/BICEPS STRETCH

Sit or stand comfortably. Clasp your hands together behind your back. Raise your arms up and back as far as you can comfortably. You'll feel both the shoulders and arms stretching. Hold for ten to thirty seconds.

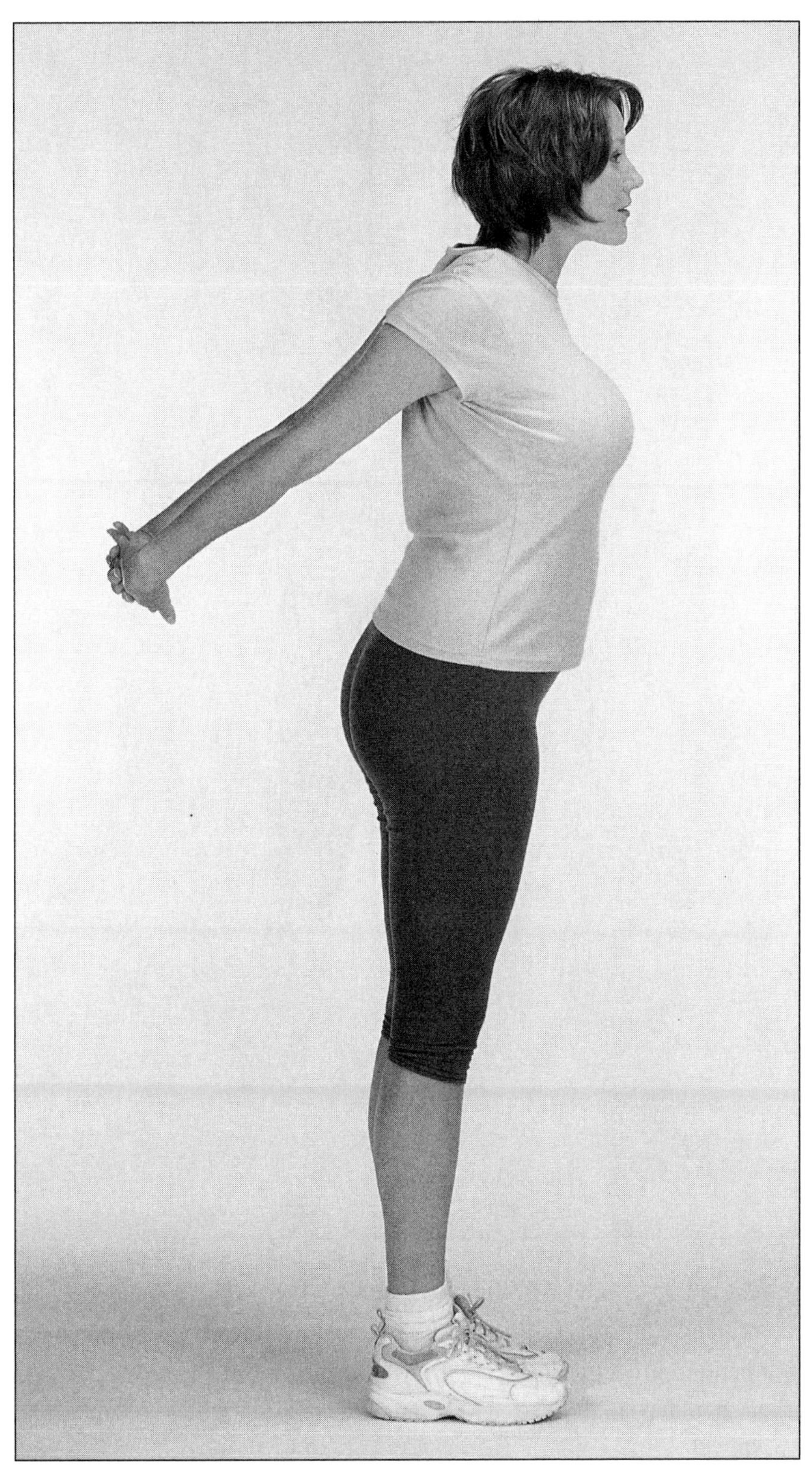

front shoulder/biceps stretch

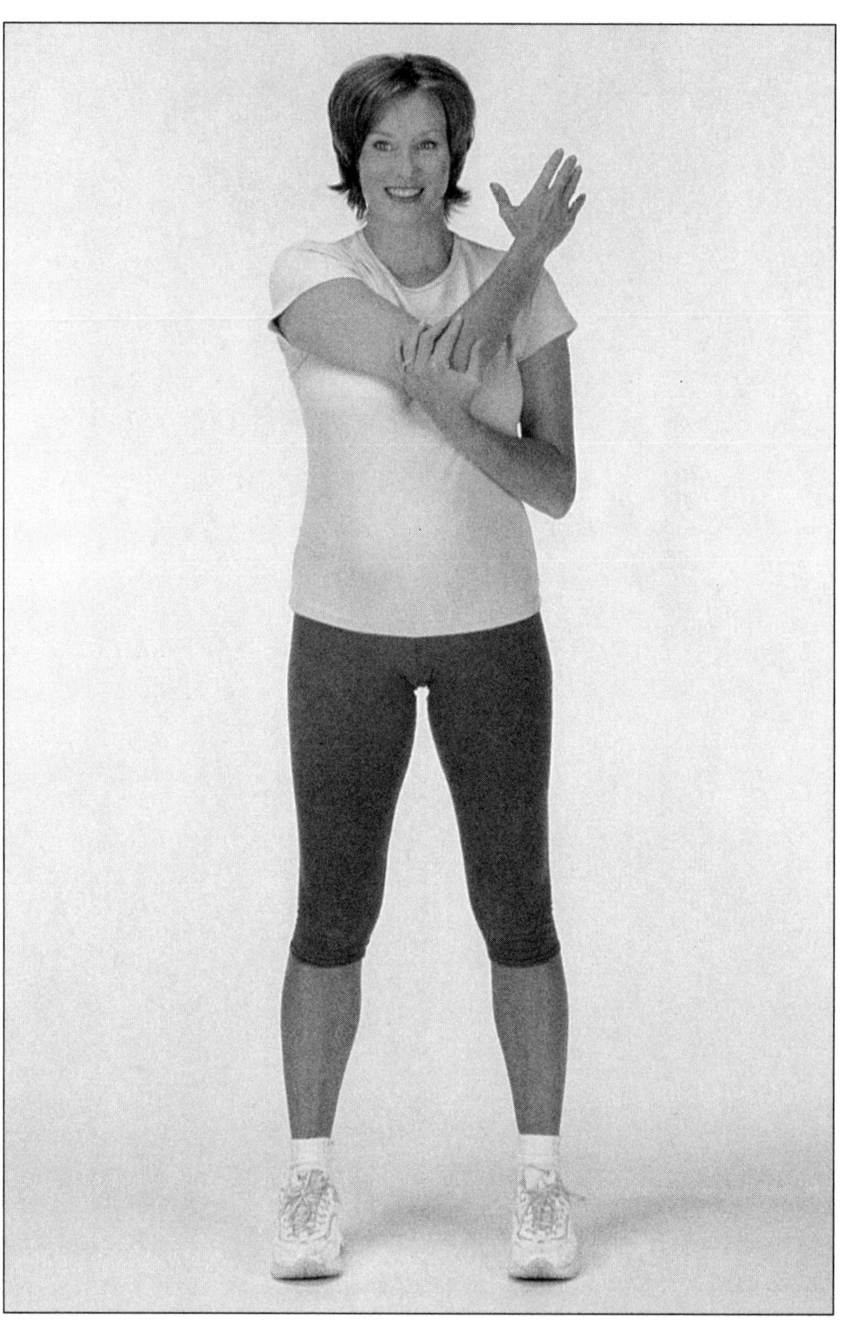

rear shoulder stretch

REAR SHOULDER STRETCH

Sit or stand comfortably. Draw your right arm across your chest, using your left hand to press the elbow toward you until you can feel a stretch in the right shoulder. Hold the stretch for ten to thirty seconds. Release and repeat on the other side.

TRICEPS STRETCH

Stand or sit with your right arm up and behind your head. Grab your right elbow with your left hand, pressing the right hand gently down the middle of your back, until you feel a stretch in the right triceps. Hold for ten to thirty seconds. Release and repeat on the other side. See page 168 for photo.

lower body stretches (lower back, hips, and legs)

Remember to breathe during a stretch; do not hold your breath. Always elongate your muscles gently; do not bounce. Be careful not to take a stretch too far.

PELVIC TILT

Stand, sit, lie on your side or back, or get on all fours. Tilt your pelvis up and forward, by squeezing and tucking your buttocks in and under. Also pull in and up from the lower abdominals, to round the lower back. Exhale as you hold for a few seconds. Release and inhale.

CAT STRETCH

This exercise is similar to the pelvic tilt, except on all fours. Tilt your pelvis, squeeze the buttocks, and pull in and up with the abs until your entire back is round and stretching. Exhale on the stretch and inhale on the release.

SPINAL TWIST

Tailor-sit on the floor or in bed. With your back straight, grab your right knee with your left hand and gently pull your trunk to the right to stretch the spinal muscles. Twist as far as is comfortable, aiming to look over your left shoulder. Hold for ten to thirty seconds. Release and twist to the other side. During the first trimester you can do a spinal twist lying on your back, pulling one knee across to the other side with the opposite hand.

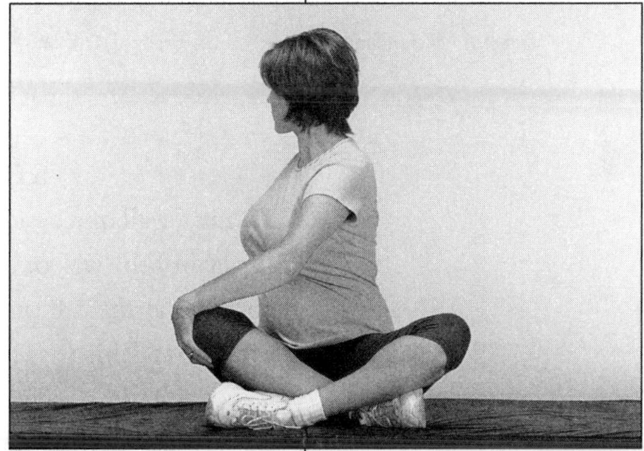

spinal twist

FORWARD BEND SITTING ON HEELS/CHILD'S POSE

Get down on your knees and sit back onto your heels, keeping your knees apart to make room for your belly. Bend forward with arms extended and stretch the spine as far as is comfortable. If sitting on your heels is uncomfortable for you, try the following version of this exercise.

FORWARD BEND TAILOR-SIT

Sit with your legs crossed. With your arms extended, bend forward gently, as far as is comfortable without crowding your uterus. It may become difficult to do this exercise later in your pregnancy. This stretch can also be done with the soles of your feet pressed together.

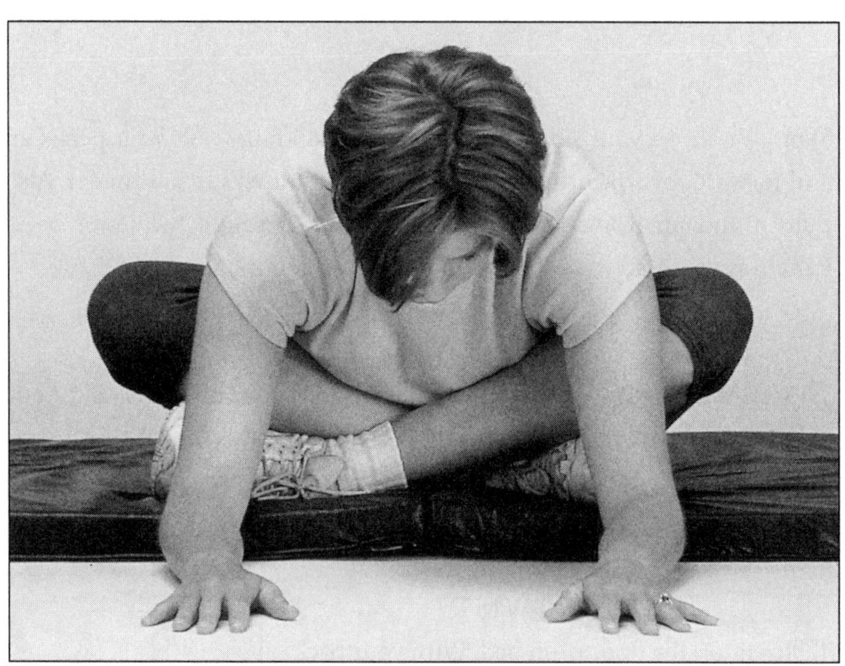

forward bend tailor-sit

STANDING CALF STRETCH

Facing a wall or a bench, turn the toes of one foot up as much as you can, up against the wall or bench. Gently move your hip forward, until you feel a stretch in the calf muscle. Hold for ten to thirty seconds. Repeat on the other foot. This stretch focuses on the gastrocnemius, the "meat" of the upper calf. To stretch the soleus muscle, the broad, flat muscle that lies underneath the gastrocnemius, stretch again but gently try to bend the knee without lifting the heel off the floor.

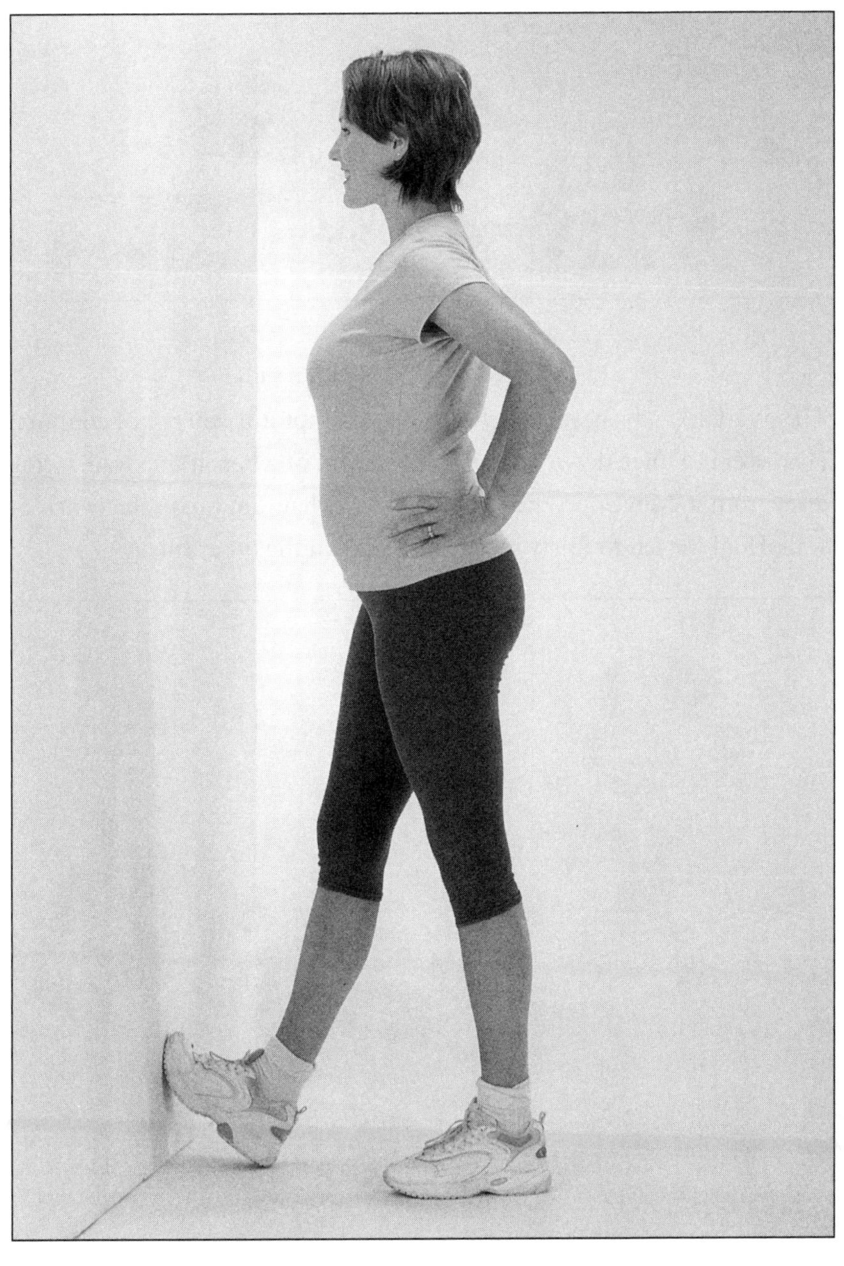

standing calf stretch

SIDE-LYING QUADRICEPS STRETCH

Lie down on a mat on your right side, with your knees bent in front of you at a 90-degree angle for support. Keep your head down. Take your left foot and bring it close to your buttock. Gently press your hip forward and flex your left buttock, but don't move your knee backward. Hold the stretch for ten to thirty seconds. Repeat on the other side.

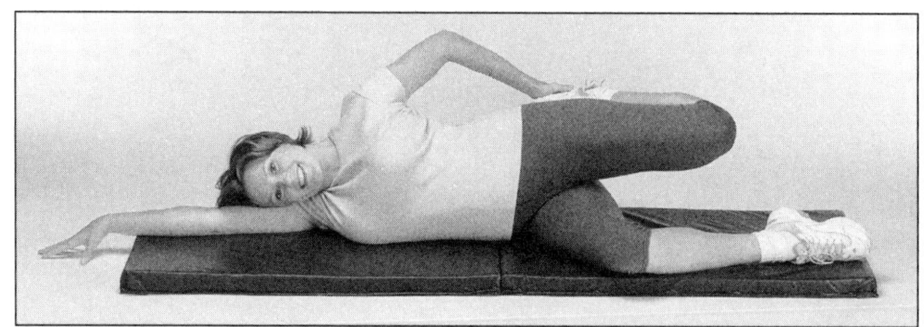

side-lying quadriceps stretch

LUNGING QUAD STRETCH

This is a fairly advanced stretch. Do not attempt it if you're not comfortable with it. Lunge down on the floor in front of a bench or a wall, facing away from it. Move one knee back and place that foot up on the bench or wall. Hold for ten to thirty seconds. Repeat on the other side.

lunging quad stretch

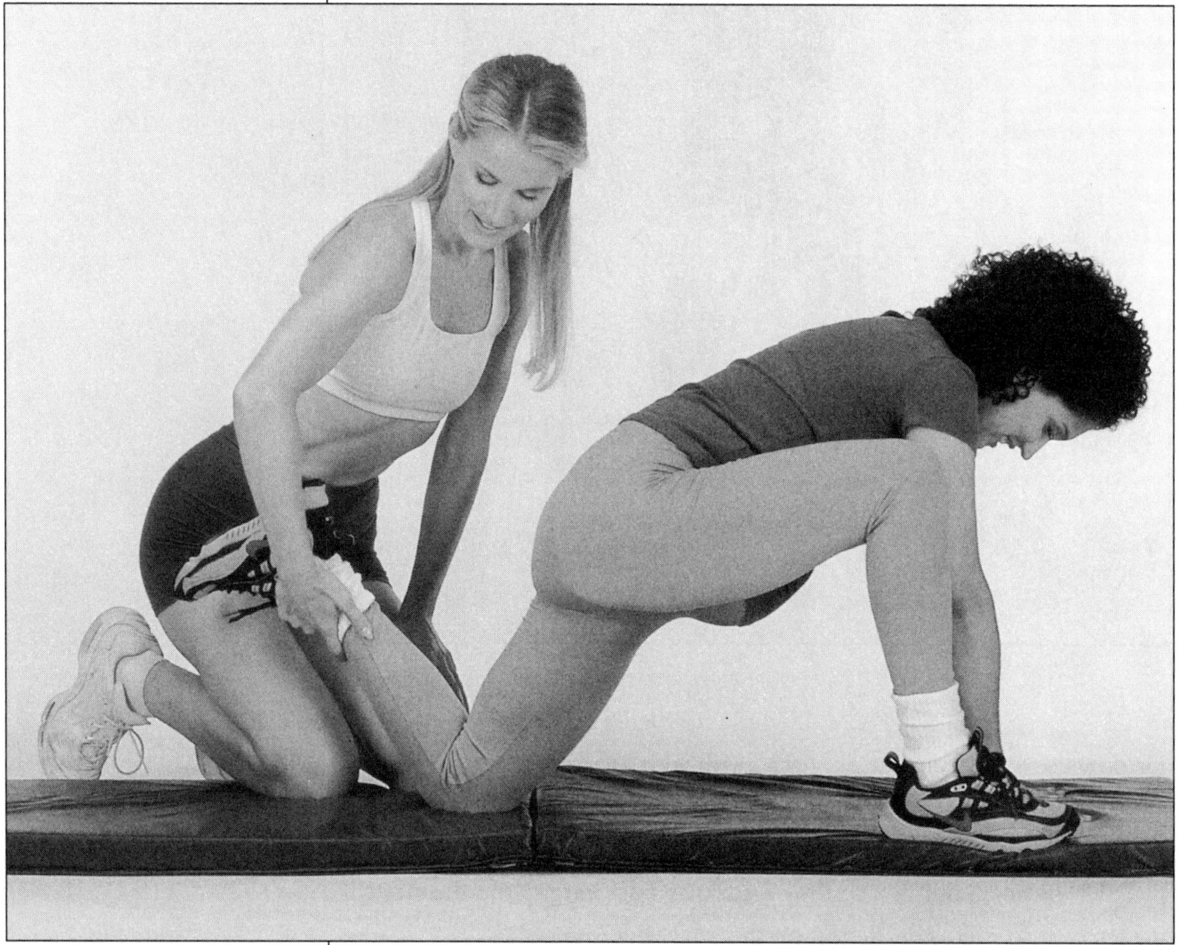

SEATED HAMSTRING STRETCH

Sit down on a mat, with the left leg extended in front and the right knee bent. Hold a short towel in your hands and wrap it around the left foot. Aim for a straight leg and a straight back, rather than rounding your back to bend forward. If you do not already feel a stretch, pull on the towel. Be careful not to take the stretch too far. Hold the stretch for ten to thirty seconds, and repeat on the other side. This stretch can also be performed sitting on a bench, with the other foot on the floor.

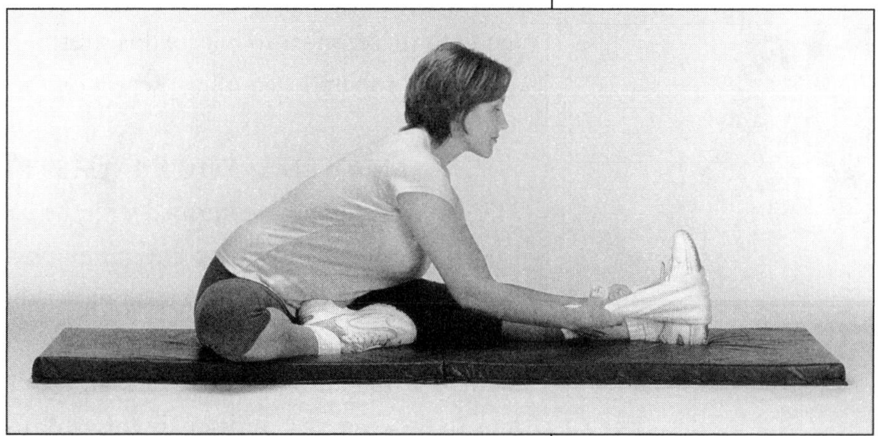

seated hamstring stretch

SIDE-LYING HAMSTRING STRETCH

Lie down on a mat or in bed on your right side, with the right leg bent for support. Grab your left calf, ankle, or foot (depending on how flexible you are), and slowly extend the leg as straight as you can. Gently pull the leg closer toward you, until you feel a stretch. Hold for ten to thirty seconds. Repeat on the other side.

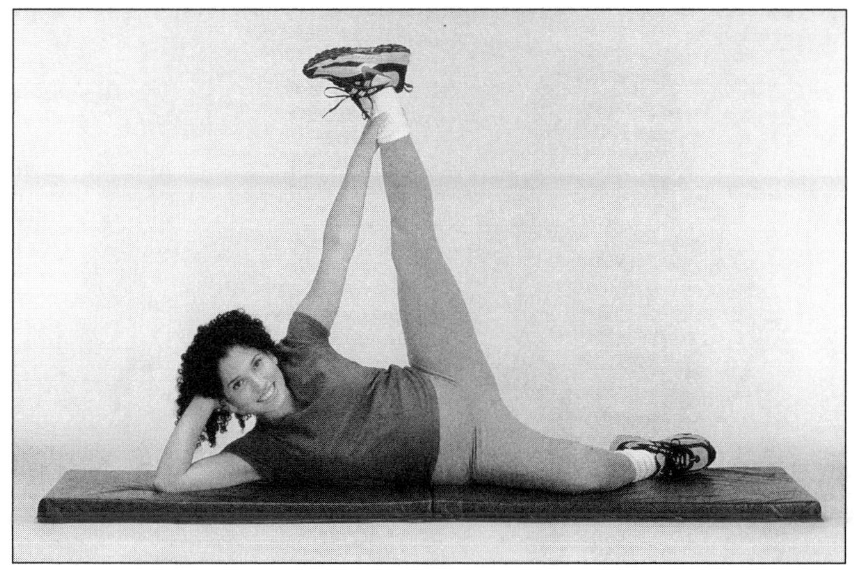

side-lying hamstring stretch

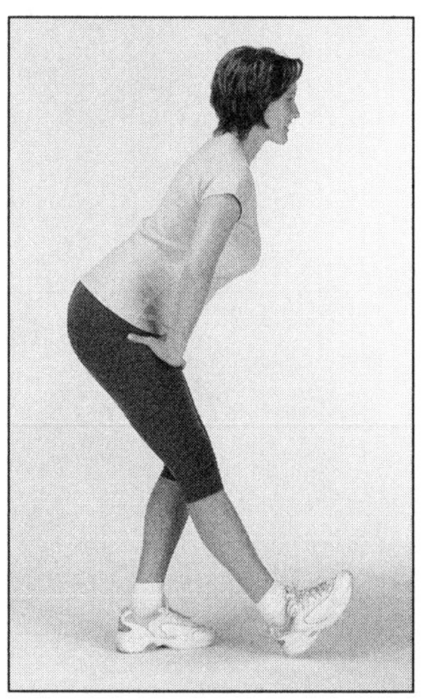

standing hamstring stretch

STANDING HAMSTRING STRETCH

This one comes in handy if you're outdoors. Place your right foot about a foot in front of the left one. Bend your left knee and place both hands on your thigh. Make sure that your back is straight. Gently lift the toes of the right foot up until you feel a stretch in the right hamstring. Hold for ten to thirty seconds. To release this stretch, pull in with your abdominals and slowly roll up to standing. Repeat on the other leg.

MODIFIED YOGA HAMSTRING STRETCH

This stretch is usually performed with the hands placed on the floor, but I do not recommend doing anything upside down during pregnancy. With your hands or arms on a chair or bench, place your right foot two to three feet in front of the left foot, a bit away from the chair or bench. Bend forward at the hip with a flat back and abdominals pulled in. Align the hips so they are even and square forward. You should feel this stretch in the right hamstring. Hold for ten to thirty seconds. To release, pull in the abdominals and roll up slowly. Repeat on the other side.

STRADDLE STRETCH

This stretch lengthens the hamstrings and inner thighs. Sit on the floor with your legs spread apart in a "V" as far as they will comfortably go. Either hold on to the inside of your legs, or if you're more flexible, place

straddle stretch

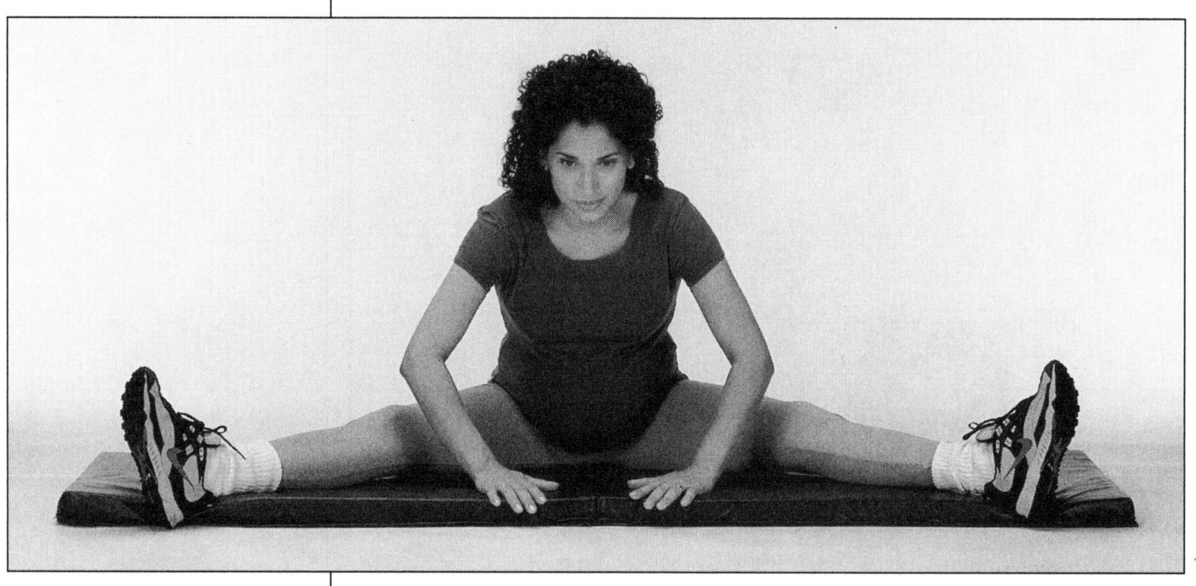

your hands on the floor in front of you. Using the muscles in your lower back, aim to straighten your back. If your back and legs are straight and you still don't feel a stretch (you're very flexible), walk forward with your hands until you do. Be careful not to take the stretch too far, and avoid pressing your belly into the floor. Hold the stretch for ten to thirty seconds. To release, pull in your abdominals and roll up.

INNER THIGH STRETCH

Sit on the floor with the soles of your feet together. Hold on to your ankles or feet, place your elbows on the inner thighs, and press down gently on the knees. Don't force the legs down. If you feel any strain on the inner thigh where it attaches to the pubic bone, discontinue this stretch.

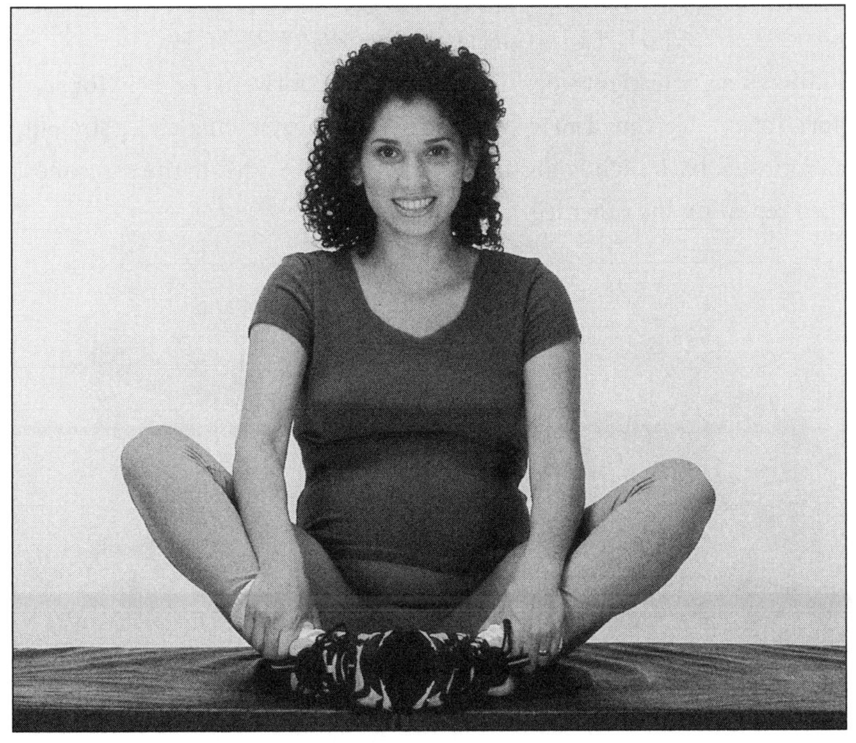

inner thigh stretch

LUNGING HIP FLEXOR STRETCH

Because the hip joint and lower back are so interdependent, you may also find the following hip flexor and piriformis stretches to be beneficial in loosening up a tight lower back. Lunge with the right foot forward. The right knee should be directly over the ankle, not protruding over the toes.

Place your hands on the floor on the inside of the right leg. Gently sink the left hip down toward the floor as far as is comfortable. If you still don't feel a stretch in the left hip flexor, flex the left buttock. If this is not enough, slide the left foot further backward into a longer lunge. Hold for ten to thirty seconds. Repeat on the other leg.

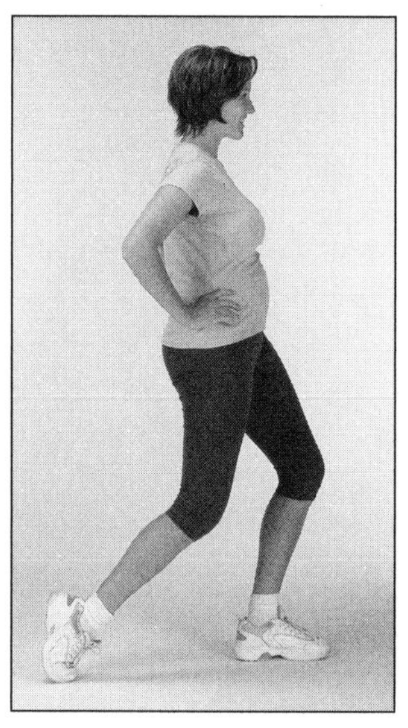

standing hip flexor stretch

STANDING HIP FLEXOR STRETCH

Begin by placing your left foot about one foot in front of the right. Next, slowly raise your right heel off the floor, bending the knee slightly. As you would do for a pelvic tilt, tuck the buttocks under and gently press the left hip forward. Hold this position for ten to thirty seconds. Repeat on the other leg.

SIDE-LYING HIP FLEXOR STRETCH

Lie down on your right side with the right knee forward and bent for support. You can use your arm to support your head. Extend the left leg straight, and move it back slightly to stretch the hip. Hold for ten to thirty seconds, then repeat on the other leg.

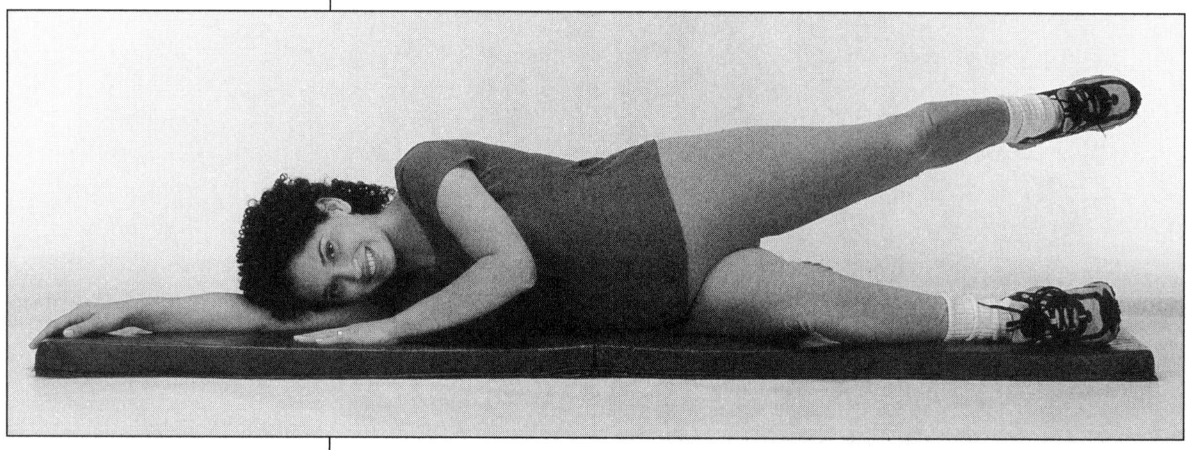

side-lying hip flexor stretch

SEATED FIGURE 4

The Figure 4 stretches the piriformis and outer thigh. Sit on a bench, chair, or bed. Place the right ankle over the left knee. If you do not feel enough of a stretch, lean forward a little without crowding your belly, or try the pretzel stretch (opposite page). Hold for ten to thirty seconds, and repeat on the other leg.

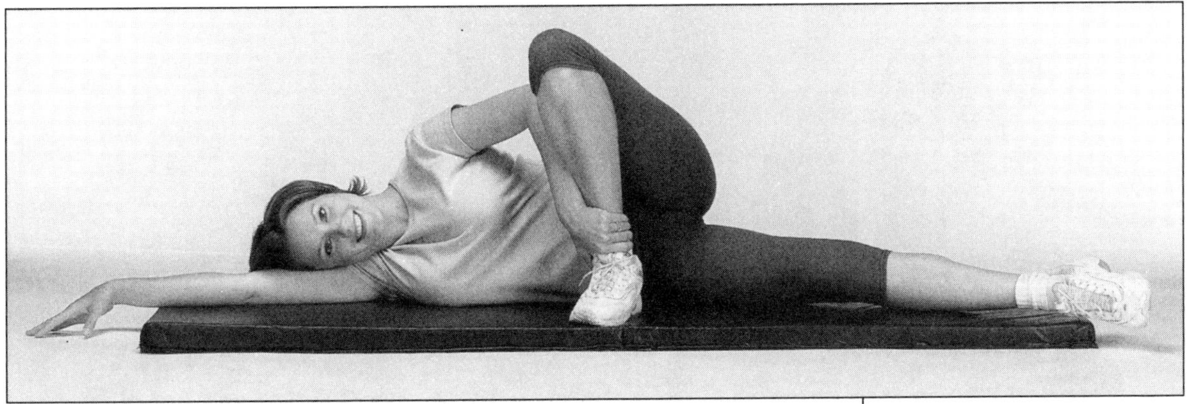

side-lying figure 4

SIDE-LYING FIGURE 4

If the seated version is too difficult, this one should be easier. Lie down on your right side, extend the right leg straight or keep it bent. Bend the left knee and bring the foot toward your belly, and hold it as close as is comfortable for you with your hand, if you can reach it, for ten to thirty seconds. Repeat on the other side.

PRETZEL STRETCH

This is a great stretch for the hip rotators and outer thighs, but it may get too difficult to do at the end of your pregnancy. Sit on the floor with both legs bent, one on top of the other. The feet should be pointing in opposite directions. Aim to get the knees on top of each other, by moving the feet out to the sides as far as you can. This may be enough of a stretch; if it's not, bend forward slightly for a deeper stretch. Do not crowd the uterus. Hold for ten to thirty seconds. Repeat on the other side. When your belly gets too big for this, do the Figure 4 stretches instead. Postpartum, lean your chest forward as close to your knees as possible.

pretzel stretch

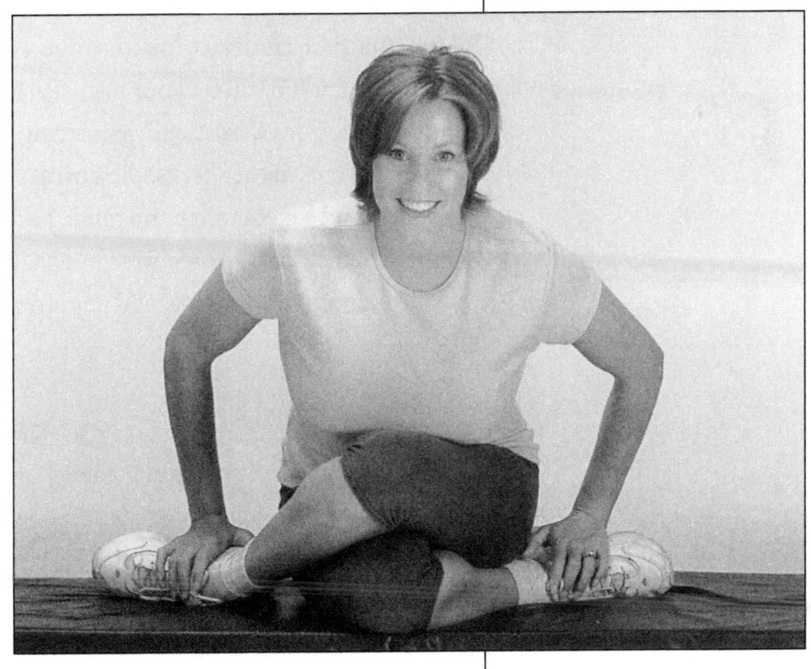

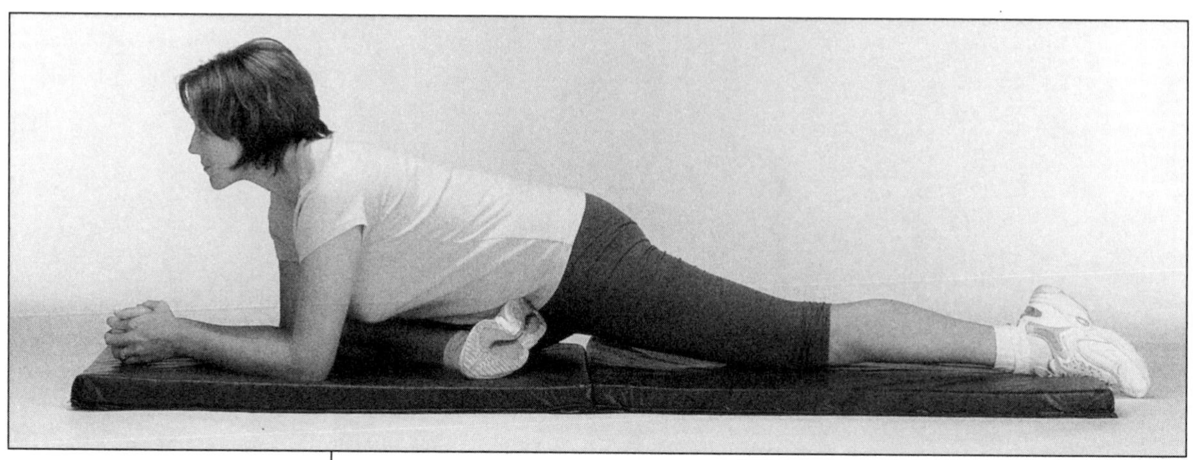

piriformis stretch

PIRIFORMIS STRETCH

Kneel on the floor. Put your hands down and extend the left leg backward. Slide the right foot to the left under your hips, and gently lower yourself onto the right ankle. Lean as far forward as you can, without crowding the uterus. You'll feel a stretch through the outer thigh and deep in the hip under the buttock. Hold for ten to thirty seconds and repeat on the other leg. When your belly gets too big, discontinue this stretch.

stretches to avoid

After the first trimester, discontinue stretches that crowd the uterus or require you to lie still on your back. Particular stretches to avoid are standing or seated forward bend hamstring stretches with both legs straight, which will crowd the uterus; the hurdler's stretch, which could injure softer cartilage and ligaments in the pubic bone, knee, and ankle; and the forced inner thigh stretch, which may injure the pubic bone and hip joint. Also avoid abdominal stretching and any stretches that cause pain or discomfort.

yoga

Yoga has gotten very popular lately, and rightfully so. To many people, yoga conjures an image of Eastern religion, weird gurus, chanting, incense, and impossible contorted poses. To enjoy the benefits of yoga, one does not need to practice a different religion, be a vegetarian, or be double-jointed. Yoga is more spiritual than religious. It is a type of exercise that focuses on a body–mind connection and balance, using concentration to teach you awareness, alertness, relaxation, peacefulness, and joyfulness—all of which would be beneficial to pregnant women.

Yoga has been practiced for about 2,000 years and is considered a philosophy, a science, and an art of self-improvement. The word *yoga* comes from the Sanskrit *yuj*, which means yoke, or joining together. It was introduced to the Western world from India in the 1960s as hatha yoga. Hatha (physical) yoga includes a series of postural exercises called *asanas*, breathing exercises called *pranayamas*, and meditation techniques. Yoga is mind and body therapy; the exercises are believed to benefit the internal bodily functions by improving circulation and increasing flexibility, while the breathing and meditation techniques create inner peace and soothe the mind.

The more you practice yoga the more pliable and capable your body will become.

Yoga can calm your mind, relieve stress, improve muscle tone, flexibility, coordination, circulation, posture, digestion, respiration, energy levels, and physical and mental well-being. Practicing yoga exercises during pregnancy can alleviate muscle stiffness, while the meditative effects and breathing techniques—which are very similar to what is taught in childbirth education classes—make it beneficial for labor and childbirth preparation.

The exercises consist of muscle contractions and stretches and can be aggressive or slow. Some postures may be more difficult than they look, and you may not be able to execute them perfectly, but be patient and your body will improve. You may not be able to do all of the poses perfectly during pregnancy. Like any exercise, yoga should be a challenge, but each pose should be done only to the extent of your body's capability and comfort level. It should not be painful to hold a pose. The more you practice yoga the more pliable and capable your body will become. To get the full benefit, try to practice daily if possible, whether for ten minutes or an hour.

As with most sports and activities, pregnancy requires modifications to yoga. Advanced yoga positions that require extensive twisting, inversion, or balancing should be avoided. If your balance is off, try holding onto a chair while doing the standing postures. If you're a beginner, do not hold a pose for as long. As you improve, you can increase the duration of each pose. When moving upward or moving your limbs away from your body, inhale. When moving downward or moving your limbs toward your body, exhale. Never hold your breath when holding a pose—keep breathing slowly and consciously. Yoga usually teaches you to breathe in and out

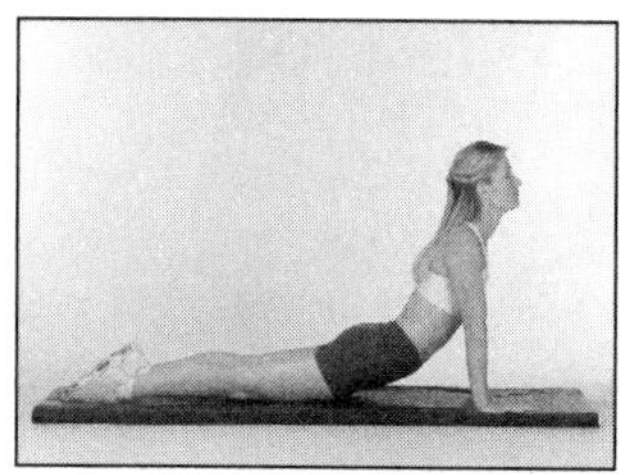

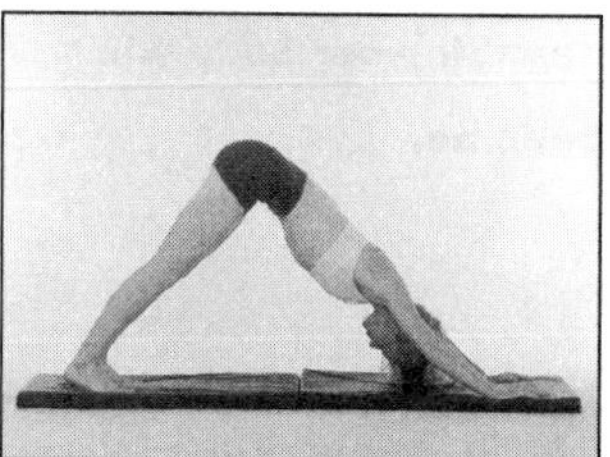

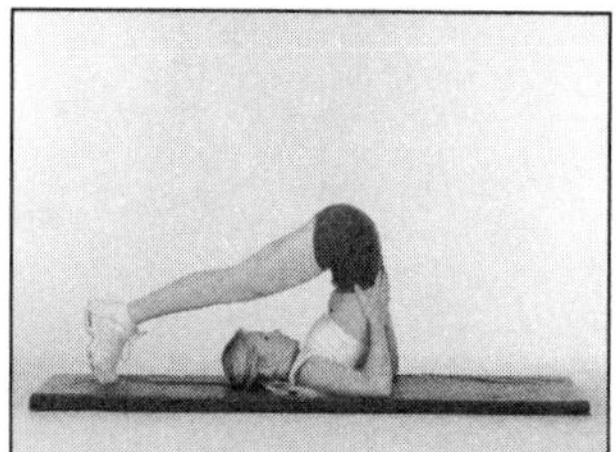

Birgitta demonstrates pregnancy no-nos: up dog (top), down dog (middle), plow (bottom)

through your nose only, but if you're not accustomed to this and you are pregnant, breathe any way you can (mouth, nose, or both). Oxygen is too important to risk restricting your intake.

Other contraindicated conditions besides pregnancy that may require modification of yoga exercises are: seizure disorders, hypertension, detached retina, Ménière's disease, multiple sclerosis, myalic encephalomyelitis, physical handicaps, migraines, headaches, and post-operative patients. Yoga has been proven to be beneficial for respiratory problems, arthritis, diabetes, heart disease, stress, and back and neck problems.

YOGA POSES TO AVOID DURING PREGNANCY

- Avoid any inverted (upside down) exercises (head-, hand-, and shoulder stands, down dog, and inverted hamstring stretch). Many people believe that inverted poses during pregnancy may distort the baby's sense of direction, so it does not know which way to turn when it is time. There has been no scientific evidence to support this belief, but there have been incidents of babies in breech position whose mothers practiced inverted exercises during pregnancy. Until this theory is proven (or disproved) conclusively, it's best to be on the safe side—right-side up.
- Avoid arching your back by stretching in an upward/backward motion such as back bends and the up dog. The warrior pose may be okay if you reach up only.
- Avoid any exercises that crowd the uterus—such as prone exercises, seated forward bends (see photo page 83), and the plow pose.
- In the lotus position, never force your inner thighs down to touch the floor with your knees. If you can't sit in the lotus pose, modify it to a tailor-sit.
- Avoid any pose requiring too much twisting.
- Avoid balancing on hands or one foot.
- Avoid taking any stretch into pain or to your physical limit.

relaxation

Although pregnancy is a very special time, it is by nature a very emotional one. Hormonal changes can cause mood swings and make you more irritable, which in turn may place tension on your relationships with your spouse, family, friends, and coworkers. Your work may demand too much of you on days when you're fatigued, or you may demand too much of yourself, thinking that you can do it all without slowing down.

Continued stress can cause further emotional and physical problems such as insomnia, ulcers, even heart disease. Worse, the mother may be tempted to turn to alcohol, cigarettes, or drugs instead of relaxation techniques.

Relaxation slows your brain waves and will ultimately help you relieve stress, tension, cramps, muscle and joint stiffness, back pain, headaches, and insomnia—to mention just a few benefits. The better you become at relaxing during your pregnancy, the more you will be able to release tension during labor. Your delivery will feel easier, and you're less likely to need any medical intervention. It may or may not reduce the actual level of pain you experience, but it can help change your perception of and threshold for pain.

For some women, the prospect of giving birth is a terrifying one. Unfortunately, this fear in itself can be more dangerous than the act of labor. The adrenaline that is produced by prolonged stress and fear (like the fear of flying) tends to decrease the amount of blood and oxygen that is transported to the fetus during labor. Also, when we tense up, our muscles tighten. Fatigue and fear from tension and stress interfere with the relaxation of your muscles and could result in muscle cramps. Very extreme cases of prolonged stress during pregnancy may slow the baby's growth and development. The few childbirth education classes that most women attend toward the end of their pregnancies may be too little and too late with regard to breathing, relaxation, and stress relief techniques. For your health, and your baby's, you need to learn to relax—even in the face of this life-changing event.

To release tension properly requires muscle awareness. Learning how to relax your body—specifically the pelvic floor muscles in between contractions—will help ensure a smoother descent of your baby through the birth canal, and it will decrease the likelihood of an episiotomy or tearing of the perineal muscles. Delivering a baby is naturally very tiring, hence the apropos name "labor." Being tense could protract the labor process and cause you unnecessary pain. It could also increase your need for epidurals and anesthetics. These medications can slow down labor and make you weak and tired. However, anesthesia, especially epidurals, can reduce and sometimes prevent the harmful effects of stress.

MEDITATION

Meditation is an easy way to calm your mind and body. If you have other children, the hardest part may be finding a quiet, dark place where you won't be disturbed for ten to twenty minutes. You can meditate lying down or sitting comfortably. Just close your eyes and empty your mind by either focusing on your breathing (in through your nose and out through the nose, unless you have a respiratory problem), listening to music or guided meditation audio tapes, imagining a beautiful place or environment, repeating a calming word in your mind on each exhalation, or practicing a full-body relaxation technique (see following). You may have a tough time at first trying to clear your mind to achieve total relaxation or a blissful state of mind. Many beginners allow their minds to wander in different directions, with distractions. The more you practice, the better you will get.

TOTAL BODY RELAXATION TECHNIQUE

Totally relaxing your body, or even putting yourself to sleep, can be achieved by systematically relaxing one body part at a time, from head to toe, or the reverse. If you're just looking for relaxation, start with your face and head, and work your way down. If you are having trouble falling asleep at night, start with your toes and work your way up to your face (if you don't fall asleep before you get that far up), this will help you out tremendously.

Lay down comfortably. If you haven't passed your sixteenth week of pregnancy, you may stay on your back, with your hands comfortably by your sides. After the sixteenth week, prop yourself up in an inclined position, or lie on your side with lots of pillows. Take a few deep breaths, concentrating on your breathing. Be aware of the inhalation through your nose, and the oxygen filling up your lungs and diaphragmatic area all the way down into the abdominal area. Feel your stomach rise and then slowly sink as you exhale every ounce of that oxygen back out through your nose. When you are comfortable breathing in this manner, start repeating the word *relax* (or any other calming word) slowly on each exhalation, and visualize your tension flowing out with it. Repeat at least ten times.

Then visualize and concentrate on your toes in your mind, telling them to relax. Visualize them relaxing, and as soon as you feel them relax, move to the balls of your feet, then to your arches, heels, and ankles, relaxing each before proceeding to the next part. Imagine the feet falling out to the side and becoming very heavy, as if they would go through the mattress. Slowly move up through your lower legs and calves using the same technique, continuing with the knees and up to your thighs. Visualize and feel your thigh muscles becoming so heavy and relaxed that they fall off the bones. Relax your pelvic floor muscles before you continue up through the abdominals and pectorals. Then similarly relax your buttocks, moving up through the lower back, middle, and upper back, making your whole body feel really heavy and relaxed, breathing continually.

If you're still awake, or shall we say *aware,* slowly relax your shoulders, and feel this relaxation flow down through the arms and forearms, into your fingers, which should feel all tingly by now. Go back up through the arms and into your neck, making it relax to such a state that it feels as if the cervical spine is flattening (if you are on your back). Gently move up the back of your head and imagine it feeling as heavy as a bowling ball. Imagine your head falling through the bed or backward onto the pillow. Then imagine a serene and soothing feeling flowing through your temples, relaxing the facial muscles in your cheeks, jaw, and chin. Imagine they become so heavy that they almost fall off your face. Concentrate on your lips and feel them relax, before moving up through the nose, and lastly, concentrate on relaxing your eyes and eyelids. Your eyes should feel so heavy that you couldn't open the lids if you tried. But you're probably already asleep by now. If you're not, keep concentrating on your breathing technique.

If your only aim is to relax rather than fall asleep, completely reverse this process, starting with your eyes instead of your feet. In the beginning, your mind may distract you or you may feel an itch somewhere. When this happens, just start over from the beginning again. If you don't think you'll be able to remember this process, tape record yourself as you describe the steps, slowly, in your own words, for a personalized relaxation tape. There are, of course, several relaxation and meditation tapes commercially available, which you can try.

If you're busy or working and don't have even ten minutes to spare, try a real quickie, by sitting, standing up, or lying down and stretching your whole body out with your arms overhead. Close your eyes and take two to three really deep breaths. Or, if your upper back is tired and sore from office and computer work, or just from carrying this pregnancy, squeeze your shoulder blades and upper back muscles as tightly as you can, for as long as you can, then drop and slowly release them. Repeat this four to five times and feel the difference.

VISUALIZATION

Visualization is the ability to conceive and create a clear image or picture in your mind. During your pregnancy, you may visualize your baby inside of you, kicking, sleeping, growing. You try to picture its face, toes, fingers, and so on. You can combine visualization with breathing by visualizing the oxygen of a deep breath, flowing with the blood through your body, through the placenta and umbilical cord to your baby, and visualizing how the baby grows from this nourishment. Visualize your happy, healthy baby inside your womb. To prepare for giving birth, you can visualize the process of delivery, your baby descending down the birth canal, and your body opening up to let it out.

You may visualize what it will be like to be a mother, caring for your child. Whether this is a first, second, or third child, imagine what it will feel like. These images can be calming, joyful, relaxing, or stressful depending on the situation, but they can help you prepare for motherhood. If for whatever reason, this pregnancy is not a pleasant occurrence in your life, visualization may make it less stressful and possibly help you bond with your unborn. Remember, whatever your mind can conceive, your brain can believe, and your body can achieve.

MASSAGE

A massage can be very soothing and relaxing for both body and mind. With all the changes that your body goes through during pregnancy, physically and mentally, a massage may just be the best medicine. If your mate is not willing or capable of giving you a nice massage, it's well worth the investment to get a professional one. In addition to being very relaxing, a massage will revitalize your circulation and ease water retention. Unfortunately, no matter what anyone tries to tell you, massage cannot rid your body of cellulite or toxins.

During pregnancy, of course, your position during a massage needs to be modified. You cannot lie on your belly, or on your back after the sixteenth week. If lying on your side doesn't work for you, try sitting in bed propped up with pillows, or straddling a chair backward, leaning over the back. Or kneel/sit in a special massage chair. Some masseuses have specially designed massage chairs or tables with a hole for the belly, enabling pregnant women to lie on their stomachs. Call around your neighborhood and see what's available to you.

A deep tissue or shiatsu sports massage may not help you relax much, unless you're used to them. The lighter Swedish efflourage massage technique may ease your tension better. Ask to have any sore areas, such as your feet, neck, upper and lower back, massaged a little extra. A foot massage or reflexology session (in which pressure is applied to nerve endings and pressure points in the feet) will probably send you to heaven, as, to a lesser degree, will hand reflexology. Avoid having your belly or any varicose veins massaged. Spinal adjustment (such as neck twists or cracks) is not recommended during pregnancy. Your spouse could help you alleviate headaches by massaging your face, temples, and head.

During pregnancy, oxygen has an even more important task to accomplish—it is your baby's single most important nourishment.

breathing

Oxygen is the most important component of life. It doesn't just sustain life, it also gives life. Without oxygen, you will die. It sustains and maintains your body, including your muscles and respiratory and cardiovascular systems. It also helps your body burn calories, by making the fat-burning process more efficient during and after exercise. That's why the more oxygen you inhale, especially during exercise, the more calories your body will burn.

During pregnancy, oxygen has an even more important task to accomplish—it is your baby's single most important nourishment. Without it, cells will not divide and your baby will not develop and grow to full term. You must do your best to supply your baby with sufficient oxygen. That means abolishing any habit that could cause oxygen deprivation, such as smoking or inactivity. The more you exercise, the more oxygen your body takes in. This makes your body more fit and capable of taking in even more oxygen. All this extra oxygen will help your baby grow better.

It is therefore important to learn and practice good breathing habits and techniques, to optimize your oxygen supply during pregnancy. It will even help you in the delivery room. Insufficient breathing can disrupt your ability to relax, especially if you are hyperventilating, which you will need to avoid during labor. Hyperventilating in labor will give the mother too much oxygen, possibly causing her to faint, which in turn would reduce the oxygen supply for the fetus. Breathing easily and deeply helps you relax and save energy.

Deep breathing techniques may take some practice, but they will improve and expand your lung capacity, ensuring proper oxygen exchange. By practicing these techniques, you will also improve your circulation, increase your energy level, relax better, and give your abs a workout at the same time.

DIAPHRAGMATIC BREATHING

Deep breathing is called diaphragmatic breathing. Your diaphragm is a sheath of muscle that divides the chest cavity from the abdominal cavity. It aids you when you breathe, cough, sneeze, sing, eliminate waste, and deliver a baby, by moving downward to let the lungs fill up with air, and then upward to expel the air. Breathing during pregnancy will become harder and harder, because the diaphragm will have less and less space to move in, until the baby "drops" (turns into the head-down position in preparation for delivery).

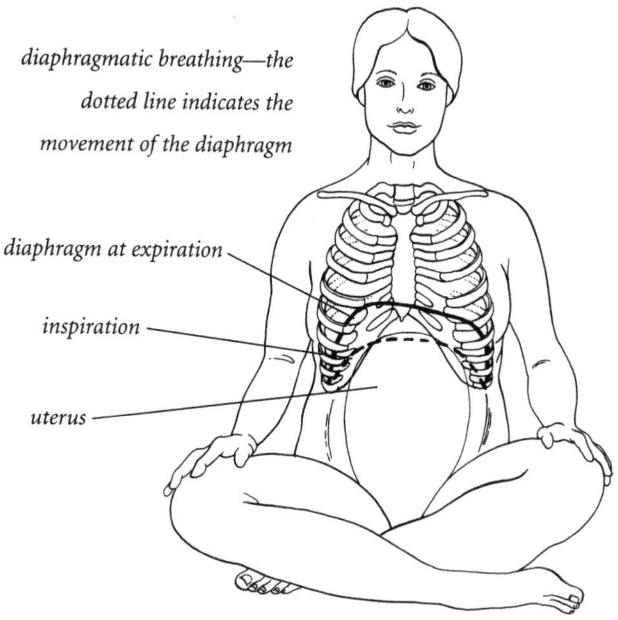

diaphragmatic breathing—the dotted line indicates the movement of the diaphragm

This type of breathing is similar to the abdominal pulse exercise described on page 167, but much slower. Sit comfortably in a chair and hold your belly with your hands. Focus on your breathing and concentrate on the slow inhalation, letting your chest and abdominal cavity fill with air. You should feel your belly expand. Then expel the air out *slowly,* and you'll feel your abdomen deflate a little. Practice this throughout your pregnancy. It will get more and more difficult the further your pregnancy progresses, as your growing uterus pushes up on your diaphragm, limiting your breathing capacity. Once you are used to this kind of breathing, you can be more forceful on the exhalation, by pulling your stomach in tight. Postpartum, you can do this lying down.

LATERAL BREATHING

Another form of breathing that can help you during pregnancy, especially in the last trimester, is lateral breathing. This kind of breathing is practiced in Pilates. Lateral breathing stems from ballet and dance, where I'm guessing it was probably practiced to prevent the waistline from expanding when breathing during a dance number, for aesthetic reasons.

Sit comfortably, either in a sofa or bed, or tailor-sit on the floor. If this is your first time learning lateral breathing, place your hands on your rib cage and point your elbows out to the side. As you slowly inhale, flare your rib cage laterally, expanding the chest cavity out sideways and backward, slightly lifting your elbows up and out to the side, to make room for the expansion. Your abdominals and rib cage should not expand forward as they did in the diaphragmatic breathing. Slowly exhale and notice your elbows naturally returning back down.

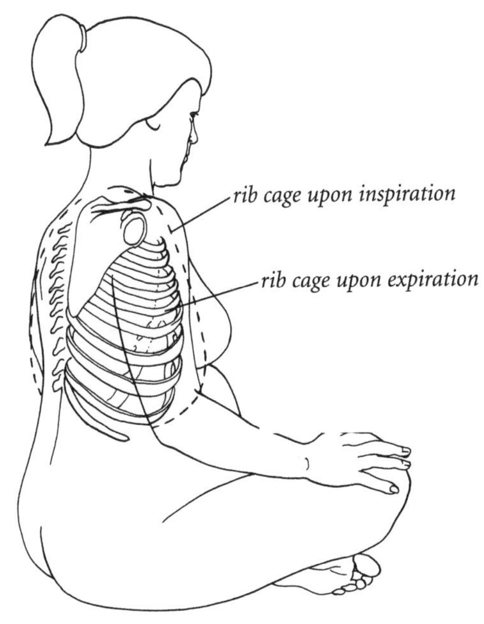

lateral breathing—the dotted line indicates the expansion of the rib cage

Many pregnant women find this type of breathing much easier and more comfortable to do in late pregnancy, before the baby drops. At this time the diaphragm has a very limited range of movement up and down. When you can do this without your abdominals and rib cage expanding forward, lift your hands and arms out sideways while breathing laterally. It will give your lungs even more breathing room. You may be tempted to walk around with your arms lifted to the side for the rest of your pregnancy! More likely though, you will become so good at it that you won't need to raise your arms. If you have trouble mastering this technique, look up your nearest Pilates studio or instructor for help.

BREATHING AND EXERCISE

When you exercise, your breathing technique is very important. It is vital to prevent hyperventilation. During cardiovascular exercise, move at a steady pace without alternating intervals of higher and lower intensities. You will probably find that moving or swinging your arms a little up and out to the side (similar to lateral breathing) will help you during cardiovascular exercise. Always exhale on muscle contraction or exertion and inhale on muscle release. Inhale when you stretch a muscle; exhale on the release. Try to be very aware of your breathing at all times. Exercises that make proper breathing easier to learn are the cat stretch (see page 131), body stretch (pages 178), doing arm circles or breast strokes with your arms, and yoga.

There are, of course, special labor breathing techniques, including pant breathing and feather blowing. These methods are taught in Lamaze and childbirth education classes, which you should consider participating in along with your partner. These classes typically run for about six to eight weeks.

All of these breathing techniques will enhance and aid your labor experience. The more mind–body awareness and trust in your body's capabilities you have, the more confident you'll be in the delivery room, knowing that you can control your body, and the birth of your baby, to some extent. Practice makes perfect, so get started early.

Chapter Eight

nutrition and pregnancy

IN THIS CHAPTER

- *Sample daily menu for active moms*
- *The dangers of dieting during pregnancy*
- *Weight gain chart*
- *Important guidelines for vegetarians*

You've heard the saying, "You are what you eat." That's true, but when you are pregnant or nursing, *your baby* is what you eat (or don't). A *healthy* baby doesn't just happen. Your diet during pregnancy affects not just your health, but also your baby's physical, mental, and behavioral well-being for the rest of its life, and the health and well-being of your future grandchildren.

You may know women who supposedly ate only "junk food" and even drank alcohol or smoked throughout a pregnancy, and still had an apparently healthy baby. If it's true, they are lucky indeed. But did you ever investigate that "healthy" child's *real* health? Does he get sick often, have allergies, injure easily, is accident prone, or have any mental, behavioral, or learning problems? Is he in a high-risk category for cancer heart disease? And what effects will the mother's unhealthy behavior have on babies born to future generations in the family?

The questions are endless. There is no insurance policy that will guarantee you an absolutely healthy child, but by eating and exercising properly throughout your pregnancy, you can prevent many of these possibilities. Remember: While you are in almost total control of your child's health during the pregnancy and the nursing period, you have no control over possible genetic defects and health problems that your parents or grandparents may have passed on to you. However, with proper nutrition, you may be able to minimize or at least delay the onset of some genetic problems, including immune disorders, cancer, and heart disease.

You are in almost total control of your child's health during the pregnancy and the nursing period.

Though vitally important, exercise alone is not enough. Good nutrition optimizes your chance of having a perfectly healthy child, a safer and easier pregnancy and labor, and a speedier return to your original shape.

the mother-child connection

The fetus shares all available nutrients with the mother, who is in charge of what, when, and how much is consumed. Nutrients and oxygen travel through the mother's bloodstream into the placenta, before continuing through the umbilical cord to the fetus. When the fetus has used what it needs, it returns any waste material back through the umbilical cord to the mother's bloodstream for excretion. For these exchanges to happen, the placenta must be healthy. If the mother's nutrient stores are not sufficient in the first trimester when the placenta is developing, the baby's development could be compromised.

don't delay—begin today!

It is important that you begin practicing good nutritional habits as soon as possible, even before you are pregnant or know you are pregnant. Most fetal tissues and organs develop within the first two months of pregnancy. Proper nutrition is vitally important to fetal development, especially at this crucial time. Do not wait until your pregnancy is confirmed to begin eating right. In fact, for the best possible results, your nutrient stores should be at optimal levels at least one month before you conceive. Unfortunately, 60 percent of all pregnancies are unplanned.

The possible risks of poor nutrition to the fetus begin at conception. If the mother isn't healthy, the fertilized egg may not implant in the uterine lining, resulting in miscarriage. The embryo requires the right balance of nutrients to develop properly. If the folic acid supply is deficient, the fetus may develop a spinal or brain deformity. The spinal cord starts to develop by the seventeenth day, before many women even know that they are pregnant. Folic acid is vital for this process. By the eighth week, the cardiovascular, digestive, and central nervous systems develop.

As pregnancy progresses, each individual organ, tissue, and body part follows its own growth pattern. They develop at different stages of the pregnancy, and they need optimum nutrition in certain amounts at all times.

Some of the most common effects of poor nutrition during pregnancy are children with smaller brain cells, poor dental health, reduced height, behavioral and learning disabilities, late sexual development, and a weak immune system. These facts are not meant to scare you, but to show how insufficient nutrition at any time could have irreversible negative effects on the baby's development.

Some deficiencies affect both mother and child. If a mother's nutritional intake is too high in fat and cholesterol, she may place herself and her baby at greater risk for heart disease, cancer, and obesity. If the mother is significantly overweight, the delivery may be difficult or a Cesarean section (C-section) may be required. Consuming too much sugar or not enough chromium may increase the risk of receding gums and diabetes in both mother and child. (Too much sugar consumption reduces the chromium supply, which, with a genetic disposition, can result in diabetes.) A lack of calcium, protein, and vitamin C can cause bleeding gums in the mother; add to that a lack of vitamin D and the baby may be born with teeth and bone malformations.

The fetus will almost always be ensured enough calcium—it will draw calcium from its mother's bones if there isn't any available. The mother, however, may end up with osteoporosis later in life if she doesn't consume enough calcium, as her bones will become weak from this depletion. If she doesn't consume enough fiber, she may suffer from constipation, hemorrhoids, and, in the worst case scenario, develop intestinal cancer later in life. If she's short on zinc, the child could have an increased risk of eye malformations. Other risks for the mother include anemia—caused by insufficient folic acid and iron—and premature labor, which can be caused by dehydration or a lack of iron or zinc.

don't diet

Pregnancy is not a time for trimming and slimming. Dieting during pregnancy can be detrimental to the baby, causing brain damage and metabolic problems. When your body doesn't have enough glucose to burn for energy, it will start to burn fat and then protein tissues like muscles and organs instead. The metabolic process that transforms fat or muscle during weight loss produces ketones, a toxic by-product. Ketones are chemically related to acetone, which is found in solvents such as nail polish remover. If excessive amounts of ketones accumulate in your body, it could be fatal to both you and your child.

Furthermore, if you are too skinny with very low body-fat levels, your level of estrogen production may decrease, which in turn could cause miscarriage and infertility. In cases of severe fat and carbohydrate deficiencies, protein is used for the mother's energy, which inhibits the proper development of the baby.

Eating too little during pregnancy can be more harmful than eating too much. Don't ever restrict your food intake during pregnancy, except under a doctor's direction and close supervision. Do not limit carbohydrates and fiber-rich grains such as brown rice, whole wheat bread, and especially fruits and vegetables.

Even when you're not pregnant, dieting slows down your metabolism, putting you on an evil roller-coaster ride of yo-yoing up-and-down weight fluctuations. Protein speeds up your metabolism; excess fat and carbohydrates slow it down. The high carbohydrate diet that was long favored won't help you lose weight. If you want to lose weight (and you are not pregnant), a diet consisting of high protein, medium carbohydrate, and low fat intake—combined with exercise—will do the trick. Never completely eliminate fat or carbohydrates from your diet—every nutrient has its own function in maintaining overall health.

weight gain

The recommended weight gain during pregnancy is approximately twenty-five to thirty-five pounds. Keep in mind that some women may gain more or less weight. Your exact weight gain may vary, depending on your age, race, height, build, fitness level, lifestyle, and other considerations. The average weight gain during the first trimester is three to six pounds. You should continue to gain about one-half to one pound per week over the latter two trimesters.

The following two charts will help you to determine your weight gain goal during pregnancy. First, use the Prenatal Weight chart to locate your height (in inches) in the left-hand column. Then follow that row to find your approximate pre-pregnancy weight. The range in this column will tell you if you are underweight, a normal weight, overweight, or very overweight. Finally, the chart at the bottom illustrates the desirable weight gain for your build.

PRENATAL WEIGHT

(HEIGHT IN INCHES, WITHOUT SHOES, AND WEIGHT IN POUNDS, WITHOUT CLOTHES)

height	*underweight*	*normal*	*overweight*	*very overweight*
58"	*94 (or less)*	*95–127*	*128–143*	*144 (or more)*
59"	*97 (or less)*	*98–131*	*132–147*	*148 (or more)*
60"	*100 (or less)*	*101–135*	*136–151*	*152 (or more)*
61"	*102 (or less)*	*103–138*	*139–155*	*156 (or more)*
62"	*106 (or less)*	*107–143*	*144–161*	*162 (or more)*
63"	*109 (or less)*	*110–147*	*148–165*	*166 (or more)*
64"	*112 (or less)*	*113–151*	*152–170*	*171 (or more)*
65"	*116 (or less)*	*117–156*	*157–176*	*177 (or more)*
66"	*119 (or less)*	*120–161*	*162–181*	*182 (or more)*
67"	*123 (or less)*	*124–166*	*167–187*	*188 (or more)*
68"	*126 (or less)*	*127–171*	*172–192*	*193 (or more)*
69"	*131 (or less)*	*132–177*	*178–199*	*200 (or more)*
70"	*134 (or less)*	*135–182*	*183–204*	*205 (or more)*

DESIRABLE GAIN

(HEIGHT IN INCHES, WITHOUT SHOES, AND WEIGHT IN POUNDS, WITHOUT CLOTHES)

height	*underweight*	*normal*	*overweight*	*very overweight*
all	*28–40*	*25–35*	*15–25*	*15 (or less)*

Adapted from the California Department of Health Services, Maternal and Child Health Branch and WIC Supplemental Foods Branch: *Nutrition During Pregnancy and the Postpartum Period: A Manual for Health Care Professionals.* Sacramento, CA, Department of Health Services, 1990; and *Nutrition During Pregnancy and Lactation: An Implementation Guide.* Institute of Medicine. Subcommittee for a Clinical Application Guide, Committee on Nutritional Status During Pregnancy and Lactation, Food and Nutrition Board: Washington, D.C., National Academy Press, 1992.

Things to Consider

In reading this chart, keep the following points in mind:

- *Teenagers should aim for the upper limit of their weight-specific goal.*
- *Women less than sixty-two inches tall should aim for the lower limit of their weight-specific goal.*
- *Women with twins should aim for a weight gain of thirty-five to forty-five pounds.*
- *If you are carrying more than two babies, add an additional ten pounds per baby.*

Weight Distribution

The following table represents the approximate distribution in pounds of a twenty-four- to twenty-eight-pound weight gain during pregnancy:

THE BABY	
fetus	*6–9*
placenta	*1–2*
amniotic fluid	*2*
THE MOTHER	
fat and protein stores	*4–6*
fluid volume	*2–3*
enlarged uterus	*2*
enlarged breasts	*1–2*
increased blood volume	*3–4*
TOTAL	*24 to 28 lbs.*

Wonder where all that weight goes? Approximately 40 percent of the weight gain is accounted for by the fetus; the other 60 percent is maternal change. Most of the weight gain is water.

Most of the necessary maternal fat gained is deposited internally and externally in the pelvic and abdominal region during the first trimester. Most of the fluid is retained in the second and third trimester. The baby accumulates its own fat and fat cells during the last ten weeks of the pregnancy and during the first year of its life. By eighteen months of age, an infant's total number of fat cells is set, which determines weight control ability. The more fat cells, the more of a weight problem that child will have later in life. You can avoid subjecting your child to a weight problem by watching what you eat (and exercising) during pregnancy and lactation, and feeding him/her properly in infancy.

You have to gain enough weight, but keep in mind that *just* gaining weight isn't enough—it should be a steady weight gain, gained by eating healthy foods. Junk food and empty calories will not feed your baby's development, only your fat cells. You can be overweight and still malnourish the fetus. Proper nutrition is vital for human growth, maintenance, repair, energy, and physical performance. The basic rules during pregnancy include cutting down on all fats, sugars, and caffeine, and increasing intake of protein, complex carbohydrates, fiber, water, and calcium. Eating for two doesn't mean doubling the food, but doubling the *nutrients.*

recommended daily allowances

Later in this section, you'll find an easy-to-use menu plan. But first, the following breakdown of the recommended daily allowances for each food type will give you some general guidelines to follow. Of course, it's not practical for you to walk around with a scale and measuring cup, weighing everything you eat. This breakdown will give you a general idea of how the sample menus were derived and allow you to make your own substitutions.

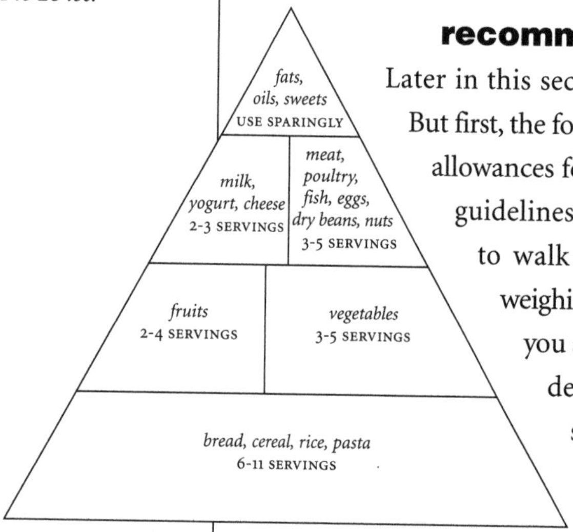

fats, oils, sweets
USE SPARINGLY
milk, yogurt, cheese
2-3 SERVINGS
meat, poultry, fish, eggs, dry beans, nuts
3-5 SERVINGS
fruits
2-4 SERVINGS
vegetables
3-5 SERVINGS
bread, cereal, rice, pasta
6-11 SERVINGS

From the U.S. Department of Agriculture, U.S. Department of Health & Human Services

RECOMMENDED DAILY ALLOWANCES DURING PREGNANCY

Food category	*Servings per day*
protein	*4–5 (75–100 grams)*
carbohydrates	*6+*
calcium	*4–5 (1,200 milligrams)*
iron-rich foods	*1–2 (40 milligrams)*
vitamin C	*2*
green leafy or yellow vegetables and fruits	*3*
other vegetables and fruits	*2*
water	*8–10 glasses*
fat	*1*

HOW MUCH IS A SERVING?

One serving of *protein* is approximately equal to:

- 3–3½ ounces of meat, chicken, fish, or cheese
- 3 glasses of milk
- 3 whole eggs, 5 egg whites, or 1 small Eggbeater® carton

For vegetarian protein combinations, combine one of the following:

- 3 cups soy milk
- 4 ounces tofu
- ¾–1 cup legumes or beans
- ½ cup nuts

with either:

- 1 cup of pasta
- 1–1½ cups rice, cereal, or corn
- 4 slices of bread

One way to satisfy the daily protein RDA is to eat a large (6–8 ounces) piece of meat (fish, steak, or a medium-sized chicken breast) for lunch and dinner. Another is eating either cereal or toast for breakfast with milk or soy milk, and drinking a few additional glasses of milk or soy milk during the day. Or mixing either type of milk with protein powder before it is poured on cereal (almost all powders are made with cow's milk, in one form or another, but there are a few delicious soy-protein powders now available, including Spiru-tein). This would cover the daily protein and fat serving requirement, as well as some of the iron and carbohydrate requirements.

One *carbohydrate* serving is approximately equal to:

- 1 slice of bread
- ½ of a pita bread
- 1 small tortilla
- ½ bagel or English muffin
- 2 rice cakes
- a few crackers
- 1 ounce of any cereal
- 2 tablespoons of wheat germ
- ¼–½ cup grains (such as rice, wheat flour, soy flour, rye flour, kasha)
- ½ cup beans

As you can see, these servings are only half of what most people would eat in one meal, so getting enough carbohydrates should not be a problem.

One *calcium* serving is approximately equal to:

- 1 cup milk, yogurt, or goat milk
- 1¼–2 ounces cheese
- ¼ cup Parmesan cheese
- 1¾ cup cottage cheese
- 1–2 cups very green vegetables (such as broccoli, collard greens, romaine lettuce, or kale)
- 3 tablespoons blackstrap molasses
- 3–4 ounces seafood
- 9 ounces tofu
- 1–3 cups soy milk (depending on the brand) or soy protein

Try to get your calcium from a variety of sources, not just from dairy products. Other good sources are dried figs, apricots, fruits, vegetables, grains, and meat. See more on calcium and dairy on pages 246–248 and 254–257.

Try to get your calcium from a variety of sources, not just from dairy products.

Iron-rich foods are readily available, but they vary in terms of iron absorption. Iron from meat and animal sources is very easily absorbed by our bodies, whereas iron from vegetable and grain sources is not as easily assimilated. Much of it goes to waste. You need twice as much iron when pregnant, and your doctor will probably prescribe an iron supplement to ensure that you consume an adequate amount.

Foods that are high in iron include liver, meat, chicken, clams, tuna, blackstrap molasses, toasted wheat germ, mixed grains, wheat bread, bagels, granola, rice, potatoes, beans, bran, dried fruit, millet, soy foods, some nuts, pumpkin seeds, and tomato paste.

One *vitamin C* serving can be found in:

- 1 cup or piece of most fruits, especially citrus fruits, berries, and melons
- 1/2 of a papaya, mango, or guava
- 1 glass of most fruit juices
- 1/2–1 cup of most vegetables
- 1/2 of a bell pepper (yellow and orange bell peppers contain the most vitamin C, red is next, and green contains the least)

One *green leafy or yellow fruit or vegetable* serving includes:

- 2 pieces of small fruit, such as apricots, plums, or nectarines
- 1 medium-sized fruit, such as a peach
- 1/2 of a large fruit, such as a mango, papaya, or a banana
- 1 cup cooked green leafy vegetables such as broccoli, kale, or asparagus
- 10 leaves of lettuce (romaine, butter, bibb, etc.)
- 1/4 cup cooked spinach or squash
- 1/4 yam or sweet potato
- 2 roma tomatoes or 1 large tomato
- 1/2 red or yellow bell pepper
- 1 glass of vegetable juice

One serving of *other fruits and vegetables* would include:

- 1 apple or pear
- 1 cup cherries, berries, cranberries, pineapple
- 1/4 cup dried fruit (or a few large pieces)

Many pregnant women can better tolerate a higher food intake if it's spread out in six smaller meals over the course of the day.

- 1 cup sprouts, beans, beets, cabbage, celery, eggplant, artichoke, or onion
- $^1/_2$ cup mushrooms, cucumber, squash, zucchini, or water chestnuts

One serving of *fat* is equivalent to:

- 1 tablespoon butter, margarine, oil, mayonnaise
- 2 tablespoons peanut butter
- 2 tablespoons salad dressing

You will probably consume enough fat without having to add any supplementary fat to your diet. One steak, for example, will supply you with ample fat for the day. Even if you consume mostly low fat foods, it is highly unlikely for you to become "fat deficient."

easy-to-use daily menu plan for active moms

There is no need to worry about measuring and weighing everything you eat. Just eat a little more than you normally would. If you're normally a light eater, eat a *lot* more. The following daily menu plan is meant to serve as a guideline; modify it to suit your needs, wants, environment, and lifestyle. For vegetarian combinations, see pages 220–222.

This daily menu plan was designed for active moms and it involves a lot of food. If you can't eat it all in one sitting, split it into smaller portions and reserve some for later. Remember, even if you're not hungry your baby is, and you're eating for two. Depending on your exercise level, you should consume an extra 300 to 500 calories per day while pregnant (up to 800 if you are extremely active or a professional athlete). A mere 300 to 500 calories may not seem like much, but you're not just concerned with calories—your daily requirements for nutrients doubles. Most of the foods you should eat are of the nutritious low fat variety, such as lean meat, fruits, and vegetables, rather than high caloric foods.

Many pregnant women can better tolerate a higher food intake if it's spread out in six smaller meals over the course of the day. If you have lower daily caloric needs or are unable to fit your daily food requirements into one day—as may occur in the case of severe morning sickness—you may need to take supplements to ensure adequate nutrition. Discuss it with your doctor and possibly a nutritionist.

If you dine out in a restaurant, try to find a similar meal, and if the menu doesn't offer exactly what you want—just ask, they will probably accommodate you. No matter how you modify your meals, do not modify in the water department—unless you drink *more.* Drinking adequate amounts of water is essential to prevent dehydration, which can predispose you to premature labor. If you are drinking enough water, your urine will be light yellow in color, not dark yellow.

SAMPLE MENU

Breakfast

- Two glasses of water before you eat (keep a glass by your bed)
- A bowl of oatmeal or cereal (the whole grain, low sugar kind)
- 3–4 spoonfuls of toasted wheat germ
- A sliced piece of fruit or berries
- A full glass of milk or soy milk (if it's too much for the cereal bowl, drink the rest on the side)
- One glass of pure fruit juice
- One cup of herbal tea, or some kind of health-food-store coffee substitute, or plain water—no caffeine

Breakfast Alternative

- A bagel, 2–3 pieces of wheat or mixed grain bread, or pancakes with a little low-sugar jam, syrup, or honey (no butter)
- Plus the same amounts of fruit, milk, juice, and tea listed previously

If you're suffering from morning sickness and can't possibly get all this down in one sitting, divide it and eat the second half later in the morning. If you work during the day, bring the juice and the fruit to your workplace.

Snacks

- One glass of milk or soy milk
- A handful of dried fruit, such as apricots, figs, or raisins

Workout

- Drink water before, during, and after your workout—a total of at least two to three 8-ounce glasses

Lunch

- Two glasses of water before you eat
- 6–8 ounces fish, chicken, or eggs (either 1 egg and 4 egg whites, or 6 egg whites, or 1½ Eggbeater containers)
- A cup of rice or pasta, a baked potato, or two slices of bread if you're having a sandwich
- A green salad or a side of green vegetables
- One piece of fruit
- One glass of juice
- One cup of herbal tea or decaffeinated coffee (optional)

Snacks

- One glass of milk or soy milk
- A handful of dried fruit

Dinner

- Two glasses of water before you eat
- 6–8 ounces fish, chicken, or lean meat
- A cup of rice, pasta, or potatoes
- A cup-sized portion (⅓ of your plate) of green, red, and yellow vegetables or a side salad
- One glass of juice
- One piece of fruit
- One cup of herbal tea or decaffeinated coffee (optional)

Evening Snack

- Two glasses of water or two cups of herbal tea if you didn't have tea after lunch or dinner
- Dried or fresh fruit (optional)

vegetarianism

There are various forms and degrees of vegetarianism; depending on the level, vegetarianism can be a concern during a pregnancy. People who consider themselves vegetarian because they avoid red meat, but still consume a fair amount of poultry and/or fish should not have any special nutritional concerns during pregnancy. They will get enough nutrients and protein in their diet. Fish is actually one of the best protein foods available.

Lacto/ovo vegetarians consume dairy products and eggs as their only animal protein source. To get enough protein in your diet during pregnancy from just these sources, you would have to eat *a lot* of eggs and dairy foods. This can be problematic in terms of caloric and fat intake levels. The high ratio of fat to protein and calcium in cheese and other high-fat dairy products may not be worth it postpartum, when you have to work it all off. Eggbeaters are a great low-calorie, low-fat substitute for regular whole eggs. Even if you restrict your fat intake, a high protein lacto/ovo vegetarian diet may still require too much food intake for most women.

Wheat germ has more protein, vitamins, and minerals per ounce than any other food.

Then there are the strict vegetarians or vegans, who will have special nutritional concerns during a pregnancy. It may upset some people to read this, but vegetable and plant protein is just not good enough during pregnancy. A complete lack of animal protein will leave you void of vitamin B12 and deficient in zinc, iron, and folic acid—all absolutely essential for a healthy pregnancy. It is crucial to supplement your diet with extra vitamin B12, iron, calcium, magnesium, and vitamin D.

Unlike animal protein, plant proteins are not complete proteins and are not absorbed by the body as well. Vegans must be very careful to mix their protein properly (legumes such as soy, beans, peas, or nuts with grains such as wheat, corn, rye, or oats) to get complete proteins. Legumes have only some of the twenty-two amino acids that make up protein; grains have the remaining amino acids. When combined in the right amounts, the two sets of amino acids complement each other to make a complete protein. Why is this so important? Without all of the twenty-two amino acids present together, none can be absorbed or utilized properly. Babies are made of protein—their organs, muscles, skin, and so on. Additionally, proper protein consumption is vital for a healthy immune system, so that we can fight off illness and slow down the aging process.

Keeping track of amino acid combinations can be difficult if not tedious. You may want to consider giving up your vegetarian lifestyle during pregnancy. If you do remain a vegetarian or vegan, adding wheat germ to any meal will help increase your protein intake because wheat germ has more protein, vitamins, and minerals per ounce than any other food. Sprinkle it on your breakfast cereal, soup, pasta, or salad. You can also add soy protein powders to soy milk. Egg whites (cooked, never raw) are another great protein source.

Mixing Protein

A complete protein serving can be achieved by mixing legumes with:

- 2/3–1 cup of lentils, beans, chick peas, split peas, or soybeans
- 1/2 cup of nuts
- 1/4 cup of seeds

Grains

- 1/3 cup of wheat germ
- 1 1/2 cup rice or pasta
- 4 slices of bread

Or dairy

- 2 ounces cheese
- 1/2 cup cottage cheese or dry skim milk
- 1 1/4 cup milk, buttermilk, or yogurt

SAMPLE MENU FOR LACTO/OVO VEGETARIANS

Breakfast

- 1 slice whole wheat toast
- 1 teaspoon margarine
- 1/2 cup Wheatadena
- 1 cup nonfat milk
- Sugar*

Lunch

- 1 1/2 cups lentil soup
- 2 whole grain rolls
- Salad (1 fresh tomato, 1 cup romaine lettuce, 1 hard-boiled egg, 1 tablespoon Italian dressing)
- 1/2 cup nonfat milk

Dinner

- Stuffed Pita (1 whole wheat pita, 1/2 cup kidney beans, 6 oz. tofu, 1/2 cup hummus, 1/2 cup mushrooms, 1/2 cup tomato puree, 1/2 cup raw carrots, 1 teaspoon olive oil)

Snacks

- Smoothie (4 oz nonfat milk, 1/2 cup yogurt, 1 banana, honey*)
- 8 whole wheat crackers
- 1/2 cup frozen yogurt

* Indicated foods that provide extra calories are used only for seasoning. Stricter vegetarians, and those not consuming any dairy foods, can substitute the milk and frozen yogurt with soy milk and frozen tofu dessert (may be difficult to find in some parts of the country).

From the California Department of Health Services, Maternal and Child Health Branch and WIC Supplemental Foods Branch: *Nutrition During Pregnancy and the Postpartum Period: A Manual for Health Care Professionals.* Sacramento, CA, Department of Health Services, 1990.

Morning sickness is not a psychological condition; it is a physical reaction to the hormonal influx and other changes your body is experiencing.

nutrition-related discomfort and symptoms during pregnancy

Morning Sickness

Up to 70 percent of all pregnant women will suffer from the misnamed "morning sickness." Morning sickness is widely misunderstood. The feeling of nausea, vomiting, and fatigue does not just appear in the morning, but throughout the day. Most women will experience it only in the first trimester, but as many as 10 to 20 percent will continue to experience these symptoms well into the third trimester. In severe cases, morning sickness can lead to dehydration and starvation, which requires hospitalization.

Morning sickness is not a psychological condition; it is a physical reaction to the hormonal influx and other changes your body is experiencing. It is believed that increased estrogen levels may enhance your sense of smell and sensitivity to certain odors. Everything suddenly smells a lot stronger, and you may develop aversions to many odors. Frequent offenders include perfume, coffee, nail polish, alcohol, bad breath, and cigarette smoke. Because inhaling these elements is not good for you or your baby, the nausea you feel may be nature's way of protecting your fetus. Estrogen levels and morning sickness are also increased by a high-fat diet. According to a Brigham and Women's Hospital study, nausea is three times higher for every twenty-five grams of fat and five times higher for every fifteen grams of saturated fat.

If you suffer from morning sickness, you may not feel like eating, but it is even more important that you do. A high intake of complex carbohydrates and protein can help decrease your nausea. Eating smaller meals more often will also help, because acid production increases in an empty stomach. This acid will eat into the stomach lining, creating more nausea, not to mention low blood sugar. Eat before you feel sick, as often as six times a day if possible. Avoid eating greasy or spicy foods. Keep snacks—such as saltine crackers or other complex carbohydrates—available at your bedside and other places you spend a lot of time. Eat something before you get out of bed.

Vitamin B6 has been shown to help diminish morning sickness. Though it is not known why, ginger, fresh grapefruit peel tea, and bitter foods are also believed to reduce nausea. In my experience, exercising prior to conception and throughout pregnancy tends to reduce the occurrence of morning sickness.

If you are vomiting, it is essential that you replenish your fluids. Drinking fluids may make you feel worse, but it is vitally important to prevent dehydration, which can cause premature delivery.

CRAVINGS AND AVERSIONS

During pregnancy, your body has many surprises in store for you. For one, you may begin to experience strange cravings or aversions you've never felt before. For the most part, cravings and aversions are perfectly normal and pose no reason for concern. Cravings can be caused by a number of things. A craving for red meat, fruit, or other "good" food is common and is probably nature's way of telling you that your body needs the protein in the meat, the vitamins in the fruit, or special nutrients from whatever other foods you are craving. Your body has a neat way of taking care of itself.

However, try to avoid sweets when you crave them. Eating artificial sweets will exacerbate any morning sickness or mood swings you may have by sending your blood sugar levels on a roller-coaster ride. Stick with dried or fresh fruit, apple sauce, cereal, raisin bread, or other foods that are naturally sweet and nutrient rich.

STRANGE CRAVINGS

We've all heard about women who crave ice cream and pickles during pregnancy. Such bizarre cravings *usually* have more to do with your psychological needs than a need for those foods. Let's face it, who needs salty pickles and sugar and fat-loaded ice cream? It's bound to increase your sugar, water retention, and body-fat levels unnecessarily all at the same time—without giving you or your baby a single nutrient worth absorbing.

Some of these cravings can come from feeling a lack of support, affection, or love from loved ones, during a time when you need much more support than normal. What you really need may be a good hug.

Chocolate has a lot of caffeine in it, which prevents absorption of iron and folic acid. These nutrients are needed to transport oxygen to the growing fetus.

CHOCOLATE CRAVINGS

Severe chocolate cravings tend to be more of an addiction than a craving. If you're a "chocaholic," you need to be careful during pregnancy—it could pose a bigger problem than you'd think. Chocolate has a lot of caffeine in it, which prevents absorption of iron and folic acid. These nutrients are needed to transport oxygen to the growing fetus. Caffeine also interferes with calcium absorption.

Instead of going gung-ho on chocolate binges every day, buy chocolate squares that can be broken off into smaller pieces, and eat only one small piece a day, or a couple of fat-free chocolate cookies to satisfy your addiction. Or even better, go to your nearest health food store and buy "carob" chocolate, which comes from a bean. It is totally natural, but it still has the same high 50 to 80 percent fat level as regular chocolate.

NON-FOOD CRAVINGS

Cravings for things other than food—such as mud, clay, dirt, sand, or detergent—is a condition called Pica. Such cravings could indicate an iron deficiency or imbalance. Consult your doctor immediately. Your doctor will do a blood test to check your iron level, and will probably prescribe extra mineral supplements. No matter how strong the craving, do *not* consume any non-food item, it could seriously harm both you and your baby.

AVERSIONS

Aversions are as common as cravings and may sometimes result in morning sickness. As you become more sensitive to scents, tastes, sights, and the environment, you may suddenly experience a dislike or even repulsion toward certain odors and products, such as coffee, alcohol, drugs, smoke, perfume, nail polish and remover, spicy or fatty foods, raw meat or fish, or

Aversions are usually just another way that Mother Nature sees to it that you avoid things that could harm your baby.

even certain movements. Driving over a small road bump or dip may feel like traversing a rocky mountain, and you may feel ill from it.

Aversions are usually just another way that Mother Nature sees to it that you avoid things that could harm your baby. For example, one common aversion is the sight or smell of raw fish or poultry. (If you can't even look at it without shivering, make somebody else cook it for you.) That goes for any other food that you become averse to. If frying onions or garlic bothers you, omit the cooking fat (use Pam spray). If it still bothers you, don't cook it at all until the aversion goes away.

CONSTIPATION

Constipation is a very common problem during pregnancy. It results from the mechanical obstruction of the colon by the uterus, the slowing down of your intestines due to pregnancy-induced hormones, and increased water absorption from the colon. Food moves through your body at a slower pace to allow for better absorption of nutrients. Additionally, the hormone progesterone decreases the tone and the movements of the gastrointestinal tract. These changes may result in constipation, difficult or infrequent bowel movements. Iron supplements may also aggravate the problem.

You can prevent or alleviate constipation by eating more fiber, drinking more water, and exercising. Water and fiber will soften the stool, and exercise increases circulation and bowel movements. Eat smaller meals more often and eat slowly to ease digestion. The following may also help alleviate constipation: prune juice, B vitamins, lemon juice, cider vinegar, mint, garlic, fennel, anise, papaya, and caraway seeds. Stool softeners can also be helpful. Laxatives are not recommended during pregnancy as they cause the excretion of valuable nutrients.

Avoid foods that you know will cause you to feel bloated. These may include milk, beans, cucumbers, cabbage, apples, fried/fatty foods, very spicy foods, dried fruit (soak it before eating), coffee/tea, alcohol, and certain mineral supplements, such as calcium carbonates and iron. Also avoid eating too much in one sitting, eating too fast, and swallowing air.

DIABETES

Diabetes can be genetic, but is often gestational. The reason is not yet clear. The fetus begins producing its own insulin after twelve weeks, but hyperglycemia can be detrimental to the development of the fetus in the first trimester, so check your glucose levels before conception if possible. If you're an insulin- or non-insulin dependent diabetic, the best thing for your baby is preconceptional glucose control, which will help prevent severe fetal abnormality of the cardiovascular and nervous systems. You can prevent and treat gestational diabetes with exercise and proper nutrition, but if your diabetes is severe you will probably also need insulin medication. Your diet should consist mainly of protein, some complex carbohydrates, a small amount of fruit and vegetables, and no refined sugar at all. Your meals should be small and frequent.

FATIGUE

Fatigue comes and goes, especially in the early and late stages of your pregnancy. In the first trimester, your body is busy trying to get used to being pregnant, sapping all your energy and leaving you tired. In the third trimester, your body is just plain exhausted from carrying this heavy load around.

The physical and emotional stress associated with pregnancy is significant and unavoidable. You may not be able to eliminate it, but you can reduce the amount of fatigue you experience to a certain extent. Getting plenty of rest, eating as nutritiously as possible, taking your supplements, and exercising regularly will optimize your energy level. Avoid sugar and fatty foods. However, particularly in the last trimester, don't shy away from animal proteins that are higher in fat, such as red meat or whole eggs—not only will they increase your energy level, but your baby's brain needs the protein and cholesterol for proper development. If your fatigue is severe or seems chronic, have your doctor check your iron level to make sure you're not anemic.

HEARTBURN

In the latter half of your pregnancy you may experience heartburn. Your growing uterus is pushing up on your stomach, and the sphincter muscle that separates the esophagus and the stomach softens. As a result, food or stomach acid may be pushed back up, causing you to feel a burning sensation in your chest.

Eating smaller meals, slowly, can help prevent heartburn. To ease digestion, avoid mixing too many kinds of foods at one meal. Stay away from spicy foods, coffee, and chocolate. Don't lie down right after eating as this can accentuate heartburn. For relief of heartburn, try a natural antacid like a calcium supplement. Liquid antacids may be necessary if heartburn becomes severe.

HEMORRHOIDS

Hemorrhoids are enlarged bundles of blood vessels—similar to varicose veins—located in a really awkward spot around the anus. During pregnancy, the combination of higher nutrient absorption, dryer feces, constipation, and hormonal factors can all contribute to the development of hemorrhoids. Straining during bowel movements and labor can also cause veins to dilate and lead to hemorrhoids.

Though not foolproof, preventative measures include: avoiding constipation, straining, and prolonged sitting; practicing your Kegels; and exercising in general to improve your circulation. Irritation can be relieved by keeping the area clean, using soothing ointments containing vitamins A, E, and D, dabbing on witch hazel or topically applied anesthetics, and soaking in warm water. Consuming vitamin E and bioflavinoids (found in some vitamin C supplements) are also believed to help.

Hemorrhoids may occasionally bleed during a bowel movement, if this happens persistently, alert your doctor. Postpartum, pregnancy-induced hemorrhoids will regress but probably not disappear. If they are severe, you may need to have them removed surgically.

LEG CRAMPS

Leg cramps are usually the result of a calcium or potassium deficiency. If you experience leg cramps, talk to your doctor—you may need to increase your calcium supplements and/or lower your intake of phosphorous-rich foods. Avoid pointing your toes and flexing your calf muscles, as this action can bring on cramping. When cramps occur, flex your foot to stretch the calf muscle.

SKIN PROBLEMS

Usually during a pregnancy the last thing you have to worry about is your wonderfully glowing skin, but there are exceptions to all rules. If you're suffering from acne, a little extra vitamin B6 may help, but talk with your doctor first. Do not self-administer any vitamin A, orally or externally. Products containing Accutane® or Retin-A® could result in severe birth defects. If your skin is very dry, try a topical moisturizer with vitamin E, jojoba, or even good old Vaseline.

dangerous substances to avoid

According to the *American Journal of Public Health,* just a glass of alcohol may render you infertile.

Alcohol

Alcohol consumption can cause FAS—Fetal Alcohol Syndrome—which causes brain damage, physical and mental retardation, and stillbirth. Even moderate drinking has been shown to cause fetal alcohol effects in the offspring, as well as miscarriage, placenta abruption, and low birthweight babies. Even a glass per week is not recommended, because alcohol interferes with folic acid absorption and folic acid is essential for proper development of the fetus. If possible, stop drinking before you get pregnant, especially if you're trying to conceive. According to the *American Journal of Public Health,* just a glass of alcohol a day may render you infertile.

Caffeine

Caffeine in all of its forms—coffee, tea, chocolate, colas—reduces your body's capacity to absorb calcium and iron. Caffeine consumption can decrease your baby's oxygen and nutrient supply, and in severe cases can result in weaker bones in the offspring due to calcium malabsorption. It is associated with low birthweight infants, prematurity, stillbirth, anemia, inflamed gums, future osteoporosis, and other problems. As little as one-half cup of coffee per day could result in miscarriage, and a study by Johns Hopkins University showed that consuming more than three cups of coffee per day reduces your chance of conception by 26 percent.

Douching

Douching is not recommended because it disrupts the natural vaginal hormonal environment, which could lead to bacterial infections. In rare instances, it can push air into your bloodstream, causing a deadly air embolism.

Drugs

Drugs, legal or illegal, should be avoided. There is no such thing as a safe drug or safe dosage during pregnancy. To prevent severe complications, birth defects, and stillbirth, do not take any drugs while pregnant.

Hair coloring and chemicals can be toxic to your unborn baby.

Hair coloring and chemicals

Hair coloring and chemicals can be toxic to your unborn baby. Be careful not to inhale or come into contact with such chemicals. Avoid coloring your hair during pregnancy. Some hair salons offer a "vegi-color," non-peroxide and non-ammonia coloring technique, but I also recommend that you pass on these non-natural processes. If you absolutely must highlight your hair with chemicals, the chemicals must not make any contact with your skin or scalp, and you must wear a mask during the process to prevent inhalation. (Michael Canale, a Beverly Hills celebrity hair-coloring specialist, has developed a 100 percent "Natural Color" hair coloring, from ancient Asian, Egyptian, and American Indian dying methods, plants, and herbs. To inquire, call the Canale Salon at 310–273–8080.)

Medications

Medications should be discussed with your doctor prior to conception and throughout your pregnancy. Do not self-administer any prescription or over-the-counter medications, including aspirin, ibuprofen, diet pills, laxatives, and cold or allergy pills. Your doctor may allow you to take certain medications, such as Tylenol®, some antibiotics, and blood pressure medication, but discuss it first.

Raw and Smoked Animal Foods

Raw and smoked animal foods are often contaminated and should not be consumed when you are pregnant. Avoid raw oysters, sushi, sashimi, rollmops, steak tartare, raw milk, raw eggs, grav lax, smoked salmon, mackerel, trout, or sausage. Eat everything well done—forget the word *gourmet* for the time being; after all, pregnancy is not a permanent condition.

Smoking

Smoking restricts oxygen and nutrient flow to the baby, causing retarded development and growth, miscarriage, stillbirth, and SIDS (sudden infant death syndrome). According to a study published in the *Journal of Pediatrics,* a child will have a 50 percent greater chance of mental retardation if her mother smokes one-half a pack of cigarettes per day during her pregnancy. If she smokes a full pack per day, the risk is 85 percent higher.

Many studies have shown that secondhand smoke is just as detrimental as smoking yourself. So do not let anybody smoke near or around you during your pregnancy. Don't be shy, tell them that they are choking your baby.

DON'T FORGET ABOUT DAD

The father's habits can affect your baby, too. If Dad smokes, the baby's risk of cancer, leukemia, heart defects, and learning disabilities increases. Any past or present drug use can seriously affect the child's mental, learning, and behavioral development. If he has been exposed to chemical radiation at work, it can have harmful effects on his sperm. Studies have not yet been done that I know of, but it wouldn't be a surprise if the father's nutritional habits also affect the offspring.

never too late

If you are reading this halfway through your pregnancy and are only now realizing that your diet may not be what it should be, it is never too late to start. Improving your eating habits now can reduce the risk for future problems or prevent existing problems from worsening. Do it for your baby, if not for yourself. You are solely responsible for supplying your baby with vital growing material every day.

For a lack of a better comparison, if you were building a house, would you build it without the foundation or without some of the bricks? If you were sewing a dress, would you leave out some of the supporting seams? If you were baking a cake, would you leave out some of the ingredients? And if you did, what would happen to that house, dress, or cake? They would all fall apart.

Simply stated: Think before you eat! Is the food going to satisfy your baby's nutrient requirements, or your own appetite and taste buds? Also, think before you *don't* eat. If you skip a meal, your baby will lose out on vital nutrients. If you're suffering from indigestion, pregnancy discomfort, or a smaller stomach capacity and feel full, your baby still needs to eat—no matter how difficult it may be. Food-wise, you shouldn't think of yourself during a pregnancy, your priority should be your unborn child.

If you have some bad eating habits, you can break them if you want to and if you believe that you can. Never doubt the old saying, "Whatever your mind can believe, your body can achieve." There is no need to be super strict. You may experience strange food cravings and moods at times, or even every day. Don't get frustrated if you want red meat instead of the fish that you're cooking for dinner. Have the meat so long as it's lean, and not a greasy sausage. Remember that your baby doesn't have the choice of when, what, and how much to eat, but you do.

For more detailed information on what foods to eat during pregnancy, please refer to *The Nutrition Almanac* by L. J. Dunne and *What to Eat When You're Expecting* by Eisenberg, Murkoff, and Hathaway.

Chapter Nine

essential vitamins and nutrients

The sample menus in the previous chapter gave you basic guidelines for what to consume each day. This chapter will give you a further understanding of the vitamins and nutrients that are essential during pregnancy. We'll explore the benefits, the effects of consuming too much or too little, and the best sources of each. We'll also discuss alternative food sources and herbal remedies.

Out of the six essential nutrients, only three are caloric—protein, carbohydrates, and fat. Protein and carbohydrates supply four calories per gram; fat supplies nine calories per gram. One pound of body weight is universally known to be equivalent to 3,500 calories, but the real caloric values are: 1,800 calories for one pound of carbohydrates, 1,800 calories for one pound of protein, and 4,100 calories for one pound of fat. The other three (non-caloric) nutrients that are vital for energy production are water, vitamins, and minerals.

IN THIS CHAPTER

- *The essential vitamins and nutrients explained—what they are, how much you need, and your best sources*
- *Exposing the myths about milk*
- *Herbal remedies—the good and the bad*

protein

Protein is the most important caloric nutrient for your baby. It is the main component of all cells and it is necessary for cell growth. Twenty-two amino acids make up what we call protein. Insufficient protein can contribute to fatigue, moodiness, low birth weight, and other complications. Protein is also very important for fetal brain development in the last trimester.

Good News about DHA

According to the American Dietetic Association, DHA Omega-3 fatty acids—found in cold-water fish like salmon, trout, and tuna—may help prevent premature labor. DHA seems to help birth weight, full-term delivery, and the neurological and immunological development of the baby during nursing.

During pregnancy, your protein requirement doubles reaching 75 to 100 grams a day, which you should try to eat without padding your hips with excess fat. Choose foods that are higher in protein than fat, such as lean meat, skinless poultry, fish, egg whites or Eggbeaters, non-fat dairy foods, and properly mixed vegetable proteins (see page 220). Avoid cooking or frying with added fat. Stay away from high-fat protein sources such as fatty red meats, which range from 35 to 95 percent fat; cheese and dairy foods, which can total 50 to 80 percent fat; so-called "low-fat" and "2 percent" dairy foods, which actually contain 37.5 percent fat; peanut butter and nuts, which contain about 75 percent fat.

Poultry, with its skin, has 50 to 60 percent fat. Instead, choose skinless poultry, which has only 8 to 15 percent, depending on the body part. Fish is another good choice. Most fish vary between 6 and 20 percent fat content. Some, such as salmon and mackerel, can contain 40 to 50 percent fat content. However, the "Omega fatty chain acids" in the fish oil is very good for you. Most beans and lentils are very low in fat (around 0.5 to 5 percent), except for soybeans, which measure in at around 50 percent. However, there are low-fat soy products you can choose instead.

High fat meats	*Lower fat meats*	*Lean meats*	*Other protein sources*
pork ribs *t-bone steak* *lamb chops*	*pork tenderloin* *lean fillet mignon* *veal chops* *salmon* *mackerel*	*skinless poultry* *fish*	*beans* *lentils*

Some proteins are more readily absorbed by the body than others. Protein from animal sources (especially eggs) is more easily assimilated than from vegetable sources. The reason is that animal and dairy proteins contain a complete set of twenty-two amino acids. Without all twenty-two amino acids present together, none of them can be properly absorbed. Separately, legumes, vegetables, and grains are not complete sources of protein. Beans and lentils have only some aminos; they must be complemented with a grain source that has the missing amino acids to make a complete set.

Most people in America get enough protein in their diets. If you don't, adding wheat germ and egg whites or Eggbeaters (cooked, never raw) to your meals will add a tremendous amount of protein, vitamins, and minerals without many calories or fat. (Don't exclude all egg yolks, your baby needs some cholesterol for proper brain development.) Add protein powder to milk or juice drinks for another protein boost.

However, be careful not to go overboard. Too much protein (more than 100 grams a day) could cause your body to excrete too much water, calcium, and other minerals.

carbohydrates

Carbohydrates are your (and your baby's) life and energy sustainers. They are the simple refined sugars and unrefined sugars—yes, carbohydrates and sugar are more or less the same. When a food product label lists sugar, it could be either refined, unrefined, or both—you have to read the ingredient list to figure out whether the sugar is "good" or "bad," so to speak. Simple refined sugars offer neither you nor your baby any benefits. They may provide you with a temporary burst of energy, but when it wears off (typically in one to three hours), your energy level will be even lower than before.

On the other hand, unrefined, high fiber carbohydrates will give you sustained energy. They can also reduce morning sickness, indigestion, constipation, and other pregnancy-related discomforts. Unrefined carbohydrates include whole grain foods such as bread, pasta, brown rice, and cereal (made of wheat, rye, corn, oats, rice, barley, millet), legumes (dried beans, sprouts, and peas), fruits, and vegetables. Eat them often in small amounts throughout the day. The closer to their natural state you can consume these foods, the better. Products that are fortified with certain nutrients are so fortified because their original nutrients got lost during processing. All of the lost nutrients are never replaced, nor is the all-important fiber.

A high complex carbohydrate intake is very important in the first and second trimesters, as these carbohydrates play a big part in the development of the fetus. During the first trimester, most of the carbohydrates you consume will be absorbed for the pregnancy, which will leave you feeling tired and lethargic. In the third trimester, the fetus uses fewer carbohydrates and more protein for growth and brain development. This leaves more energy for you, which will be a nice change.

Getting enough fat is rarely a problem in our society.

fat

Fat has many functions, which is why we have to work so hard to burn it off—our bodies don't want to let go of it. Fat is our energy storage, it's our safety protection, it's what we would live on in case of a famine, to keep our bodies from burning protein for energy. Fat also cushions our internal organs, protects a baby during pregnancy and labor, and insulates us from cold weather.

When *not* pregnant a person needs only 5 percent of their total food intake to come from fat to stay healthy. Getting enough fat is rarely a problem in our society. Unless you are suffering from an eating disorder such as anorexia nervosa or bulimia, you don't have to worry about fat deficiency. Such a deficiency would initially cause skin problems and advance to a state when the body has to burn muscles and tissue for protein to generate energy for life sustainment.

The average American diet consists of an astonishing 37 percent fat. The standard recommended level is 30 percent level, which many experts believe is still too high. A fat intake level of 20 percent is gaining acceptance as a much healthier goal, to prevent obesity, heart disease, and cancer. Even when you're pregnant, 20 percent is plenty. So don't pig out on pizza and ice cream just because you think you need to create a comfy cushion for your baby. Adding oil and butter in the preparation of your meals only pads your hips and waist unnecessarily.

In the first trimester, your body will deposit little fat "pillows" to protect the pregnancy. Both you and your baby need some "essential fatty acids." However, you don't need to worry about not getting enough—it would be impossible on a well-balanced diet to consume too little fat, no matter how hard you tried. Everything has fat in it: fruit has 3 to 14 percent, vegetables have 1 to 10 percent fat, grains have 3 to 10 percent, beans have 0.5 to 5 percent, soybeans have 50 percent, fish has 7 to 50 percent, skinless chicken 8 to 15 percent (with skin up to 60 percent), meat has 25 to 95 percent, eggs have 75 percent, milk and dairy 5 to 80 percent. You see how difficult a truly "fat free" diet would be? Even if you tried to eliminate fat from your diet completely, your body would convert any excess carbohydrates into fat. That's why "fat free/high carbohydrate" diets don't work.

FOOD LABELS

Don't believe that a food product is "fat free" just because the label says so. There are loopholes in the land of food label laws, which are taken advantage of by food manufacturers. One such rule states that for a food to be called "low fat," it has to be less than 30 percent fat. But "2 percent low-fat milk" actually has 37.5 percent fat. The 2 percent is measured by weight, not caloric value, which is what really counts. Another major loophole is that a food can be called fat free if one serving contains less then 0.5 grams of fat (4.5 calories from fat), but the size of one serving is left to the discretion of the manufacturer. Thus we have serving sizes in tablespoons! There is a certain "fat free" coffee creamer that is really up to 60 percent fat, while its "low-fat" counterpart is 75 percent fat (if you were to use this as your cereal milk, you might as well pour on heavy cream), and there is a "fat free" margarine that may be lower in calories due to water dilution, but all 5 calories are still 100 percent fat calories.

Companies can also round off the total calories up or down to the nearest 10—sometimes they lie and print 0 fat calories, even though the item may contain 4 to 6 fat calories. Consumers are being taken for a ride both legally and illegally. You almost need a degree in nutrition to figure it all out.

Due to such misleading labeling practices, changes in the label laws are pending. But to be on the safe side, you should read food labels carefully and calculate for yourself. It can be tricky—the aforementioned "fat free" creamer conveniently omits on the label where 60 percent of its calories are coming from.

The following chart will help you figure out the fat percentages for different products. On the food label, look for the "calories per serving" and "total grams of fat." Find the total calories per serving along the top row, and the grams of fat on the left column. Where the two rows intersect, the figure listed is the percent of fat calories that product contains.

FAT PERCENTAGES

calories per serving

grams of fat	60	70	80	90	100	110	120	130	140	150	160	170	180
1	15.0	12.9	11.3	10.0	9.0	8.2	7.5	6.9	6.4	6.0	5.6	5.3	5.0
2	30.0	25.7	22.5	20.0	18.0	16.4	15.0	13.8	12.9	12.0	11.3	10.6	10.0
3	45.0	38.6	33.8	30.0	27.0	24.5	22.5	20.8	19.3	18.0	16.9	15.9	15.0
4	60.0	51.4	45.0	40.0	36.0	32.7	30.0	27.7	25.7	24.0	22.5	21.2	20.0
5	75.0	64.3	56.3	50.0	45.0	40.9	37.5	34.6	32.1	30.0	28.1	26.5	25.0
6	90.0	77.1	67.5	60.0	54.0	49.1	45.0	41.5	38.6	36.0	33.8	31.8	30.0
7	—	90.0	78.8	70.0	63.0	57.3	52.5	48.5	45.0	42.0	39.4	37.1	35.0
8	—	—	90.0	80.0	72.0	65.5	60.0	55.4	51.4	48.0	45.0	42.4	40.0
9	—	—	—	90.0	81.0	73.6	67.5	62.4	57.9	54.0	50.6	47.6	45.0
10	—	—	—	—	90.0	81.8	75.0	69.2	64.3	60.0	56.3	52.9	50.0
11	—	—	—	—	99.0	90.0	82.5	76.2	70.7	66.0	61.9	58.2	55.0
12	—	—	—	—	—	98.2	90.0	83.1	77.1	72.0	67.5	63.5	60.0
13	—	—	—	—	—	—	96.9	90.0	83.6	78.0	73.1	68.8	65.0
14	—	—	—	—	—	—	—	96.9	90.0	84.0	78.8	74.1	70.0
15	—	—	—	—	—	—	—	—	96.4	90.0	84.4	79.4	75.0

calories per serving

grams of fat	190	200	210	220	230	240	250	260	270	280	290	300	310
1	4.7	4.5	4.3	4.1	3.9	3.8	3.6	3.5	3.3	3.2	3.1	3.0	2.9
2	9.5	9.0	8.6	8.2	7.8	7.5	7.2	6.9	6.7	6.4	6.2	6.0	5.8
3	14.2	13.5	12.9	12.3	11.7	11.3	10.8	10.4	10.0	9.6	9.3	9.0	8.7
4	18.9	18.0	17.1	16.4	15.7	15.0	14.4	13.8	13.3	12.9	12.4	12.0	11.6
5	23.7	22.5	21.4	20.5	19.6	18.8	18.0	17.3	16.7	16.1	15.5	15.0	14.5
6	28.4	27.0	25.7	24.5	23.5	22.5	21.6	20.8	20.0	19.3	18.6	18.0	17.4
7	33.2	31.5	30.0	28.6	27.4	26.3	25.2	24.2	23.3	22.5	21.7	21.0	20.3
8	37.9	36.0	34.3	32.7	31.3	30.0	28.8	27.7	26.7	25.7	24.8	24.0	23.2
9	42.6	40.5	38.6	36.8	35.2	33.8	32.4	31.2	30.0	28.9	27.9	27.0	26.1
10	47.4	45.0	42.9	40.9	39.1	37.5	36.0	34.6	33.3	32.1	31.0	30.0	29.0
11	52.1	49.5	47.1	45.0	43.0	41.4	39.6	38.1	36.7	35.4	34.1	33.0	31.9
12	56.8	54.0	51.4	49.1	47.0	45.0	43.2	41.5	40.0	38.6	37.2	36.0	34.8
13	61.6	58.5	55.7	53.2	50.9	48.8	46.8	45.0	43.3	41.8	40.3	39.0	37.7
14	66.3	63.0	60.0	57.3	54.8	52.5	50.4	48.5	46.7	45.0	43.4	42.0	40.6
15	71.1	67.5	64.3	61.4	58.7	56.3	54.0	51.9	50.0	48.2	46.6	45.0	43.5

water

We can survive for weeks without food, but water is so important that without it you would die within days. It's second only to oxygen in importance for human survival. Our bodies are made of approximately 70 percent water. It lubricates our joints, fills our muscles, tissues, organs, and blood, and helps us maintain our body temperature. About seven pounds of your pregnancy weight gain will consist of excess water.

We need about ten cups of water a day on average (if it's hot and humid, we need more). Ideally, most of your water intake should be plain water, but some may come from fruit and vegetables, juice, soup, or herbal tea. During pregnancy, stay away from caffeinated drinks (coffee, tea, soda) and alcohol. Cool water is better absorbed than hot or cold water. It's better to drink water all day than to wait until you get thirsty. Thirst is a signal that something is wrong; by the time you get thirsty, you are overdue. When pregnant, you must prevent dehydration, which will increase your body temperature and slow blood and nutrient flow to your baby. *Dehydration is the number one most preventable cause of premature labor.*

Dehydration is the number one most preventable cause of premature labor.

A sufficient water supply also prevents constipation, dry skin, and urinary infections. Even if you suffer from diarrhea in the first and third trimesters, do not restrict your fluid intake. The easiest way to gauge if you're drinking enough water is to look at the color of your urine. If it's dark yellow, you're deficient; if it's pale yellow, you're doing fine. When you work out it is even more vital that you remain hydrated. Drink two glasses of water before exercise, one glass every fifteen minutes during, and two glasses after your workout.

EDEMA

Water retention is common in pregnancy. You may retain water all over or only in certain areas. Edema can be caused by extremely high-carbohydrate diets, prolonged standing or sitting, excessive sodium, poor kidney function, heart failure, varicose veins, or a protein deficiency. If your feet are swollen, elevate your legs, exercise, loosen your clothes, and avoid sitting cross-legged. If it's chronic, increase your intake of calcium and vitamins D, C, and B6; modify your sodium intake only if you know that it is excessive. Activity and exercise (especially water exercise) usually minimize edema by stimulating circulation. So get into a pool and exercise.

vitamins

SUPPLEMENTS

The best way to obtain nutrients is naturally, by eating a variety of foods. However, supplementing your food intake during pregnancy with extra vitamins and minerals is very important, because it's difficult to eat enough food to gain all the necessary nutrients to make a healthy baby—particularly if you are a vegetarian or have any food allergies.

Your doctor will probably prescribe some prenatal vitamin supplements. If you are planning to become pregnant, your doctor should prescribe folic acid to you before you conceive, to establish the best possible condition for conception, implantation, and growth of a baby. Otherwise, go to your nearest health food store and buy a prenatal vitamin supplement. Choose one with no more than 5,000 IUs of vitamin A in a tablet/serving. Do not take any more than what is recommended on the bottle, because excessive supplementation may harm your baby.

ANTIOXIDANTS AND OIL SOLUBLE VITAMINS

All day we breathe in oxygen and metabolize food and nutrients, which produce oxidized byproducts and free radicals in our bodies. Free radicals are chemicals that can damage your DNA, cell membranes, and intracellular structures. This damage is part of the degenerative process that we call aging. Cancer is caused by free radical damage to cell membranes. The more oxygen you use (exercise and pregnancy both increase your oxygen exchange), the more oxidation and free-radical production will occur in your tissues, increasing your need for antioxidants. Antioxidants prevent this destructive process by neutralizing the free radicals, to keep your cellular structures healthy. It's that simple. Vitamin E is the main antioxidant vitamin, but other vitamins have some antioxidant properties as well.

VITAMIN A

This vitamin is necessary for bone and cell growth and development, and skin, hair, and mucous membrane maintenance. It lets us see in dim light and keeps our reproductive system and fat metabolism in working order. In the form of beta carotene it also has some antioxidant benefits, but not as much as vitamin E. Vitamin A is air sensitive and needs to be stored in a covered container.

RECOMMENDED DAILY ALLOWANCES (RDAS)

Nutrient	Regular	Pregnancy	Lactation
protein	45–50 gm	75–100 gm	65 gm
vitamin A	4000 IU	5,000 IU	6,000 IU
vitamin C	60 mg*	80 mg*	100 mg*
vitamin D	400 IU	400 IU*	400 IU*
vitamin E	30 IU*	30 IU*	30 IU*
vitamin K	65 IU	65 IU	65 IU
		B Vitamins	
B1—thiamin	1.1 mg	1.5 mg	1.6 mg
B2—riboflavin	1.2 mg	1.5 mg	1.7 mg
B3—niacin	13 mg	15 mg	18 mg
B6	2 mg	2.5 mg	2.6 mg
folic acid	0.4 mg	0.8 mg	0.5 mg
B12	3 mg	4 mg	4 mg
pantothenic acid	4–7 mg	6 mg	7 mg
		Minerals	
calcium	1,000 mg*	1,300 mg*	1,500 mg*
phosphorus	800 mg	1,250 mg	1,200 mg
magnesium	300 mg	450 mg	450 mg
iron	18 mg	48–78 mg	48–78 mg
zinc	15 mg	20 mg	25 mg
iodine	150 mg	175 mg	200 mg
potassium	3,500 mg	■	■
chromium	50 mcg	■	■
chloride	0.5 gm	■	■
sodium	0.5–3 gm	■	■

IU International Unit

■ *RDA not established*

* *Due to recent research showing that vitamins E and C boost the immune system, lowering risk of heart disease and cancer, new RDAs for these and other vitamins are being considered. The RDA for calcium will probably increase, to decrease risk of preeclampsia and osteoporosis.*

Too much vitamin A can cause bone, liver, and kidney damage; dry, yellow, itchy skin; hair loss; headaches; vomiting; birth defects; nose bleeds; nausea; and blurred vision. The Boston University School of Medicine found that doses higher than 10,000 IUs increases the risk of birth defects during pregnancy, and that women consuming 20,000 IUs a day quadruple their risk of having a child born with birth defects. Your prenatal multivitamin should contain no more than 5,000 IUs of vitamin A from beta carotene, not retinol. Beta carotene will convert into vitamin A, but only as much as your body needs without producing side effects.

Not enough vitamin A may cause night blindness and contribute to a poor immune system.

Your best sources are fish liver oil, liver, green leafy and yellow vegetables, and fruits. Egg yolks and fortified dairy foods are also good sources.

VITAMIN C

Vitamin C is not an oil soluble vitamin (it's water soluble), but it's part of the antioxidant group. Studies show that 250 to 500 mg of vitamin C daily could help reduce the risk of various cancers. Regular daily doses of 380 mg boost your immune system and reduce your risk of breast cancer by 40 percent. It is well known that vitamin C prevents scurvy. Many people swear it helps protect them from colds and the flu. This is probably because it works with vitamin E against the oxidative free radicals that are produced by our metabolism.

Vitamin C helps maintain bones, cartilage, muscles, and connective tissue. It helps heal wounds and aids iron in forming hemoglobin and red blood cells; this is vital to maintaining a pregnancy. Vitamin C is also needed for calcium and iron absorption as well as proper growth of your baby.

If you are under severe stress, are ill or wounded, or smoke, you will need even more vitamin C. Every cigarette that you consume destroys 25 mg of vitamin C.

Too much vitamin C can cause stomach upset, diarrhea, kidney stones, or a slow immune response. Excessive amounts can also interfere with vitamin B12 absorption and metabolism. The RDA when pregnant is only 80 mg, but most prenatal supplements contain 500 to 1,000 mg. Anything over 4,000 mg a day would be considered excessive.

Not enough vitamin C can cause scurvy (skin spots, bleeding gums, weakness), impaired immune system, and slow wound healing. A vitamin

C deficiency will also inhibit iron and calcium absorption. When you are pregnant and not absorbing iron, your body can't make sufficient red blood cells, and without these, oxygen can't be transported to the fetus, which could severely jeopardize the health, if not life, of your baby.

Your best sources are peppers (especially the yellow, orange, and red), citrus fruit, berries, melons, dark green vegetables, cauliflower, and potatoes. Vitamin C can't be stored by the body, so you need to consume sufficient amounts every day. Much of the vitamin C in foods is destroyed by heat from cooking, aging, and drying, so the best way to eat these fruits and vegetables is fresh, unpeeled, uncut, and uncooked.

Our skin actually manufactures its own vitamin D when ultraviolet light shines directly on our skin.

VITAMIN D

Vitamin D is very important for bone maintenance and formation. It helps your bones, blood, and tissues absorb calcium. Our skin actually manufactures its own vitamin D when ultraviolet light shines directly on our skin. Cold weather, rain, clouds, fog, smog, and protective sunscreen reduce this production. Due to a fear of skin cancer, many people are now in the habit of covering every inch of their bodies with sunscreen when they are exposed to the sun. As a result, they have an increased incidence of osteoporosis. The fear of skin cancer and related diseases is understandable, but you need to let some parts of your body enjoy a little sunshine, especially if you are a strict vegetarian—osteoporosis can't be reversed.

Too much vitamin D may give you an upset stomach, decreased appetite, diarrhea, headaches, kidney and cardiovascular problems, drowsiness, and excessive calcium in your tissues.

Not enough vitamin D will cause rickets in children, osteoporosis, and possibly frail bones in your baby.

Your best source is sunlight. Your body will produce its own vitamin D when it is exposed to direct sunlight. Some vitamin D is also found in fortified dairy foods (unfortunately usually the full-fat kind), fish liver oil, liver, egg yolk, tuna, salmon, and salt water fish.

VITAMIN E

Vitamin E is our main antioxidant. A deficiency in this essential vitamin is rare. While the RDA is currently only 15 to 30 IUs, a higher RDA is being considered (100 IUs) due to new studies that show it can protect you from heart disease and cancer. The experts are now recommending a daily intake of up to 400 IUs, but no more than 600 IUs.

Vitamin E works together with vitamin C to boost the immune system, slow down the aging process, and minimize the risk of cancer and heart disease. Despite the widespread belief that vitamin E increases your energy and physical performance, studies have not been able to find any proof. Applied topically, vitamin E aids in the healing of dry skin and scar tissue. It works better when used in conjunction with oral supplements.

Not enough vitamin E may cause anemia and a poor pregnancy outcome.

Too much vitamin E is only toxic to patients with high blood pressure and rheumatic heart disease.

Your best sources are wheat germ and oils from wheat germ, soybeans, corn, and cottonseed. Other sources are vegetable oils, green leafy vegetables, cucumber, lamb, asparagus, and nuts. You'll also find some in whole grains such as millet and brown rice, liver, fish, eggs, apples, mango, and believe it or not, chocolate (that's not an excuse to eat it, though—at least not during pregnancy).

Also see the antioxidant minerals zinc (page 250) and selenium (page 252).

VITAMIN K

This vitamin helps your blood to clot and is manufactured in your body, so deficiencies are uncommon. It is sometimes given to women in labor and to newborns to aid in blood clotting.

Too much of the synthetic form may cause liver damage or anemia.

Not enough may cause internal bleeding and excessive bleeding if injured.

Your best sources are dark green leafy vegetables, pork, whole wheat, bran, and oats.

B VITAMINS

B-complex vitamins are water soluble and therefore difficult to overdose on, since the body will usually excrete any excess non-usable portion. However, there are exceptions.

VITAMIN B1–THIAMIN

This vitamin helps metabolize carbohydrates. It is crucial in the first and second trimester during a pregnancy, which is the time when the fetus uses a lot of carbohydrates for growth and development. Thiamin also keeps your muscles, nerves, and heart healthy, and it minimizes fatigue and irritability. This benefit alone could make thiamin invaluable in the first trimester.

Too much may cause allergic effects, but because this is a water soluble vitamin that is quite unlikely.

Not enough thiamin can cause beriberi (disease marked by degeneration of the heart, nerves, and digestive system), fatigue, and irritability.

Your best sources are pork, peas, wheat germ, liver, yeast, sunflower seeds, and nuts.

VITAMIN B2–RIBOFLAVIN

This vitamin ensures that energy is released during the metabolism of protein, carbohydrates, and fat. It keeps your tissues, skin, hair, and nails healthy, and it helps normal cell growth.

There are no known risks of riboflavin overdoses.

Not enough of it may cause skin problems.

Your best sources are liver, dairy, meat, poultry, fish, beans, nuts, and brewer's yeast. Riboflavin is light sensitive, so store these foods in the dark.

VITAMIN B3–NIACIN

Like B2, niacin releases energy during metabolism, and it keeps your skin, nervous system, and cells healthy. Niacin is also needed for circulation and a healthy digestive tract.

Too much niacin causes flushing of your skin all over (take more than 400 mg and you'll look like a lobster and feel tingly and itchy), itchy dry skin, upset stomach, low blood pressure, and possible liver damage. Excessive niacin can also activate ulcers.

Not enough may cause pellagra, a disease whose symptoms include dermatitis, gastrointestinal disorders, light sensitivity, fatigue, loss of appetite, and a sore, red tongue.

Your best sources are meat, chicken, fish, beans, dried fruit, greens, and grains. Niacin is destroyed when foods are cooked (not steamed) in hot water.

PANTOTHENIC ACID

This vitamin is needed for healthy skin and nerves. It helps the adrenal glands produce anti-stress hormones, which could be a benefit in pregnancy.

Too much could give you edema, diarrhea, or a thiamin deficiency.

Not enough pantothenic acid could cause fatigue, nausea, sleeping problems, and poor coordination.

Your best sources are organ meats, eggs, salmon, yeast, beans, greens, and dried fruit.

*Good Sources of Folate**

PROTEIN FOODS

Beans, dry, cooked: black-eyed peas, garbanzo, kidney, lima, pinto, navy
Crabmeat, cooked
Lentils, cooked
Liver, cooked
Peas, split, cooked

BREADS, CEREALS, GRAINS

Cereals, dry fortified
English muffin, whole-wheat
Pita bread, whole-wheat
Wheat germ, plain

* *Provide a minimum of .04 mg of folate per serving.*

VITAMIN B6

B6 is a very important vitamin that helps your body properly utilize protein for tissue building. Our fat metabolism is aided by vitamin B6; it helps produce red blood cells and controls fluid balance, among other things. It also reduces PMS symptoms as well as morning sickness during pregnancy.

Way too much vitamin B6—or more than twenty times the RDA—could cause failure of your muscular and nervous system, impairing your gait, balance, and stability.

Not enough vitamin B6 can contribute to an unstable gait (common in pregnancy), numb feet, poor coordination, and brain function.

Your best sources are blackstrap molasses, wheat bran or germ, soybeans, brown rice, poultry, liver, greens, bananas, and dried fruit.

VITAMIN B12

Vitamin B12 is vital for red blood cell formation (these cells transport oxygen to tissues, and in pregnancy to the fetus), fat and protein metabolism, and nervous system functioning. It also helps children grow.

There are no known ill effects of megadoses of vitamin B12.

Not enough vitamin B12 could severely affect your protein metabolism and muscular performance, as well as your unborn baby's growth and well-being.

Your best sources are animal products such as meat, fish, poultry, eggs, and dairy foods. Strict vegetarians cannot get enough of this vitamin naturally, because it is not present in any plant food. They must take vitamin B12 supplements, especially during pregnancy.

FOLIC ACID (FOLATE)

Folic acid is probably *the* most important vitamin to stock up on before conceiving. Your body needs to have enough folate in storage before implantation of the fertilized egg to prevent spinal and brain deformations called neural tube defects. These defects occur in the first trimester between the seventeenth and thirtieth day. Most women don't know that they are pregnant during this crucial time. Any woman capable of becoming pregnant should supplement her diet with 0.4 mg of this vitamin every day.

Your growing baby will deplete your folic acid stores, leaving at least one-third of pregnant women deficient in this vitamin. A deficiency in the first trimester may cause spina bifida (a spinal cord deformity), cleft palate, and in the last trimester, brain damage or learning disabilities in the child.

Folic acid works in conjunction with vitamin B12 and iron. It is essential in hemoglobin production, red blood cell formation, and cell growth/division. It also helps circulation and protein metabolizing. It's important for brain function and mental and emotional health, and it can help remedy diarrhea, and menstrual and circulation problems. Folate can even prevent low birth weight.

The good news is that the FDA approved folic acid fortification to all bread, rice, pasta, cereals, and flours in 1998. Some orange juice companies are even fortifying their juice with folate. This will help not only pregnant women, but the rest of the population as well, because folic acid also prevents or reduces the risk of some chronic diseases, such as coronary heart disease and cancer.

Too much folate may hide a vitamin B12 deficiency.

In addition to the aforementioned effects, *not enough* folic acid can also cause anemia, gastrointestinal problems, impaired circulation, mental sluggishness, and graying hair. A deficiency can also stunt growth. Birth control pills and alcohol can interfere with folic acid absorption.

Your best sources are liver, dark green leafy vegetables, beans, asparagus, whole wheat bread, peanuts, grains, and fruit.

BIOTIN

Biotin is needed for protein, fat, and carbohydrate metabolism.

There are no known effects of biotin megadoses.

Not enough biotin may cause dermatitis, depression, and muscular pains. Eating raw egg whites may deactivate biotin. Of course, you should not consume raw eggs anyway, due to the risk of salmonella.

Your best sources are cooked egg yolks and organ meats. Biotin is available in most foods, and it is also produced by your intestinal flora.

GOOD SOURCES OF FOLATE *

Fruits and Vegetables

Artichoke, cooked
Asparagus, cooked
Beets, cooked
Brussels sprouts, cooked
Cauliflower, cooked
Corn, cooked
Grapefruit juice
Lettuce: chicory, escarole, romaine
Mustard greens, cooked
Okra, cooked
Orange juice
Parsnips, cooked
Peas, green, cooked
Spinach, raw or cooked
Turnip greens, cooked

* *Provide a minimum of .04 mg of folate per serving.*

From the California Department of Health Services, Maternal and Child Health Branch and WIC Supplemental Foods Branch: Nutrition During Pregnancy and Postpartum Period: A Manual for Health Care Professionals. *Sacramento, CA, Department of Health Services, 1990.*

Without exercise, calcium won't stay in your bones, no matter how much you consume naturally or through supplements.

minerals

CALCIUM

Calcium is one of the most important minerals. It is especially important for a pregnant woman. Calcium is needed to strengthen and maintain bone density, as well as heart, muscle, and nerve function, blood clotting, and enzyme activity. It also helps your baby grow strong bones.

Calcium and vitamin D lessen your perception of pain and reduce PMS symptoms. Taking calcium supplements during pregnancy can reduce your risk of preeclampsia by 62 percent according to the *Journal of the American Medical Association.*

Mother Nature has seen to it that your body's rate of calcium absorption doubles in the first trimester. The extra calcium is stored for your baby's use, especially in the last trimester. The fetus will draw its needed calcium from your storage first, and then from your bones, so if your stores aren't up to scratch, there may not be any calcium left for you. You could lose 5 percent of your bone density, which may result in osteoporosis later in life. You may already have an 80 percent chance of developing osteoporosis later if:

- you are Caucasian or Asian
- you have ever suffered from an eating disorder or a thyroid disorder
- you have been on any long-term medication
- you reach menopause early
- there is osteoporosis in your family

Inactivity, alcohol, and smoking make matters even worse. However, loss of bone density is preventable and fixable with extra calcium supplements and exercise. Omega-3 fatty acids and the soy compounds isoflavone and ipriflavone can also aid bone density. Weight-bearing exercise (walking, jogging, and weight training, as opposed to cycling, swimming, or other activities in which your weight is supported) is crucial for proper calcium absorption. Without exercise, calcium won't stay in your bones, no matter how much you consume naturally or through supplements. It's like pouring water into a cracked glass. Only during pregnancy does special estrogen and progesterone production prevent maternal bone loss without exercise. Exercise will, of course, enhance calcium retention even further, and prevent bone loss postpartum.

Usually we can absorb and use only about 20 to 30 percent of the calcium we consume. As soon as calcium gets into the stomach and digestive system, its first job is to neutralize acids (for heartburn, calcium helps tremendously). What's leftover will go to your growing fetus if you're pregnant, then on to your bones and muscles. Certain nutrients help our bodies absorb calcium better, such as vitamins D, C, and B6, magnesium, zinc, and phosphorus. You can also maximize your calcium retention by spreading out your intake over the course of the day, and consuming some at night, because the highest rate of bone loss occurs when you sleep.

To get the required 1,200 to l,300 mg (this RDA may increase soon to 1,500 mg) during pregnancy, you have to consume a lot of calcium. If that's not difficult enough, you also have to keep it from seeping out. Smoking, alcohol, laxatives, diuretics, and caffeine all pull precious calcium out of your bones and excrete it. A very high salt and beef intake can have the same effect. Extremely high fiber diets can also prevent calcium absorption.

For these reasons, calcium supplementation is very important, as is your choice of supplement. Read the labels well. Calcium carbonate has the highest absorption rate at 40 percent (calcium carbonate may cause some gas), calcium citrate at 24 percent. Choose Tums®, Os-Cal®, or a supplement with a 2:1 magnesium ratio and a vitamin D content. Avoid dolomite and bone-meal, which may contain lead; anything chelated; or oyster-shell, which won't absorb very well.

Too much calcium may leave you with calcium deposits in softer tissue, particularly if you are inactive or bedridden, such as during pregnancy or postoperative recovery.

Not enough calcium can be caused by an inadequate supply of vitamins D or C, magnesium, or phosphorous in your diet, or a shutdown of your hormonal estrogen production such as occurs during menopause or amenorrhea. These elements all assist in the bone absorption of calcium. Certain foods contain acids that also interfere with this absorption, such as spinach, beet greens, and rhubarb.

Your best sources are tofu, calcium-enriched orange juice, dry figs, soy milk, soy protein, milk, and other dairy foods (please choose non-fat dairy products). Other great sources of calcium are canned fish containing bones, green vegetables, blackstrap molasses, oatmeal, pinto beans, and soups made from bones cooked with vinegar or tomato.

Foods Equal to about 1 Cup of Milk for Calcium Content:

- 3 ounces sardines (if the bones are eaten)
- 1–3 cups soy milk (depending on the brand)

Foods Equal to about 1/2 Cup of Milk for Calcium Content:

- 3 ounces canned salmon (if the bones are eaten)
- 4 ounces tofu (if it has been processed with calcium sulfate)
- 4 ounces collards
- 1 waffle* (7 inches in diameter)
- 4 corn tortillas (if processed with calcium salts)

Foods Equal to about 1/3 Cup of Milk for Calcium Content:

- 1 cup cooked dried beans
- 4 ounces bok choy or turnip greens or kale
- 1 medium square cornbread* (2 1/2 x 2 1/2 x 1 1/2 inches)
- 2 pancakes* (4 inches in diameter)
- 7 to 9 oysters
- 3 ounces shrimp

* A dairy product is a major contributor to the calcium content of this food.

From *Nutrition During Pregnancy and Lactation: An Implementation Guide.* Institute of Medicine. Subcommittee for a Clinical Application Guide, Committee on Nutritional Status During Pregnancy and Lactation, Food and Nutrition Board. Washington, D.C., National Academy Press, 1992.

PHOSPHOROUS

This mineral works with calcium to form bones and teeth. Phosphorous aids in metabolism and is active in building and repairing tissues and cells.

Too much phosphorus can cause leg cramps, especially if it's not in a balanced ratio with calcium. If this occurs, try taking more calcium.

Not enough phosphorus may lead to osteoporosis, among other things.

Your best sources are meat, fish, poultry, eggs, dairy, bran, nuts, grains, fruits, and vegetables.

MAGNESIUM

Magnesium, along with calcium, builds bones. It also helps to maintain normal body temperature, protein metabolism, cardiovascular health, and nerve and muscle contraction.

Too much magnesium may cause diarrhea and problems with the nervous system.

Not enough magnesium is rare except in alcoholics, but the incredible growth that your fetus undergoes during the second to fourth months of pregnancy has a tendency to deplete your magnesium stores. Make sure your supplements are adequate and in balance. The ratio of calcium and magnesium should be 2:1, and they need vitamins D and C for proper absorption.

Without iron there would be no pregnancy, in fact there would be no you.

Your best sources are wheat germ, grains, nuts, dried fruits, green leafy vegetables, beans, tofu, fish, and lean meats.

IRON

Without iron there would be no pregnancy, in fact there would be no you. Iron doesn't just help produce the hemoglobin and red blood cells that carry oxygen in the blood to you and your baby, it also helps the body manufacture all the extra blood in a pregnancy. Normally, as much as 90 percent of the iron we eat doesn't get used, but the rate at which your body absorbs iron triples in early pregnancy. As the fetus takes what it needs, your stores may get very low. Therefore, you need twice as much iron as usual.

Iron deficiencies are very common in non-pregnant women, especially those who exercise strenuously. (This is another reason why you shouldn't and usually can't work out too hard when pregnant.) A pregnancy depletes your iron stores further, making supplements a necessity. It is difficult to get iron in sufficient quantities from your food during pregnancy. Iron supplements should be consumed with some vitamin C–rich food, such as fruit or juice, for better absorption. Iron can't do its work properly without its coworkers—folic acid, B12, and copper.

Most colorless foods, such as white bread and sugar, are also iron-less. Plant sources of iron, such as spinach and grains, are very difficult for our bodies to absorb. Vegetarians, pregnant or not, should always take supplements.

Calcium and magnesium compounds (such as antacids), caffeine in coffee, and tannin in tea can inhibit iron absorption.

Too much iron is rare, but could cause cramps, vomiting, liver damage, shock, heart failure, and death.

In addition to the aforementioned complications, *not enough* iron could cause anemia, decreased immune function, reduced circulation, and weakness.

Your best sources are animal sources, especially liver, red meats, fish, poultry, and eggs. The iron from these sources is very easily absorbed by your body. Oysters are very high in iron, but they are not recommended for consumption during pregnancy. Other sources such as green vegetables, beans, nuts, and grains are fine, but not as easily absorbed. Cooking your meals in iron cookware however, will add iron to your food, and vitamin C–rich foods such as tomatoes and fruit will help iron absorption.

ZINC

Experts have come to a new realization of the importance of zinc, particularly during pregnancy. Zinc maintains tissues, regulates insulin activity, and is essential in blood formation, the immune system, growth, and DNA and RNA integration and construction. Zinc also aids digestion and wound healing, and possibly affects diabetes and male infertility. It's also starting to be viewed as an antioxidant. These factors are all very important during a pregnancy.

Too much zinc may cause nausea, vomiting, diarrhea, dehydration, fatigue, kidney failure, or fever.

Not enough zinc can cause male infertility and reduced immunity to disease.

Your best sources are oysters (however, these are not recommended for consumption during pregnancy) and wheat germ. Other good sources are grains, meat, poultry, fish, seafood, eggs, legumes, beans, and popcorn.

IODINE

Iodine is important for your thyroid function, but it's rare to find anyone with a deficiency or an overabundance of iodine.

Not enough iodine may enlarge the thyroid gland in the mother, which also in turn may induce goiter in the fetus. A deficiency can also cause hardening of the arteries, obesity, and slow metabolism.

Your best sources are fish, seafood, seaweed, and iodized salt.

POTASSIUM

This mineral enables muscle activity and contraction, helps the nervous system, metabolism, fluid and electrolyte balance, and is essential for your cardiovascular well being.

Too much potassium may cause cardiac arrest or weak muscles.

Not enough can cause muscular cramps and weakness, and even paralysis and cardiac arrest.

Your best sources are fresh and dried fruits and vegetables—such as bananas, yams, oranges, mushrooms, and green leafy veggies—and fish, wheat germ, meat, and legumes.

Chromium Picolinate

According to chemists at the University of Alabama, chromium picolinate (a dietary supplement purported to reduce body fat and build muscle) damages DNA, possibly causing cancer.

CHROMIUM

Chromium controls blood sugar, fat metabolism, and the health of your cardiovascular system.

Too much chromium, as in occupational exposure, can damage the lungs, skin, and kidneys.

Not enough chromium could lead to poor sugar metabolism, sluggishness, and possibly gestational diabetes. An excessive intake of refined sugar and/or excessive amounts of exercise require a higher chromium intake, or it could lead to a deficiency. (Deficiencies are common during pregnancy.)

Your best sources are brewer's yeast, whole grains, mushrooms, meat, liver, seafood, eggs, poultry, and bananas.

COPPER

Copper assists iron in the formation of hemoglobin, red blood cells, bones, and connective tissue, and keeps your nerves and blood vessels healthy.

Too much copper may damage your liver and nervous system, and is related to a poor pregnancy outcome.

Not enough copper is associated with anemia, cardiovascular and bone problems, and is also a problem during pregnancy.

Your best sources are organ meats, beans, peas, grains, leafy vegetables, dried fruits, prunes, and brewer's yeast.

SODIUM

Sodium maintains your electrolyte and fluid balance, as well as nerve function.

There are no special restrictions regarding sodium during pregnancy, but as with most things, moderation is the key. If you consume too much salt, you will retain more fluids. To minimize edema, make sure you drink

There is plenty of sodium in most foods. You should neither restrict sodium nor add extra amounts.

plenty of water. If your face, ankles, and hands swell up, it may have nothing to do with your sodium intake, but could possibly be a symptom of a more serious problem. Check with your doctor.

There is plenty of sodium in most foods. You should neither restrict sodium nor add extra amounts. However, do avoid MSG. Check your food labels, especially on stock powders and cubes, and Asian food products.

Too much sodium can cause edema and exacerbate existing hypertension, which can lead to strokes.

Not enough sodium could cause decreased appetite and muscle cramps.

Your best source, of course, is different kinds of salt, but animal meat also has a fair share. Most foods contain plenty of sodium naturally.

SELENIUM

This overlooked mineral plays an important role in the immune system as an antioxidant helper.

Too much selenium may cause nail and hair loss.

Not enough selenium can lead to a poor immune system, and heart and muscle deterioration.

Your best sources are seafood, grains, and meat.

MISCELLANEOUS

Other not-so-well-known nutrients, which may also have beneficial effects, include:

Alpha Carotene

Alpha carotene, found in pumpkins and carrots, may help prevent lung cancer.

Canthaxanthin

Canthaxanthin, in natural food colorings, may help prevent skin cancer.

Flavinoids

Flavinoids, found in tea, apples, and onions, may help prevent heart disease.

Genistein

Genistein, found in soy foods, may help prevent cancerous tumors.

Indoles

Indoles, found in broccoli, cabbage, and cauliflower, may help prevent breast cancer.

Lutein

Lutein, found in dark green leafy vegetables, may help prevent lung cancer.

Lycopene

Lycopene, found in watermelon and tomatoes, may help prevent cervical, colon, and bladder cancers.

Types of Sugar

Fructose sugar—found in fruit and pure maple syrup—has a different chemical composition than sucrose or glucose, and is more readily absorbed and used by our bodies.

fruits and vegetables

By now you probably understand how during pregnancy it will take a little more than just "an apple a day to keep the doctor away." In fact, it takes seven fruit and vegetable servings a day to ensure enough vitamins for your growing baby. By now you have hopefully learned that each fruit and vegetable is loaded with nutrients. The fresher, richer, and darker the color, the more vitamins and minerals they contain.

Unless you suffer from hyperglycemia or diabetes, do not limit your fruit intake. Unfortunately, an unfounded belief persists among some people that the fructose sugar in fruit will make you fat. Nothing could be further from the truth. Fruits are made up of 90 percent water, are very low in calories and fat, are digested within thirty to forty-five minutes, and they contain vitamins and minerals that are vital to your baby's development. Only fat and an excessive consumption of refined sugars and carbohydrates can make you fat. Most people do eat too many sugars in the form of sweets, breads, and pastas, but no one eats too much fruit. You cannot compare a nutrient-void doughnut with a nutrient-dense apple, despite a similar sugar content—it's the quality that counts.

If you consume a lowfat diet, rich in protein and complex carbohydrates, and lots of fruits and vegetables during your pregnancy, it's highly unlikely that you will gain excessive weight, especially if you exercise. Fruits are also your best pre-exercise snack. A piece of fruit will give you just enough energy to get through a workout, while sweets will give you only a temporary sugar rush, then leave you with low blood sugar levels after an hour.

The importance of eating plenty of vegetables cannot be stressed enough. Vegetables are essential to your baby's well-being. So eat a good green salad every day.

If you consume a lowfat diet, rich in protein and complex carbohydrates, and lots of fruits and vegetables during your pregnancy, it's highly unlikely that you will gain excessive weight, especially if you exercise.

dairy

What I'm going to tell you in this chapter may be contrary to everything you've ever heard about milk. We've always been urged to drink milk by our parents, and TV and magazine ads add to the pressure by claiming milk "does a body good." We've been led to believe that we can't survive without milk and other dairy products, especially during pregnancy, when it's important to consume a lot of protein and calcium. Dairy has always been considered a perfect food in regard to the protein, calcium, phosphorus, and other vitamins and minerals it contains.

However, there are quite a few not-so-well-known problems related with dairy foods that may make you reconsider your dairy consumption. For starters, the protein content in dairy is not that high, and the fat content is higher than we often think. To get a complete serving of protein from milk you would have to consume at least three to four glasses in a sitting. Most dairy products contain no more than 10 percent protein, accompanied by 5 to 85 percent saturated and cholesterol-laden fat and some sugar in the form of lactose, which many people can't digest. Non-fat dairy foods contain only half the calories, and "almost" no fat (5 percent), a little more protein and calcium than the higher fat dairy foods, and almost no cholesterol.

Food labeling laws for milk were finally instituted in 1998, but I believe they are still misleading. The so-called 1 percent milk now called "low fat" really has 10 percent fat. Two percent milk, now called "reduced fat," actually has 37.5 percent fat, and the regular full-fat milk contains 60 percent fat, which is not that far off from cream and butter at 80 percent and 85 percent respectively. The new labeling laws are more accurate, but still not perfect.

Whether a dairy food is nonfat or full fat, it may exacerbate and/or contribute to a variety of problems, such as heart disease, cancer, arthritis, migraine headaches, allergies, colds, asthma, ear infections, thyroid and metabolic problems, behavioral problems, skin problems, fluid retention, bloating, abdominal cramps, and osteoporosis (yes, keep reading). It can impede proper food digestion by lining the stomach with the milk protein casein, preventing absorption of other nutrients and creating a build up of mucus.

MILK CALCIUM

Cow's milk was designed by Mother Nature for consumption by calves, just as dog's milk was designed for puppies, and human milk for our babies. There is a good amount of calcium in cow's milk, but it is very coarse and much harder to digest for us humans, compared with that in human milk. Cow's milk has 300 times more casein (a milk protein) than human milk, which is designed to build very large cow bones. The enzyme that we need to digest milk sugar with, lactase, also diminishes in most people after the age of three. The casein becomes a tough curdy goo (casein is also the base for some of woodworking's strongest glues), lining the walls of the stomach, preventing absorption of all other nutrients, and thus slowing down your metabolism. The effects of this are slower weight loss, fatigue, and bloating. The coarse calcium is tied to the casein, which also reduces its absorption.

To further aggravate the problem, milk is acidic, and calcium's number one priority is to neutralize any acidity first, so there may not be much calcium left for you or your baby, thus making you susceptible to osteoporosis later in life.

OTHER MILK FACTS

The American Journal of Epidemiology says that galactose, the milk sugar, may reduce female fertility.

The added vitamin D content of milk can vary 20 percent up or down from what is actually listed on the label. If it's up, you may be overdosing on vitamin D, which would negatively affect your kidneys and cardiovascular system.

There is also the unreported use of genetically engineered growth hormones being administered to most cows to produce more milk. This contributes to infections in the cows, which then need antibiotics for treatment. These cows naturally produce milk of reduced quality (less protein, more fat) and, possibly, with added bacteria. This is acceptable by FDA standards, but is it okay with you?

When the Department of Agriculture came out with a new "Eating Right Pyramid" telling people to eat less dairy, the dairy industry objected, and the new pyramid got scrapped from distribution.

The *New England Journal of Medicine* reported that soy protein, when replacing meat, can reduce cholesterol levels by 10 to 20 percent in one month.

LACTOSE INTOLERANCE

Lactose intolerance comes in varying degrees of severity. The effects include mild to severe digestive problems, gas, bloating, indigestion, and cramping. If you have a mild intolerance, you may be able to eat dairy as long as you consume a product such as LactAid to prevent any discomforts. The worst offender, with the most lactose, is milk itself. Other products such as unflavored yogurt, buttermilk, and cream cheese contain less lactose. If you can't even eat these, avoid all dairy foods including derivatives of whey, casein, and milk solids, which are often hidden ingredients in many products. Almost every cereal, bread, protein drink, or protein bar derives its protein from one of these sources, so read the food labels thoroughly.

MILK SUBSTITUTES

Is there any other way to get that all-important calcium and protein? Well, of course there is! A glass of soy milk can have as much calcium and protein as regular milk, and it contains no cholesterol, whether the soymilk is nonfat or not, its calcium is more easily assimilated by our bodies than the calcium in cow's milk. There is also almond milk (which can be rather high in fat content), rice milk, and oat milk. Both soy and nut milk need to be combined with grains to supply you with a complete protein. Goat's milk is also more easily assimilated by our bodies, and it contains a little more calcium, the same amount of protein, a tad more fat, and less folic acid than cow's milk. But like cow's milk, it wasn't designed for human consumption, and it therefore has its fair share of problems.

Whatever milk product you use with your cereal, don't leave any of it in the bowl. The *Tufts University Diet & Nutrition Letter* published a study showing that 40 percent of the folic acid in cereal seeps into the milk. So finish your milk or you may lose out on this essential nutrient.

SOY

Soy foods are now becoming the next health craze and miracle food. Soy has been shown to prevent cancer and heart disease, and help unclog cholesterol-laden arteries. The *New England Journal of Medicine* reported that soy protein, when replacing meat, can reduce cholesterol levels by 10 to 20 percent in one month. Soy also reduces the bad LDL cholesterol, without affecting the good HDL cholesterol. Mark Messina, Ph.D., a soy industry consultant, reports that soy may also strengthen arteries and help prevent osteoporosis.

Soy also seems to prevent and stop the cancer process by destroying tumor-causing enzymes. The Chinese believe that one serving of soy a day will decrease your cancer risk by 40 percent—especially breast cancer, by decreasing your natural estrogen levels. And after menopause, when a woman's natural estrogen production ceases, the estrogen found in soy copies your human estrogen to reduce menopausal symptoms. Possibly wishful thinking, but maybe one day we won't need manufactured drugs to prevent this female syndrome.

One cup of soybeans contains about 28 grams of protein, 250 calories (half of which come from fat, but with no cholesterol), and 25 percent of your daily calcium needs. Soy comes in the form of beans, milk, tofu, flour, protein powder, tempeh, soy sauce, miso, textured vegetable protein, bacon, luncheon meat, cheese, pizza, and desserts.

The Benefits of Soy

The FDA recently approved health claims on low fat foods containing 6.25 grams of soy protein. Soy protein, as part of a diet low in saturated fat and cholesterol, reduces the risk of heart disease, and slows calcium loss.

OTHER DAIRY SUBSTITUTES

Sardines and salmon (especially with bones) are very high in calcium and protein. This kind of fish does contain some fat, but the omega fish oils are actually very good for you. Almonds, grains, beans, dark green leafy vegetables, tofu, and brown rice all have a high calcium content that is very easily digestible. With all the available alternatives, there is no reason to become deficient in this mineral. Eating the right calcium-rich foods, engaging in weight-bearing exercises or resistance training, and taking a good calcium supplement can maximize calcium absorption to keep your bones healthy. Every woman should take calcium supplements throughout her life to minimize her risk of osteoporosis.

herbs and natural remedies

During pregnancy, most women change their lifestyles and habits for the good of their baby. You are probably more conscious of what you are putting into your body during pregnancy than at any other time during your life. Perhaps you never cared about eating healthy before, but now that you are responsible for another life, you are trying new things that are good for you and your baby.

But are we always sure what's "good" for us? People are always touting the rejuvenating effects of certain herbs or herbal therapies, and it would seem only natural that these remedies would be beneficial to both mother and child—but this is not always the case. Certain herbs and herbal teas could cause serious complications during pregnancy. To be on the safe side, you should avoid most exotic herbs and natural remedies. Before you take anything, check with your doctor.

THE BAD . . .

Raspberry tea has been touted to ease pregnancy, reduce morning sickness and labor pain, and speed up delivery by stimulating the uterus. The last reason is the most important, because it may cause a miscarriage. So can *Mexican zoapatle leaf tea, slippery elm, cohosh, pennyroyal* (as little as two tablespoons of this has caused miscarriage and killed the mother in a severe case), *mugwort,* and *tansy.* Please avoid these while pregnant.

Cottonwood tree bark, fenugreek, and *goldenseal* are herbs that could agitate and stimulate uterine contractions during pregnancy.

The herbs *Ma Huang (ephedra), yohimbine, chaparral,* and *comfrey* can elevate your blood pressure and blood sugar levels, causing hypertension, hepatitis, cancer, and diabetes.

Coltsfoot is used as a cough suppressant, but it has been known to cause liver cancer. *Sassafras* can cause liver damage and lung cancer.

Kola nut, which is used for energy, acts as a stimulant due to its caffeine content, which may lead to heart palpitations or irregularities, not to mention reduced iron absorption. If you need an energy boost, take some deep breaths or go for a walk instead. Oxygen and exercise are the only natural energy generators.

Ginseng and *astragalus* are used for energy, alertness, and better concentration. They're great when you need to really put your mind to something like studying or working—but *not* when pregnant. Their stimulating effects increase your heart rate and blood pressure. Ginseng may also give you insomnia and diarrhea.

Kava is used as a sedative and muscle relaxant, and should not be taken during pregnancy or lactation.

Rue has been known to cause bleeding.

Herbal laxatives such as *senna* can cause a mineral imbalance, because they flush out valuable minerals such as potassium and calcium. These laxatives can deprive your baby of nutrients, and cause your heart to stop beating. Ingested orally, *aloe vera* may also act as a laxative, which could eliminate essential vitamins, minerals, and other nutrients from your body and baby.

Echinacea can cause allergic reactions in the mother or child.

Valerian root, a muscle relaxant, may be dangerous if taken during pregnancy.

The effects of *St. John's Wort* on pregnant women have not yet been studied. It should be avoided until research is conducted.

Gingko biloba is touted to improve memory, but it is not recommended during pregnancy.

Alfalfa sprouts can be contaminated with E. coli.

Other herbs to avoid are *dong-quai, cat's claw, casgara sagrada,* and *feverfew.*

Ginger is believed to significantly reduce the severity of morning sickness, aid digestion, alleviate headaches and toothaches, reduce cholesterol levels, and help low blood sugar.

AND THE GOOD . . .

There are some herbs and natural remedies that are believed to be safe and possibly beneficial during pregnancy. However, to be on the safe side, always check with your doctor before taking anything.

Ginger is believed to significantly reduce the severity of morning sickness, aid digestion, alleviate headaches and toothaches, reduce cholesterol levels, and help low blood sugar. *Peppermint tea* is a natural pick-me-up and digestion aid, with no known side effects. It is also known to reduce morning sickness, irritable bowels, and intestinal cramping.

Chamomile is great for upset stomachs, cramps, insomnia, and irritated skin. *Royal jelly* (the nutrient dense part of honey) is known to give a little energy, and may help you with allergies and asthma.

Garlic has always been touted to help your immune system. It has been proven to lower cholesterol and prevent blood clotting.

Grape seed extract or *oil* is a good antioxidant and may help prevent heart disease and cancer. It also improves circulation, which is beneficial during pregnancy.

Basil may relieve gas.

Rosemary aids digestion and inflammation.

Cranberry juice helps to treat urinary tract infections.

In different regions of the world, healing traditions have been passed down through generations. Some women in the South and Southwest United States drink a mixture of water and baking soda to reduce morning sickness. In New England they use a teaspoon of apple cider vinegar with water for the same reason.

Hippocrates, the father of medicine, said that the *mugwort* plant will deliver the afterbirth (placenta) easier. In China they use *ginger* and *Angelica* for the same result. After pregnancy they consume *kelp* to get the uterus back to normal, along with *seaweed* twice a day to help return normal thyroid function and body shape, by speeding up weight loss (no wonder, it contains iodine).

In Britain, some women eat garlic and onions during pregnancy for better energy and an easier birth.

Despite a lack of scientific proof, women all over the world slather vitamin E cream, coconut oil, or olive oil on their breasts and bellies to minimize stretch marks.

Chapter Ten

postnatal fitness and nutrition

The period of time just after delivery is a highly emotional one. In the aftermath of this life-changing event, you may feel euphoric over this unforgettable experience, or just numb and exhausted from the incredible effort that you have put forth. While holding your brand new baby, you may feel like you have reached the highlight of your life so far. Or you may just feel strange for a while. You may feel several different emotions at once or in rapid succession. Your hormones can play tricks on you, adding to these overwhelming feelings. All of this is perfectly natural. A nine-month-long buildup of emotions and expectations has culminated with the amazing crescendo of giving birth.

In addition to the emotional changes, your body will be going through physical transformations as well. It will take your body three to twelve months to adjust to not being pregnant. As far as exercise is concerned, you should consider yourself still pregnant for the first two to three months, except for the fact that you can finally lie on your back and belly again. Your joints will still be loose, leaving you with a flawed sense of balance and coordination. Your uterus will take about six weeks to shrink back to its normal shape. This shrinking process, which is helped along by the stimulation of

IN THIS CHAPTER

- *Postnatal exercises—including some you can do with your baby*
- *Breastfeeding versus bottle-feeding*
- *Alleviating postpartum depression and other problems*

breastfeeding, may cause "after pains," which feel like little contractions. Your perineum (pelvic floor) should recover within six weeks, and if you had an episiotomy, the incision will heal within four weeks.

You may experience hot flashes and sweats (similar to the effects of menopause) for a few weeks after giving birth, due to a decrease in estrogen levels. This is most common in women who breastfeed. Exercise can help reduce these symptoms. Your hormonal level should be back to normal in six weeks, and it may take that long to stop spotting and discharging the afterbirth. You'll get your period back in six to twelve weeks unless you breastfeed at least five times a day. Your metabolism will gradually return to normal but your cardiovascular and thermal (cooling) system may remain at elevated levels, making you more fit than before conception.

For most women, breastfeeding helps trim the waistline faster due to the extra calorie burning of milk production. But in others, it may not make a difference. The last three to five pounds do not usually come off until after you have finished nursing.

Though you will lose about seventeen pounds over the first ten days after delivery, getting your body back into shape will not be so automatic. To regain your strength, muscle tone, balance, stability, energy, and other physical and mental capabilities, you must rest. But you should not just kick back and relax all the time. Without proper exercise, your body will go to mush. Your breasts and abdominal area will sag, as will the arches in your feet. Lower back aches are common. If you did not exercise much during the pregnancy, any aches, pains, and postural problems you had during the pregnancy may not just persist, but may actually get worse.

Some women think that pain is a natural consequence of having a baby. But pain—except during labor—is not normal and should not just be accepted as part of life. Most aches and pains are preventable or fixable, or can at least be minimized through exercise.

Of course, your attitude will be a very important aspect of your recovery. A negative attitude can be very detrimental. You can effectively think yourself into aches, pains, and other problems. Being in the right mindset can work wonders.

Even if your body is never quite the same as it was before you got pregnant, postpartum exercise is vital to your well-being. Naturally, the more you were able to exercise before and during your pregnancy, the faster the postpartum process is going to be. But don't despair, it is never too late to start. And it is not just about losing weight. Toning is necessary to strengthen your muscles, joints, and bones. If your bones were depleted of calcium, strength training is the best treatment to help your bones reabsorb this mineral and lower your risk of osteoporosis.

Of course, the goal is to strengthen your entire body. But, just like in pregnancy, your pelvic floor, abdominals, and lower back will be a priority. The pelvic floor and lower back carried that extra weight for nine months, and your abdominals are probably softer from being stretched to their maximum.

How soon you resume your exercise routine after delivery depends on your physical and mental condition, exercise history, ease of pregnancy, new parental duties, and work schedule.

postnatal exercise guidelines—baby steps

Most athletes and very fit mothers want to leap back into training almost immediately after delivery. Other women feel they need—and deserve—a break. How soon you resume your exercise routine after delivery depends on your physical and mental condition, exercise history, ease of pregnancy, new parental duties, and work schedule. Remember that your joints are still loose and will not stabilize for two to eight weeks postpartum, which can interfere with your balance and coordination. So start carefully.

The most important exercise—Kegels—should be started as soon as possible. This cannot be stressed enough. Weak and flabby pelvic floor muscles cause urinary incontinence in 10 to 25 percent of women under age sixty-five and 50 percent of elderly women. It can also cause pelvic organ prolapse, a condition where the pelvic organs literally fall out through the vagina. Pregnancy, especially with a vaginal delivery, is the main cause of the weakening of these muscles. Even if you had a C-section, the pelvic floor muscles did a lot of work supporting the pregnancy and need to be revitalized.

Without Kegels, any pregnancy-related problems with the pelvic floor might end up requiring surgery. Such drastic measures are avoidable if Kegels are done regularly. If that is not incentive enough, these exercises will also enhance future lovemaking. You can start doing Kegels almost immediately after delivery. You can perform these simple but crucial exercises from the comfort of your bed.

Your abdominal muscles, which have been thoroughly stretched by your pregnancy, need strengthening and shortening. Abdominal exercise will help flatten your stomach and stabilize your spine and pelvis, which will in turn help your posture and mobility. You can begin doing pelvic tilts and abdominal contractions the day after a vaginal delivery, and two to three days after a C-section. If you had a C-section, wait for the staples to be removed and for a doctor's approval before doing any regular abdominal exercises.

Make light walking your next physical accomplishment. If you had a normal, vaginal delivery, you can begin walking short distances the next day, even if it is just around the hospital corridors. Otherwise, get up and about in a few days, and after a week, start going on little walks.

Other cardiovascular exercises and strength training can be commenced as soon as ten days after a healthy pregnancy and vaginal delivery, or fourteen days after a C-section. If you are still discharging heavily, you may want to postpone your program until the discharge stops. If you had an episiotomy, do not ride a bicycle for six weeks. If you are at risk for infections, do not swim for a while.

Only start to exercise when you feel ready and have obtained your doctor's approval. Exercise is important, but overdoing it may interfere with the postpartum recovery. Most women will feel ready to resume working out within two to three weeks. Remember, consider yourself still pregnant for at least two to three months postpartum. Take it easy, and work slowly with cardiovascular exercise, strength work, or stretching. Any weight training should be light at this point. Whatever your activity, from running to boxing to kayaking, consider yourself a beginner again. Be very aware of your form and do not rush the process. At this time you should be thinking *recover,* not *bust my butt.* A delivery is major surgery, and you know better than to jump into a strenuous regimen right after an operation, don't you?

Seasoned athletes can start light jogging after a few weeks. Do not start any serious training until at least six weeks postpartum.

Once you're ready to start, plan to exercise three days a week. You might feel a little shaky in the beginning, but you'll get stronger. Gradually increase your frequency and intensity until you reach your previous fitness level.

The exercises described in this chapter have varying levels of difficulty. The advanced versions should be done only weeks or even months after delivery, depending on your individual strength level. If you are a well-trained athlete, you may be able to do them sooner. However, your doctor and instructor should clear all exercises first.

Now that you are caring for an infant, fitting in workout time may be difficult. However, the benefits should be enough to motivate you. Even just a little exercise will prevent or decrease postpartum blues, increase your self-esteem, and give you the strength to cope with your new status as a mom. It can also give you time to yourself, away from the baby. And, as you'll see later in this chapter, there are also ways to fit your baby into your workout routine.

Even just a little exercise will prevent or decrease postpartum blues, increase your self-esteem, and give you the strength to cope with your new status as a mom.

designing your postnatal workout

Just as each woman's pregnancy is different, each woman's rate of recovery will vary. The following schedule contains suggestions of how soon after delivery it might be appropriate for you to perform certain exercises. You should proceed at your own pace and with your doctor's advice. The postnatal exercises listed below are described in this chapter.

WITHIN TWENTY-FOUR HOURS OF NORMAL VAGINAL DELIVERY, OR TWO TO THREE DAYS AFTER A C-SECTION

- Kegels
- abdominal contractions
- pelvic tilts
- walking (short walks around the hospital or at home)

AFTER ONE WEEK, YOU MAY ADD

- abdominal curls
- hip curls
- leg slides
- foot exercises
- scapular retractions
- neck exercises
- wall sit and reach
- stretches (see chapter 7)
- breathing exercises (see chapter 7)

AFTER TWO WEEKS, ADD

- abdominal pulses/plank pose (alternate or pick one)
- diagonal curl/lateral curl (alternate or pick one)
- leg lowering
- back extensions
- cardiovascular exercise: Take regular easy walks for twenty minutes at least three days a week. Increase the intensity as you see fit. Or choose another cardiovascular activity and resume slowly.
- strength training: Your routine should include two upper back exercises, one chest exercise, leg extension, leg curl, inner and outer thigh exercise, one biceps exercise, and one triceps exercise (choose strength-training exercises from chapter 5).

A couple of weeks on this program will build a foundation for your most basic needs: strong upper back and arms and stabilization of your hips and knees. Expect to feel better within a week or two, and expect to see improvements within six to twelve weeks. From there you can increase or change the exercises in your program and gradually build your strength up to previous levels. Consult with an instructor or trainer knowledgeable about the postnatal condition and its special concerns.

Your body is bound to be tired and you may want to slouch at every opportunity. Bad postural alignment from pregnancy may have rounded your shoulders, arched your back, and weakened your stomach and hips. Postpartum, your uterus and other abdominal organs may press on your weakened abdominals, giving you continued backaches. So be aware of your posture at all times. Pull in your abdominals, lift your rib cage, and keep your shoulders back. Keep your chin up, your pelvis under, and your toes pointed forward when walking. You may have to really force your body in the beginning to keep it straight.

Now that you are not just carrying your baby, but the carrier, stroller, car seat, diaper bag, extra groceries, and everything else your infant needs, you are really going to need to stay strong. Be sure to strengthen your abdominals and upper back, and stretch your lower back and chest in your workouts.

When you lift your baby or any baby accessories, lift them properly. Stay close to anything that you are going to lift, bend your knees, not your back, and stand up the same way you bent down. To avoid any further problems, avoid backward bends and rotations; double leg lifts; shoulder-, hand-, or headstands; and the Hurdler's stretch. Also, do not strain to lift anything too heavy, avoid exercise that's too strenuous or too fast, and do not attempt any ballistic (bouncy) stretching.

postnatal exercises

(If you had a C-section, skip ahead to Postnatal Exercises After a C-Section.) Be sure to check for diastasis recti—separation of the abdominal wall—before doing any abdominal exercise. If you have a separation, pull your sides together toward the middle with your hands or a towel wrapped around your back while doing any abdominal exercises.

KEGELS, KEGELS, KEGELS

Remember these? Well, what are you waiting for? Your pelvic floor muscles endured a lot of pressure for a very long time, and if you had a vaginal delivery they were also completely stretched, weakened, and possibly torn or cut. If you are just picking up this book for the first time, and haven't yet mastered this exercise, refer back to pages 124–125 for detailed instructions.

ABDOMINAL CONTRACTION

Lie on your back with both knees bent. Contract and pull your abdominals in tight. Hold the position as you exhale. Release and inhale. Repeat this ten times for three sets every day for a week. This can also be done seated.

abdominal contraction

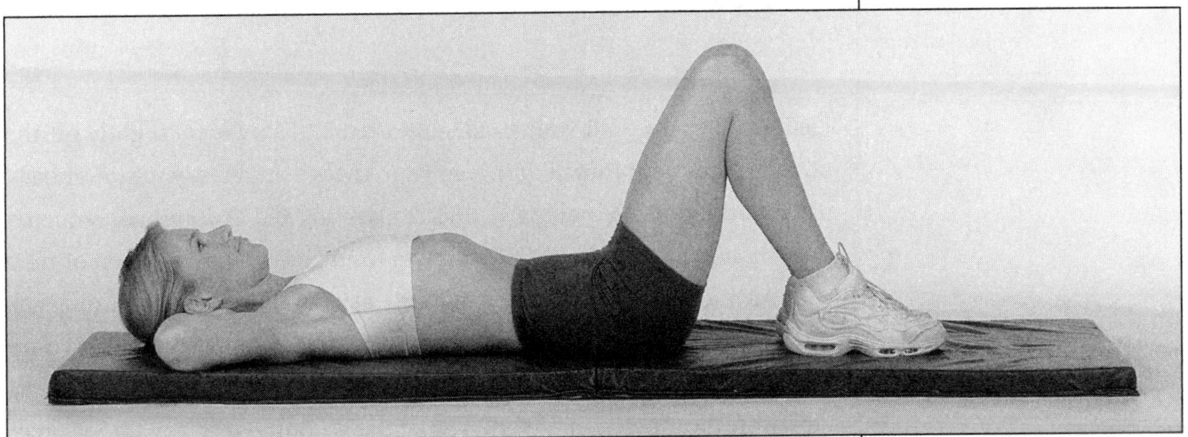

PELVIC TILT

Lie on your back with both knees bent. Pull your abdominal muscles in and squeeze your buttocks together as you tilt your pelvis upward, rounding the lower back. Hold the position and exhale. Release and inhale. Repeat ten times for two sets once a day. This can also be done while supine, seated, standing side lying, on all fours, or on a ball.

ABDOMINAL CURL

After a week postpartum, you can add this curl to your pelvic tilt exercise. Start by contracting your abdominals and tilting your pelvis. Next, lift or curl your shoulders and head off the floor about 30 degrees with your arms extended forward or behind your head, and exhale. Inhale as you lower your body back to the starting position. Repeat ten times for two sets every other day for a week.

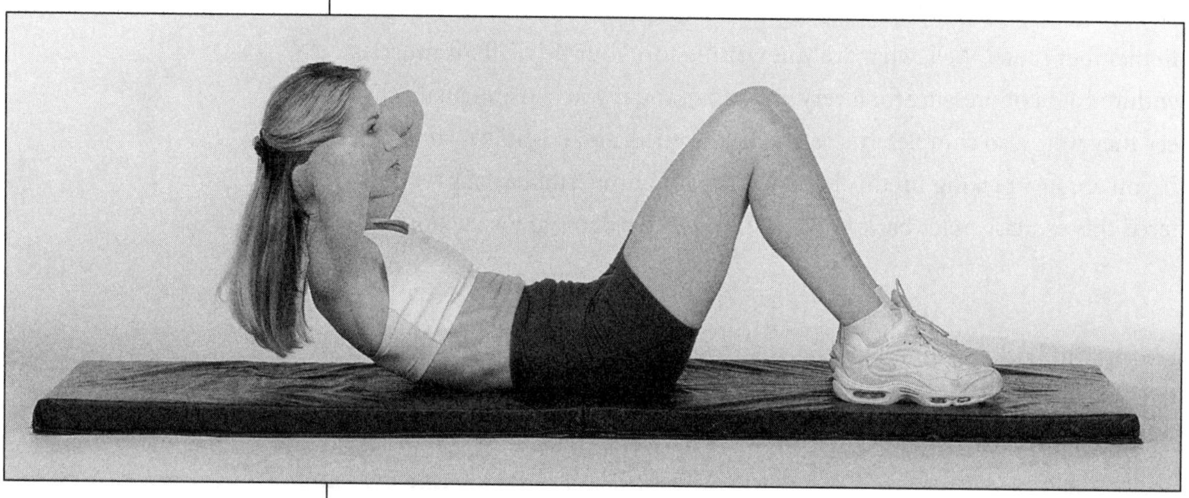

abdominal curl

LEG SLIDE

Lie on your back with your head supported and shoulders slightly off the floor. Flex the abdominals and keep your knees bent. Press your lower back flat into the floor by pulling in and contracting the abdominals isometrically (holding a muscle contraction in a fixed position for a period of time without releasing it) as you slide one leg out as straight as possible and back again. Don't hold your breath. Do two sets of five to fifteen repetitions once a day. Repeat this exercise with the other leg. If your lower back is not pressed down on the floor completely, you are not contracting the abdominals properly or hard enough. Another possibility is that your abdominal muscles may be too weak. If the abdominals aren't strong enough, discontinue this exercise and try again when your abdominals have regained strength.

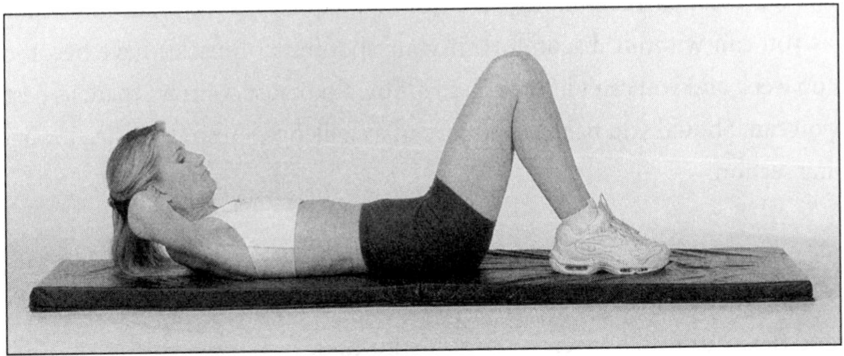

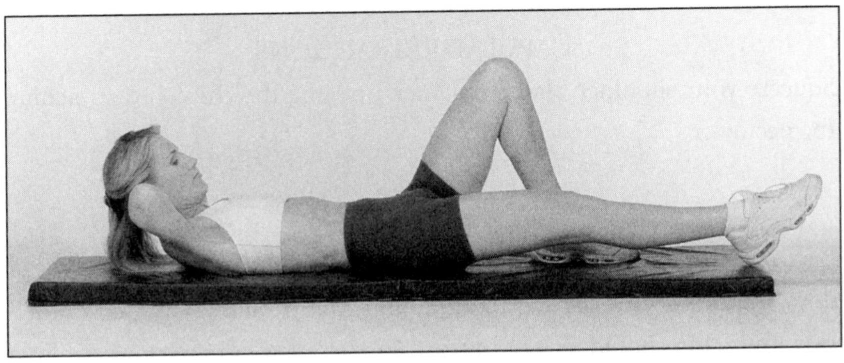

leg slide from beginning (top) to end (bottom)

Advanced Leg Slide Variations

When you have mastered the previous exercise, try these variations, which are listed in ascending order of difficulty:

Double Leg Slide—Slide both legs simultaneously.

When that gets too easy, go back to sliding one leg at a time, but lift the leg off the floor slightly as it straightens, pressing down the lower back with your abdominals.

When that becomes to simple, start with both feet lifted off the floor and your knees bent. Extend one leg straight out, and make sure to keep your lower back pressed down flat on the floor.

The most difficult way to do this exercise is to lie flat, lift both legs (knees bent) off the floor, and extend both legs out straight off the floor, pressing your lower back flat using only the sheer strength of your abdominal muscles. The level of difficulty increases the closer your legs are to the floor. This takes a long time and lots of practice to master. You should not attempt this exercise unless you are very fit, which may take several months postpartum.

Do these exercises slowly and not in a haphazard way. Lift only as far as you can without discomfort. If your abdominal muscles have become too weak and you can't lift your legs off the floor, just contract them as best you can. Should you need even more of a challenge, jump to the leg lowering section.

FOOT EXERCISES

You can do the following foot exercises seated or lying down. Circle, point, and flex your feet. Squeeze and relax your toes.

SCAPULAR RETRACTIONS

Squeeze your shoulder blades together, opening the chest and stretching the pectorals.

NECK HALF-CIRCLES

Begin with your head turned sideways to the right. Gently roll your head downward in a semi-circular motion until your head is turned to your left side. Your chin should almost touch your chest. Do not go backward for a full circle. Bending your head backward could strain your cervical spine.

ABDOMINAL PULSE

While seated, pull the abdominals in as tightly as you can and exhale hard. Relax and inhale, letting the air fill up your abdominal cavity. Repeat this exercise twenty times.

PLANK POSE

The plank pose is the best exercise you can do to regain a flat stomach. Start this yoga position on all fours, on your hands or elbows and knees. (Resting on your elbows is easier than resting on your wrists.) Your back should be straight, as if you were preparing to do push-ups. Do not let your back arch or sag. Tilt your pelvis and hold your stomach in and up for as long as you can. Try to hold this position for twenty to thirty seconds while still breathing at a normal rate. Don't hold your breath. Gradually work up to

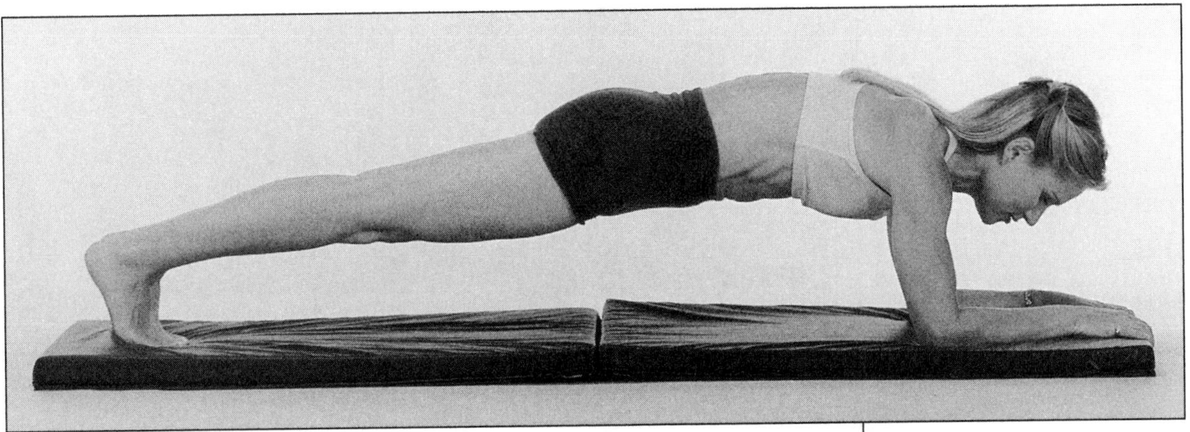

plank pose

one minute. Repeat twice. If you feel any strain in your back, you're not contracting your abdominals hard enough, or they may be too weak to do this exercise. For an advanced version of this exercise, rise onto your toes. Do not attempt this exercise if you suffer from high blood pressure.

ABDOMINAL HIP CURL

Start on your back with your knees bent and feet off the floor, close to your buttocks. Keep your arms behind your head, on the floor by your sides, or hold on to a heavy chair behind your head. Lift your hips up and off the floor an inch or so by contracting and shortening your abdominal muscles and exhale. Inhale as you lower your hips slowly as if against resistance. Don't just drop down—you lose half the exercise and could potentially hurt your back. Repeat this exercise ten to twenty times for two sets. See page 125 for photo.

LEG LOWERING

Start in the same position as you did for the abdominal hip curl. Extend one leg straight up in the air, and lower it down slowly as you press your lower back flat into the floor. When lowering the right leg, focus on pressing the right side of the lower back down really hard, and vice versa for the left side. Before the leg you are lowering reaches the floor, bend and pull in your knee. Repeat with the other leg. Keep alternating legs for two sets of ten.

This is a very advanced abdominal exercise that requires a great deal of strength and control if it is to be done safely and correctly. Do not attempt this exercise if your abdominals have separated (diastasis recti), or if your strength has not returned.

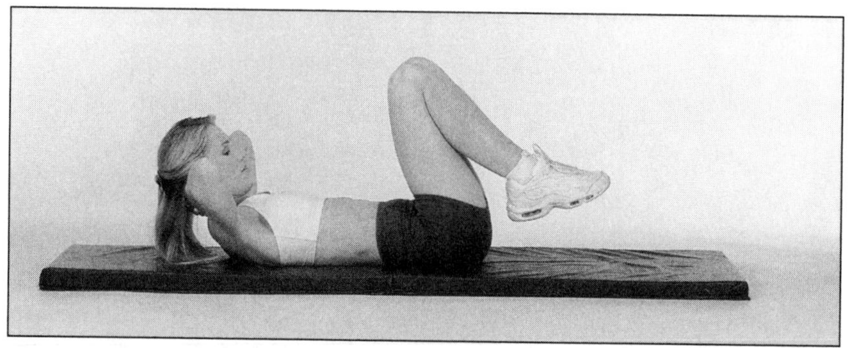

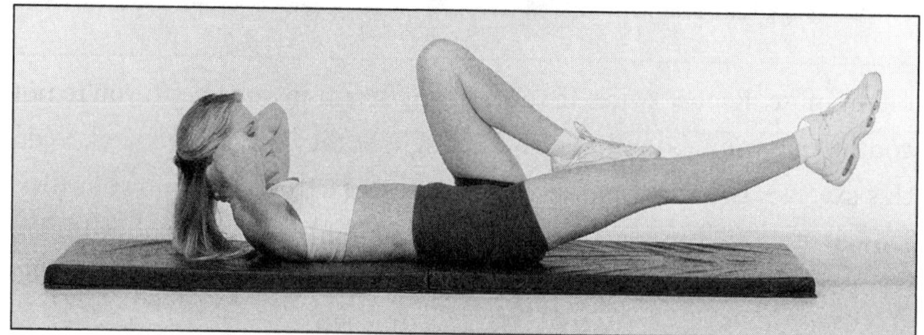

leg lowering from beginning (top) to end (bottom)

DIAGONAL CURL

The diagonal curl and the variation that follows (lateral curl) both target the obliques. Start by lying on your back with knees bent and your hands supporting your head. Slowly lift your left elbow up diagonally toward your right knee, making sure to keep your right shoulder down. Repeat this move with the other arm. If your abdominals have separated, you should not do this exercise.

diagonal curl

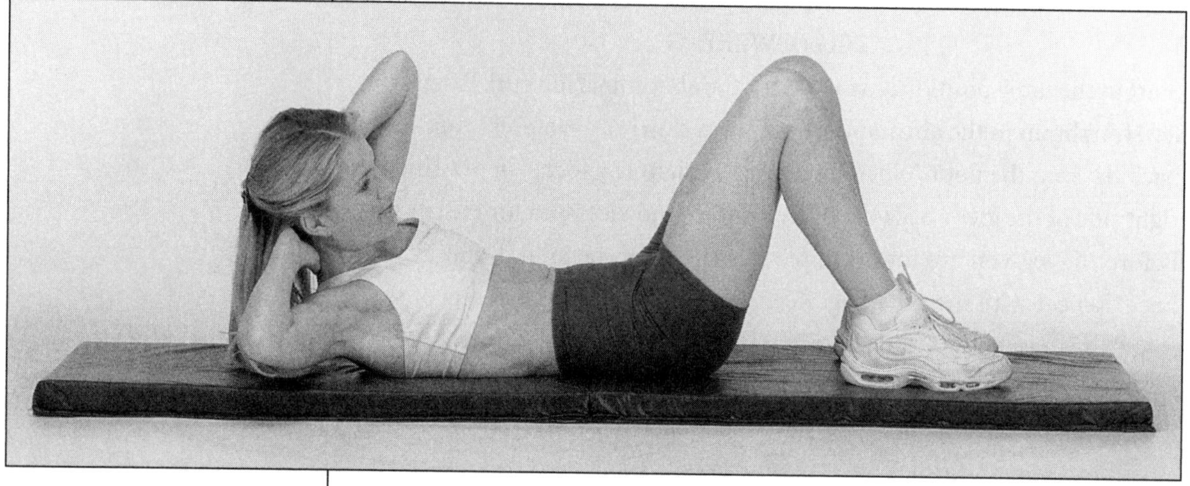

LATERAL CURL

Lie on your back with knees bent and the left hand supporting your head. Lift your head and shoulders off the floor, reaching for your right heel with the right hand, flexing the obliques sideways and exhaling. Return to the relaxed position and inhale. Repeat ten times on each side. Again, do not do this exercise if your abdominals have separated.

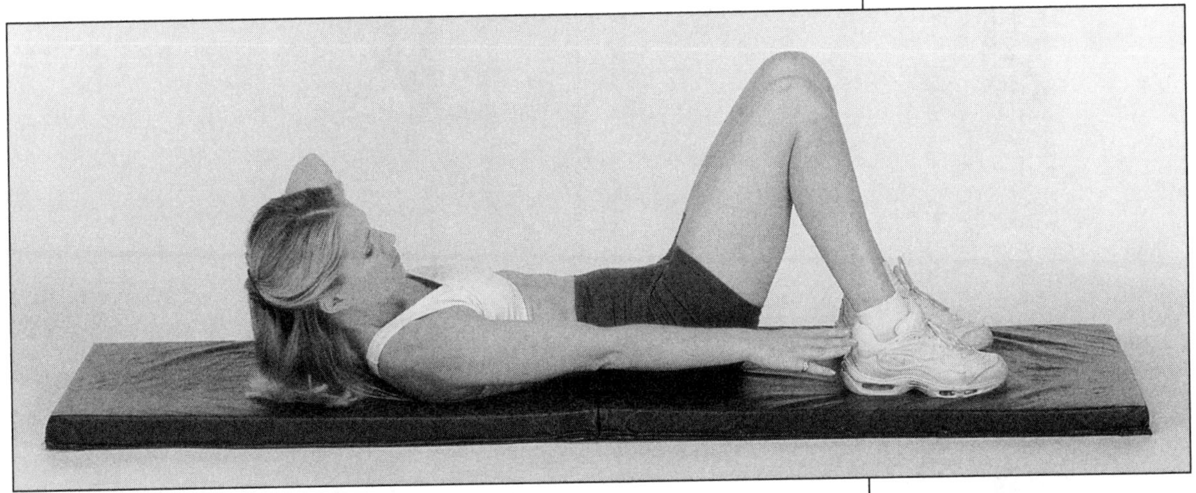

lateral curl

BACK EXTENSION

In a prone (lying face down) position with both arms outstretched forward, lift the left arm and right leg up and down ten times. Keep your head and nose down. Repeat on the other side. When this gets too easy, slowly move both legs and both arms up and down simultaneously.

WALL SIT AND REACH

This is a postural exercise that takes care of almost your entire body and should be practiced by everyone. Semi-sit against a wall with your knees bent at more than 100 degrees. Press down through your heels, not your toes. Lean forward a little first, then slowly roll and press your spine up against the wall with your stomach in tight. Your entire back, especially the lower back, should be pressed into the wall. Next, slowly raise your arms up over your head as high and straight as possible without letting any part of your back leave the wall. Reach up only as far as your body will allow comfortably, challenging yourself without straining. You should feel a lot of tension in the upper back, not in the shoulders, so keep the arms up high.

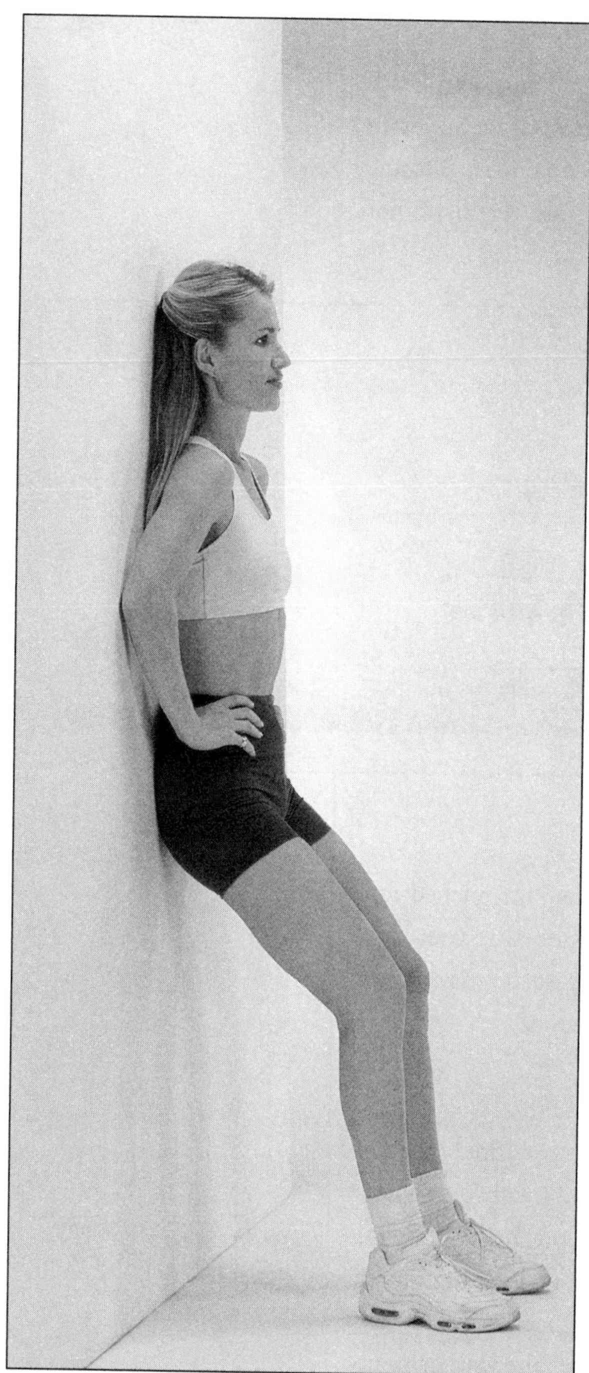

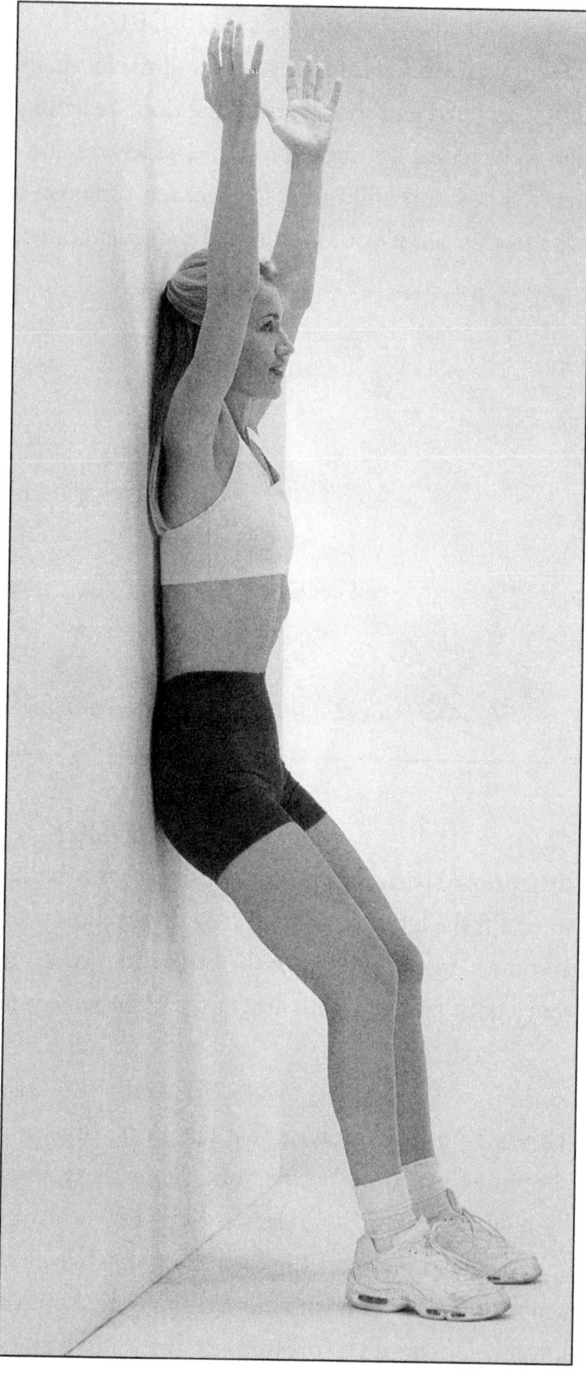

beginning (left) and advanced (right) wall sit and stretch

Hold this isometrically for as long as you can bear, up to one minute if you can, while breathing slowly. Repeat twice. Beginners can leave their arms down, since flattening the back can be difficult enough. This exercise should be avoided if you suffer from high blood pressure.

postnatal exercise after a c-section

Your muscles will quickly atrophy after a C-section if you do not exercise, so it's important to start right away. The special exercises following will help speed your recovery. They can all be performed in bed.

After your staples have been removed, you may ease into the regular postnatal exercises described previously. After about two to four weeks, you may resume a normal exercise program, but do not start until your body is ready for it and you have your doctor's approval. Of course, do not exercise if your incision hurts or becomes infected, or if you experience heavy bleeding, pain, excessive urinary incontinence (leaking), or breast infection.

Your muscles will quickly atrophy after a C-section if you do not exercise, so it's important to start right away.

two to four days after a c-section

Practice diaphragmatic breathing (see page 204–205) slowly to get your lungs back in action. While breathing, support the abdominal area around your incision with your hands. Let the lungs and chest cavity expand as you inhale, and lightly contract the abdominals as you exhale.

KEGELS

Yes, Kegels. Your pelvic floor didn't get stretched out, but it still carried all that weight for nine months and it is just as tired as you are. Besides, the Kegel exercise needs to be continued for the rest of your life, no matter what. See pages 124–125 if you need a refresher course in Kegels.

PELVIC TILT

This exercise will help relieve tightness in the lower back. Also, by squeezing your buttocks, you will help get your rear back into shape, too. Do them seated or lying in bed (with knees bent) as soon as you can. Pull the abdominals in and squeeze your buttocks together as you tilt your pelvis upward, rounding the lower back. Hold the position and exhale. Release and inhale.

five to seven days after a c-section

PELVIC HIP LIFT

Lie down with your knees bent. Do a pelvic tilt, but lift your hip up in the air and hold for a few seconds. Lower and repeat ten times.

LEG BRACING

While lying or seated in bed, gently press your knees down into the mattress.

FOOT EXERCISES

Point, flex, and circle your feet in all directions to promote circulation. Squeeze and relax your toes.

exercising with your child

Bonding with your baby is important, so never take intimacy with your infant for granted. You can bond by exercising with your child. Your baby will think it's all fun and play with mommy, while providing resistance. Repeat each exercise ten times for two sets. Wait until your child is a few months old before doing these exercises; they are not safe for brand new infants.

BABY CHEST PRESS

Lie on your back and push your child straight up and down, holding onto its sides under the arms. Your baby will love it.

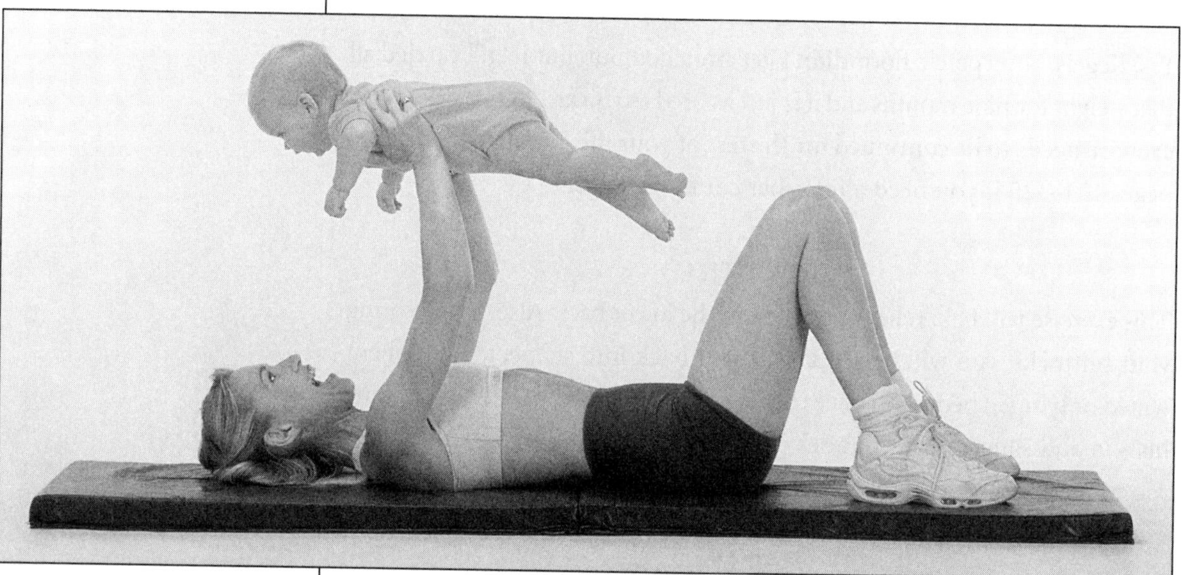

baby chest press

BABY TILT

Lie on your back with your baby sitting on top of your stomach or pelvis. Do a pelvic tilt, using your baby as resistance.

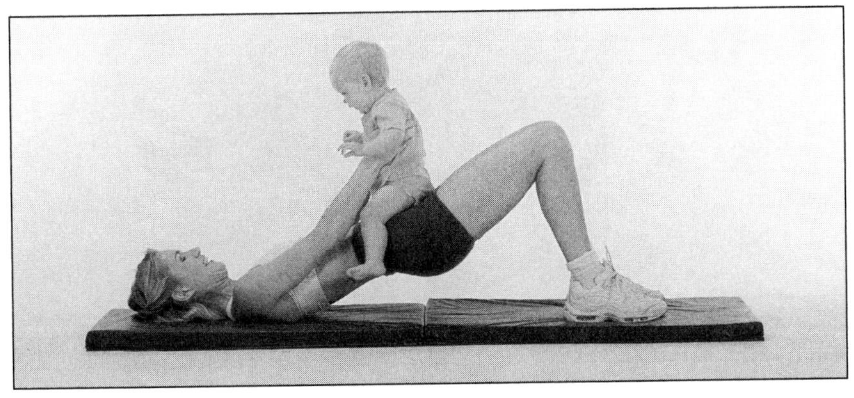

baby tilt

BABY CURLS

Place your baby either face down or seated on your stomach and curl up your shoulders and head using your abdominals.

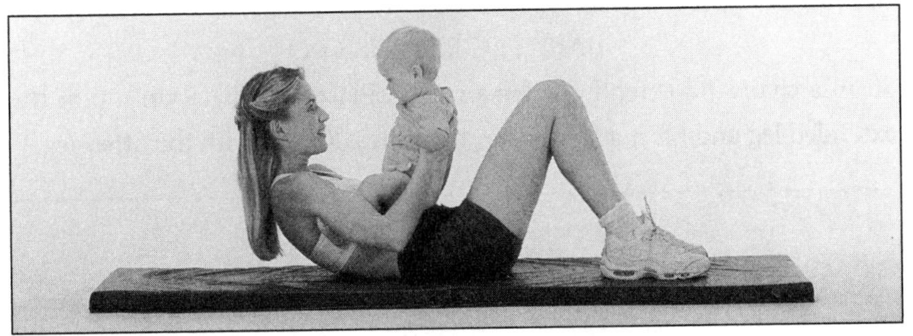

baby curls

ROCK-A-BABY

Lie on your back with your feet off the floor. Place your child face down on top of your lower legs while holding on to the baby's arms. Rock your torso forward and backward gently for an abdominal exercise.

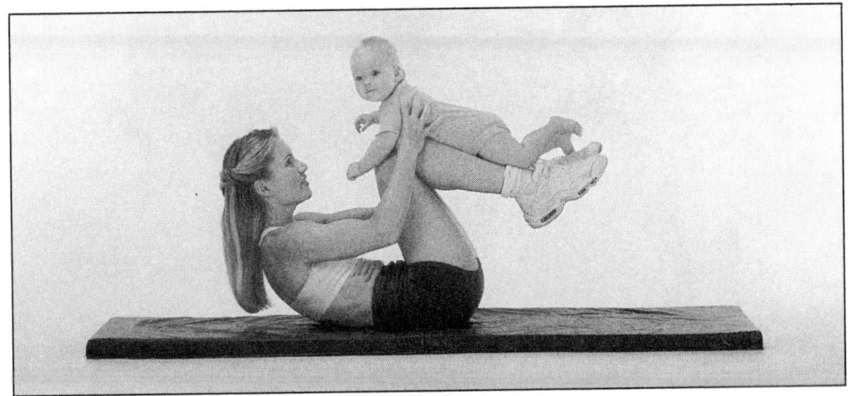

rock-a-baby

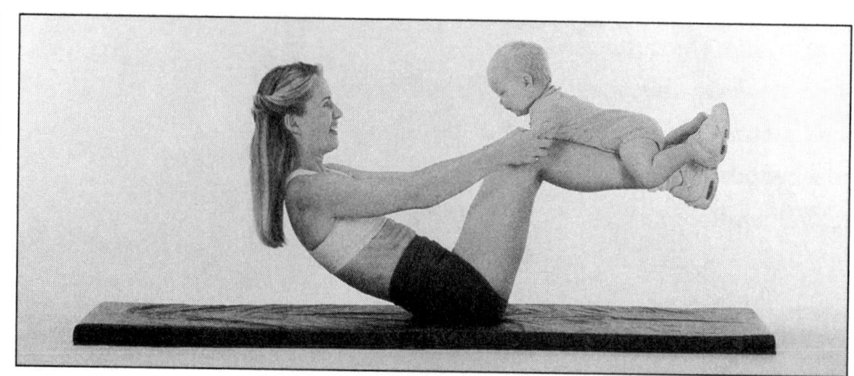

baby "v"

BABY "V"

This exercise was designed by Jane Seymour. In the same position as for rock-a-baby, extend your legs and upper body into a V-shape as well as you can. Be careful, you need strong abdominals for this.

BABY LEG EXTENSION

Sit in a chair and extend one leg straight. Place your baby on top of the extended leg and lift it a few inches ten times. Repeat with the other leg.

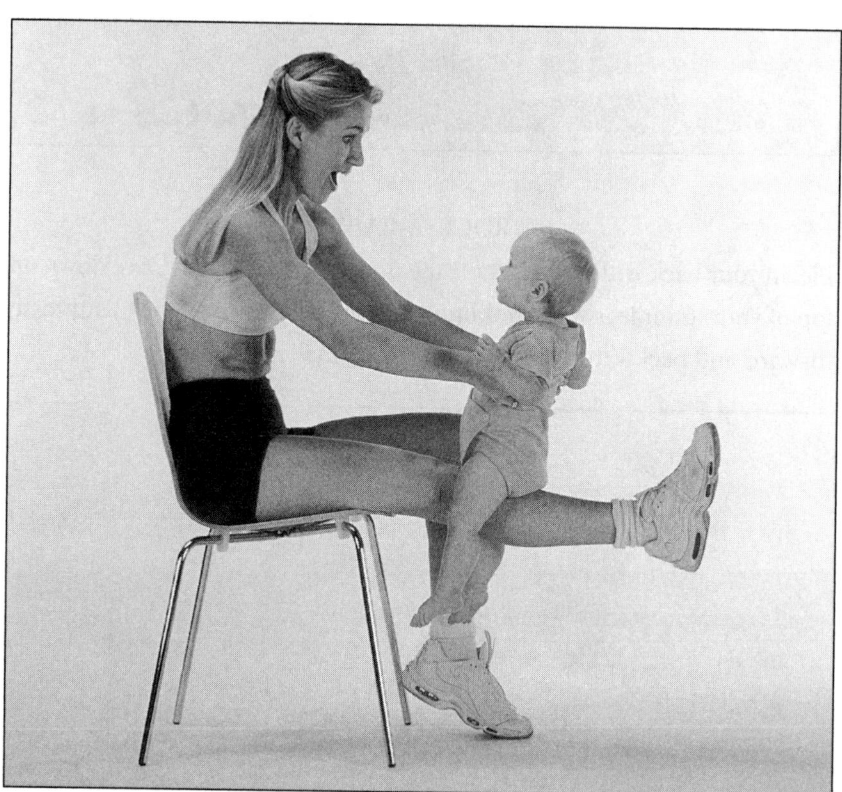

baby leg extension

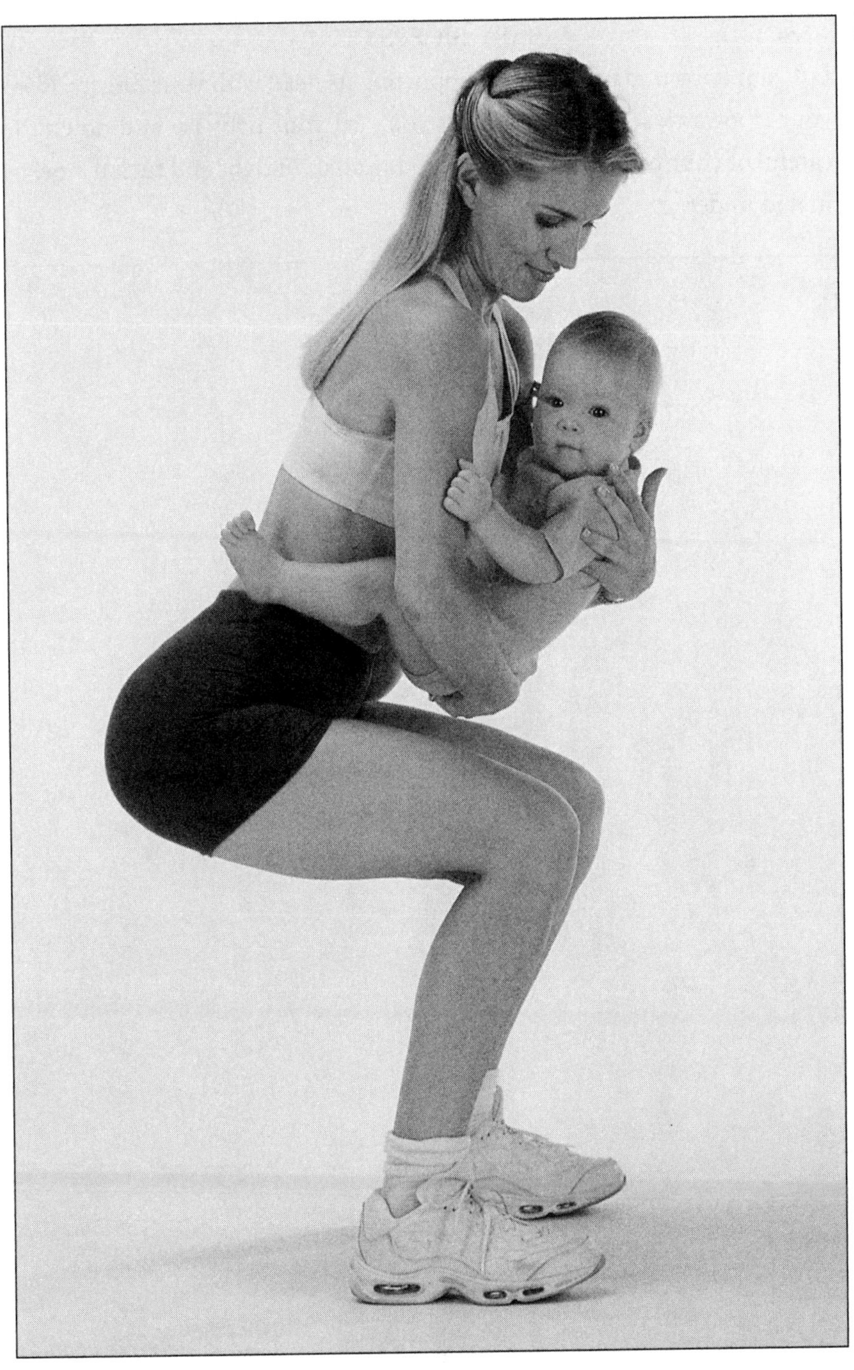

baby squats

BABY SQUATS

Hold your baby very close to you as you perform squats. Posture and form are of the utmost importance. Keep your abdominals in, your chest up, and your knees behind your toes as you squat.

BABY BICEPS CURLS

Lift your baby under the arms, supporting its head with your fingers. Keep your elbows close to your waist as you curl your baby up and down. Be careful of your posture. Keep those abdominals in tight and tuck the pelvis in and under.

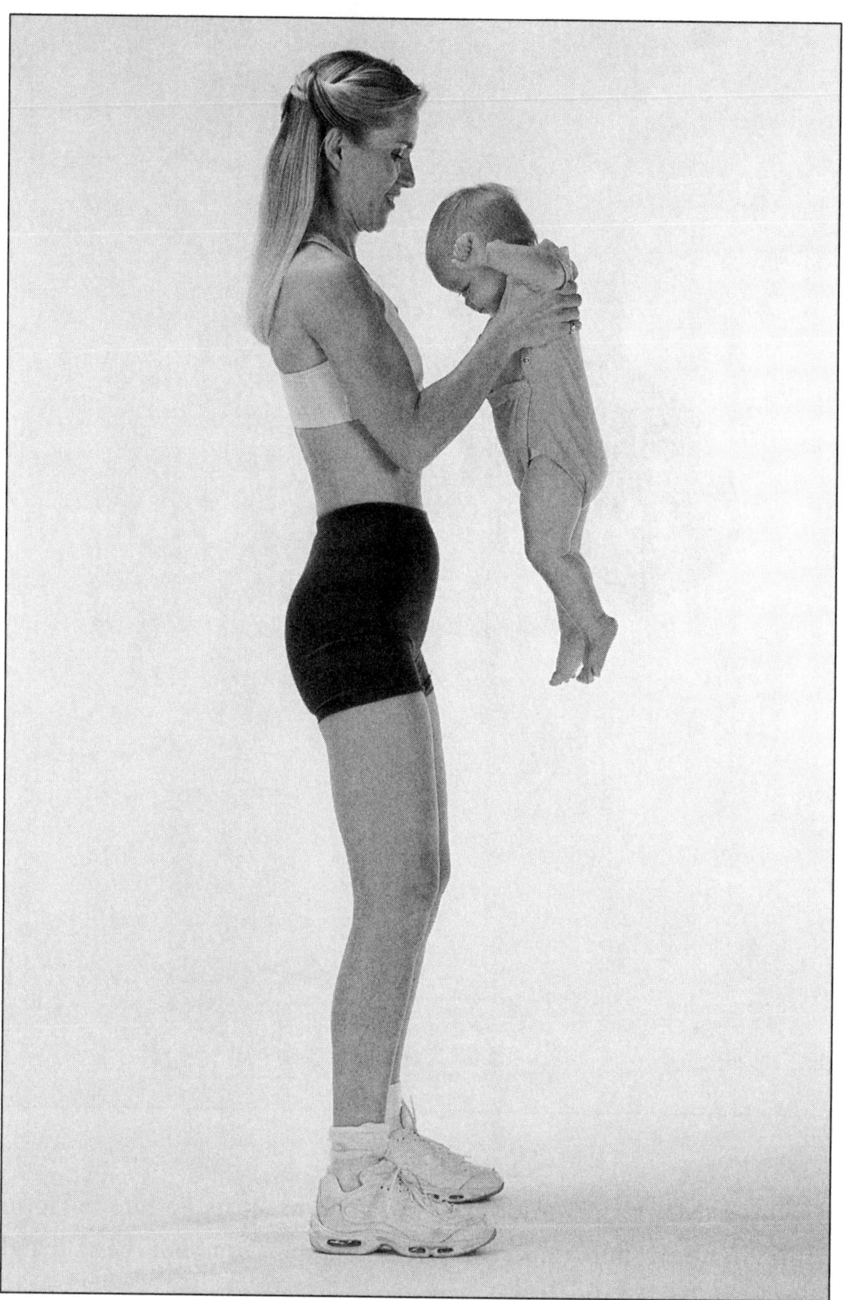

baby biceps curls

Exercising with your child will help build a stronger bond between the two of you. In addition to these exercises, you can find other ways to incorporate your child into your exercise regime. You can get a jogging stroller for walks, hikes, and jogs. If you let your child be part of your workout, you will be a great role model. Your child will grow up watching you exercise, and learn to regard it as a natural part of the day.

By letting your child participate in your workout, and perhaps later letting the child try some of the exercises without the weights, your child won't feel left out. If you happen to have a trainer who comes to your house for your workouts, your child won't hate the trainer for taking mommy away to exercise (except possibly during the terrible twos, when nothing is predictable). As a final bonus, counting every repetition out loud with your child is a great way for your child to learn how to count, even if it is only to fifteen.

After delivery, your hormones shift gears once again. This time, their priority is the feeding process.

breastfeeding versus bottle-feeding

After delivery, your hormones shift gears once again. This time, their priority is the feeding process. Hormonal changes may make you feel strange or drained because your body is still only thinking of your baby, and not of your needs. If you decide not to breastfeed, your hormones will change yet again, so don't expect to feel "normal" just yet. Readjusting takes time.

Most women yearn for the opportunity to breastfeed their child and experience the incredible bonding that is created by it. Other women would never think of it, or are not able to for various reasons. The choice is up to you. Nobody else can tell you what to do. However, an educated choice will always be the best choice, so you should know some facts.

BENEFITS OF NURSING

Breastfed children have better immune systems, less allergies and infections, straighter teeth, stronger digestive tracts, a higher rate of survival of childhood illnesses, and a lower risk of juvenile diabetes, heart disease, and SIDS (Sudden Infant Death Syndrome).

If you suffered from gestational diabetes, breastfeeding will help lower your blood sugar level back to normal in a shorter period of time than if you do not nurse. Mothers who breastfeed may have a lower risk of breast cancer as well as lower stress and blood pressure levels. According to the University of North Carolina at Chapel Hill, nursing promotes higher oxytocin levels, which helps to relieve stress.

In financial terms, there can be big savings in future medical and dental costs, not to mention current savings in food costs. Breast milk is free and conveniently available anywhere, anytime you need it. You don't have to carry it in a bag or heat it. It is conveniently stored for you at the perfect temperature "on board" so to speak.

MOTHERS WHO BREASTFEED

Ages of children	*Percentage of mothers who breast-fed their child or intend to*
0–3 months	*41%*
4–6 months	*37%*
7–9 months	*15%*
10–12 months	*5%*
13–plus	*2%*

Based on information as printed in *USA Today* (July 20, 1999) from Dr. Dennis Tootelian, Cal State University-Sacramento, for Nestle Carnation.

An ingredient found only in breast milk, called *Omega-3 long chain fatty acid* is beneficial for visual and brain development. Studies have shown a link between the consumption of breast milk and intelligence. It also reduces the risk of behavioral problems and school failure by half. The fact that more girls are breastfed than boys makes this data a bit controversial. Additionally, children raised on formula can have more nutritional and skin disorders, as well as coordination, visual, and movement problems.

Nursing is even Mother Nature's own form of birth control, as long as you breastfeed at least five times a day. Leading expert Professor R. V. Short states, "The breast has been designed by nature as the perfect push-button contraceptive. But it only works if you keep pushing the button often." Breastfeeding *alone* should not be used as your sole form of birth control after two months.

Breastfeeding also stimulates the uterus to return to its normal size and helps the body lose weight faster. The extra padding around your hips and thighs that accumulated during pregnancy is designed to be a storage bin of nutrients for your baby to draw from in the last trimester and during lactation. That's why the legs and hips shrink during nursing.

All of these beneficial effects of nursing are cumulative. The longer you breastfeed, the better off your child will be both physically and mentally. Although it may sound like a lot, the optimal nursing period now recommended by experts is a year. It takes at least four months of breastfeeding to prevent certain immunological problems, including allergies.

The longer you breastfeed, the better off your child will be both physically and mentally.

BOTTLE-FEEDING

Some women opt not to breastfeed due to personal preference or convenience factors. Others cannot breastfeed for medical reasons. For example, if you suffer from severe non-correctable retracted nipples, or are taking drugs such as antidepressants, antiseizure medication, or estrogen, you should not breastfeed.

If you bottle-feed you must either use your own pumped breast milk or commercial baby formula. Absolutely do not use cow's milk until your child is six months or older. It contains levels of protein and minerals that are too high for infants, and could have a detrimental effect on the child's growth.

With the cost of bottles, formula, and other supplies, bottle-feeding can be quite expensive. However, it can provide you with a well-deserved break, because you can let someone else handle the feeding now and then. Even mothers who breastfeed should pump their breast milk occasionally and allow Dad or others the opportunity to have this bonding experience with the baby.

postpartum nutrition for nursing mothers

If you are nursing your child, your nutritional habits are just as important postpartum as they were during the pregnancy. The guidelines for eating are more or less the same as described in chapter 8.

There are a few differences to keep in mind, however. Your baby is now much bigger than he or she was inside of you. You now need to consume even more food to be able to breastfeed your infant. You should consume at least 500 extra calories a day on top of your regular intake, compared with the extra 300 calories (minimum) per day you consumed during pregnancy. If you are breastfeeding twins, you need 500 extra calories daily *per child.* These recommendations are for non-active women. If you are working out, you need 700 to 1,000 more calories a day per child.

RDAs for Nursing Women

vitamin A—6,000 IU
vitamin C—100 mg
thiamin (B1)—1.6 mg
riboflavin (B2)—1.7 mg
niacin (B3)—18 mg
calcium—1,500 mg
zinc—25 mg
iodine—200 mg

You need to consume several nutrients in higher quantities postpartum. Compare the following postnatal Recommended Daily Allowances to the prenatal amounts in chapter 9. They are only slightly higher, so if you cannot find special postnatal vitamin supplements, take your prenatal multivitamins but increase the dosage by 25 to 50 percent. Speak to your doctor first.

Do not attempt to restrict your caloric intake if you are nursing. Your baby needs the nutrients to grow and does not need the ketones produced by your body burning up vital fuel for energy. Like everything else, the ketones will flow out into your milk. (See page 73 for more information on ketosis.) Do not worry excessively about trying to lose weight. Nursing itself will help you lose weight, in spite of the additional calories you are consuming. And if you are following a regular exercise program, you will regain your shape sooner than you think.

BREAST MILK COMPOSITION

A mother's milk is the perfect nutritionally balanced food for her baby; assuming the mother eats a healthy extra 500 calories a day, and doesn't partake of any cigarettes, alcohol, caffeine, or drugs. What goes into your body will come out in your breast milk. This makes it extremely important to abstain from the same substances that you avoided during pregnancy.

Your breast milk is what you eat. Your child is growing and if you breastfeed, every nutrient it needs is still being supplied by you. These nutrients do not just come about naturally. If you do not eat correctly, your nutrient stores will be depleted. Your milk will be only as good and healthy as you make it. In other words, if you don't eat your veggies, neither does your baby.

A recent study in the *Journal of the American Dietetic Association* found that if a nursing mom eats garlic, her child may get gas. If she eats broccoli, her child may get colicky. Eating chocolate may cause her baby to cry excessively, while drinking milk can increase the child's irritability. If you consume milk and other dairy foods while nursing, you will increase the chances of your child getting ear aches and inflammations. The fact that cow's milk should never be given directly to an infant younger than six months of age should tell you something. Don't give it to your child indirectly, either.

Like most breast milk in the animal kingdom, human milk composition changes during the feeding process. The foremilk (colostrum), which the baby will suck rapidly, is thin and watery and consists mostly of protein and carbohydrates. Toward the end of the feeding, the milk gets thicker as the fat content quadruples. This change in composition seems to act as an appetite control or trigger for the baby to stop sucking. Because a child's fat cells are still multiplying throughout the first year and a half, this mechanism prevents excessive fat cell division and acts to prevent obesity later in life. The more fat cells a child develops by eighteen months of age, the chubbier that child may become.

Many mothers try to make their baby finish the whole bottle, but doing so will only overfeed the baby.

Formula, even though nutritionally well balanced these days, has the same consistency of proteins, carbohydrates, and fats throughout, with no indication for the baby to stop sucking. (Pumped breast milk also has the same fat content throughout, because it has been all mixed up in a bottle. It will not give your child a trigger point to quit drinking either, but pumped breast milk is still a better alternative to formula.) Many mothers try to make their baby finish the whole bottle, but doing so will only overfeed the baby. By overstimulating the division of fat cells, the mother could possibly create a weight problem for the child later. A baby doesn't necessarily have to be chubby to be healthy.

Lower your fat intake to prevent a future weight problem for your child. Fat, sugar, and bottle-feeding stimulates fat cell division. A person's total number of fat cells is what determines how much that person can eat before gaining weight. Most thin people do not have very many fat cells. If someone has an abundance of fat cells, even eating small meals may cause that person to put on pounds. Your destiny was determined during your mother's pregnancy and in the first year of your life by how you were fed. Not coincidentally, obesity was never a common problem before formula-feeding became popular in the 1940s.

Some women fear that exercise will dry out their milk supply. This fear is unfounded. However, you do need to drink lots of water to replenish your fluids. Your breast milk may taste a little different or even sour to your child right after you work out. If your child doesn't like it, either breastfeed before exercise or wait a half hour afterward. The best way to know if your baby is getting enough milk is her growth and behavior. A baby who isn't getting enough milk will be very cranky.

postpartum problems and discomfort

You may feel terrific postpartum, or just completely fatigued. Every day may be different. Some women take longer to adjust to motherhood and not being pregnant. Try to be patient with yourself. If possible, find time to treat yourself to a massage, bubble bath, nap, or five-minute meditation period to just relax and be alone. Don't start working out until you're ready for it, but do not use that as an excuse to procrastinate. The endorphins produced by exercise will make you feel more energetic.

POSTPARTUM DEPRESSION

Most women experience some form of postpartum blues—a temporary feeling of sadness or anxiety following the birth of a child. It is quite common for this feeling to last from two to ten days. However, if your symptoms last longer or are severe, you may be suffering from postpartum depression. If this is the case, be sure to consult with your doctor. Postpartum blues may be caused by a combination of factors, including hormonal changes, the stress of delivery, lack of sleep, anxiety about motherhood, and changing body image.

Being able to spend time with your newborn may help prevent the blues. Vitamin B1 is known to minimize depression. But exercise is your best option to eliminate this specter.

BREAST INFECTION

An infection may leave you with extreme breast tenderness and redness on the nipples, or on the surrounding breast and tissue. You may also experience a fever and flu symptoms. If you experience these symptoms, don't exercise until you have checked with your doctor and feel completely recovered. Warm compresses may alleviate the symptoms, but antibiotics are usually needed to treat the infection.

EPISIOTOMY

Kegels will also speed up the healing process of an episiotomy if you had one. Sitz baths can help reduce swelling. The scar may become itchy. Proper hygiene will help with the healing process. Keep the area clean and avoid wearing polyester and nylon fabrics during this period. Do not ride a bicycle for at least six weeks following an episiotomy.

INCONTINENCE

If you did your Kegels, you will most likely not experience any loss of bladder control, but there are always exceptions. If you do have a bout of incontinence, to ensure that it is only temporary, work those pelvic floor muscles as much as you can. Remember it's never too late to start anything.

Exercising before and during a pregnancy will reduce the amount of stretch marks that you get.

STRETCH MARKS

The amount and severity of stretch marks that you may experience is partly due to genetic factors, partly a function of maintaining your weight, and partly skin tone achieved from good nutritional habits and regular exercise; regularly moisturizing your skin with a good lotion may diminish them. Exercising before and during a pregnancy will reduce the amount of stretch marks that you get. Some women swear by the old practice of using vitamin E cream, coconut oil, or olive oil to rub, grab, and massage the skin around their bellies and hips to prevent stretch marks. In this method, the skin is lifted or grabbed off the belly and massaged methodically without actually massaging the belly itself during pregnancy.

If your mother had lots of stretch marks, chances are you will get some too, no matter how much you work out or massage your skin. Getting rid of them is almost impossible. No vitamin E oil or cream is going to make them vanish. However, there are some products that can reduce their visibility. Please note that these products can be dangerous to use during pregnancy or while nursing.

Retin-A cream, if applied every day for at least two months, can reduce stretch marks. This works best on brand new stretch marks that may still be pink. Retin-A may sting a little when first applied, and it should not be used during pregnancy or while still nursing. It could severely harm your child. Wait until after the nursing period.

Tretinoin, a topical cream, can also treat new stretch marks. According to research by the University of Michigan, the cream works if applied over a period of six months. However, this is also a vitamin A derivative, and it is not recommended for pregnant or nursing women.

Pulsed dye laser treatments in very low levels can reduce stretch marks in some women. This is a new treatment used by a few dermatologists and plastic surgeons. It is expensive ($300–$400) and usually requires more than one treatment. Ask your doctor about its safety postpartum.

ENGORGED BREASTS

Until you stop breastfeeding, your breasts will be large and swollen, which, depending on your individual experience, may feel great, uncomfortable, or even painful. Make sure to wear a good, supportive bra, especially when you exercise. Wear jog bras in cotton or Supplex with no seam crossing the nipples. For extra support, wear two of them. If that's not enough, an ace bandage between the two bras can provide maximum support.

Avoid any exercises that require you to lie prone (face down). Exercise machines with a support pad in front of the chest may bother your breasts. But do not postpone your entire exercise program because your breasts are uncomfortable. You should do extra exercises for the upper back to prevent your back from getting too tired and your chest from drooping.

CRACKED OR SORE NIPPLES

If your nipples are reacting badly to postpartum life, expose them to air as much as you can, and protect them from your clothes by wearing breast shells inside your bra. Avoid using lotions such as Vaseline on them, except for pure vitamin E oil. Do not use any soap in the shower, only water.

Cracked or inflamed nipples may be prevented or minimized if you prepare them in advance. "Preparing nipples" is a way of roughening them up to condition them for the baby's sucking. If your breasts are sensitive or tender but you still want to breastfeed your baby, you should start preparing your nipples halfway into your pregnancy. Techniques for preparing them include massaging, squeezing, retracting and drawing them out, and rubbing a wet towel against them. Also, avoid wearing a bra at times to let your nipples rub against the fabric of your clothes. However, be careful not to overstimulate your nipples because this could bring on uterine contractions.

EXCESSIVE PERSPIRATION

You may feel very hot and sweat a lot. This is because your body is working hard to make milk for the baby. Drink a lot of water to prevent dehydration.

Chapter Eleven

baby and mother—the fit pregnancy

Now you know all the facts about the physical effects of pregnancy and the exercises that will prepare you and keep you in good shape. It is up to you to do the hard work of designing and carrying out your program to benefit you and your baby.

Every woman is different, with different needs and different circumstances. Regardless of your level of fitness or special considerations, there is always some form of exercise you can do. To use an extreme example, even if you are stuck on bed-rest, hooked up to monitors, with two broken legs, you can still stretch your lower back and contract your pelvic floor, abdominals, and upper back. If there's a will, there's a way! Usually, the more fit you are before conceiving, the more exercise you can do during and after pregnancy. The more a woman is able to do, the more she and her baby will benefit. An individualized exercise program is the base, and moderation is always the key.

The benefits of exercise and proper nutrition during pregnancy are numerous. To recap some of these benefits: a woman who stays fit and healthy while pregnant can expect to have a lower resting heart rate and training heart rate, a higher oxygen intake, greater calcium absorption, and a larger

IN THIS CHAPTER

- *Inspirational real-life stories from exercising moms*
- *How Jane Seymour regained her fabulous figure in record time*
- *Parting words of advice*

Ideally, you should embark on an exercise and nutrition program at least one month before conceiving.

volume of blood pumped with every heartbeat. She will have more energy and strength, better self-esteem and image, and better posture. She will have fewer pregnancy discomforts, a lower risk of gestational diabetes and osteoporosis, fewer stretch marks, and a shorter labor with fewer complications. Postpartum, she will get back in shape faster, have more strength and energy, and have a lower risk of future incontinence. She is also less likely to experience the "baby blues." Finally, she may find that exercise is her only sanity through it all.

If you have a good program and work out regularly throughout your pregnancy (including weight-bearing exercise), your baby should have higher Apgar scores, lower body-fat levels, and a lower risk of growth retardation. In addition, your baby should grow up leaner, have fewer health problems, and be calmer and more intelligent than children born of "unfit" pregnancies.

Women who exercise regularly also tend to get pregnant more easily. Ideally, you should embark on an exercise and nutrition program at least one month before conceiving. However, it is never too late, or too early, to begin.

real-life scenarios

The following are examples of women from different backgrounds and lifestyles, who had very different health and fitness levels. Not all of them had ideal pregnancies. I have included a variety of scenarios, including some who encountered and overcame problems along the way (problems usually not related to exercise). They shared one thing in common, though—and because you were motivated to read this book, I assume you share it too—the desire to give their babies the best possible start.

RENEE GREIF

Renee, thirty-five and a mother of two, asked me to help her develop a fitness plan before conceiving her third child. At first, she was a bit apprehensive about becoming pregnant for the third time. Throughout her other two pregnancies, she had felt weak and had suffered badly from morning sickness.

Her fitness level was quite low when we started, but her background in gymnastics helped her regain strength and fitness quickly. After eight months of working out, her cardiovascular fitness level had gone from 20 to 77 percent of her maximum potential. It was at this point that she conceived.

We modified her workout monthly as her pregnancy progressed. Toward the end of her very healthy pregnancy, she was walking, doing step-training, occasional pool aerobics, weight training, childbirth preparation exercises, abdominal and lower back exercises, Kegels, and general stretching. The result of all this work was a very healthy eight-pound, eleven-ounce baby boy delivered at term.

This pregnancy gave Renee very little grief. She felt energetic, strong, and fit. The few symptoms she did experience during pregnancy—light morning sickness, some sciatic pain, and varicose veins—all disappeared postpartum.

Postpartum, she was full of energy and ready to work out after three weeks, instead of feeling weak and lethargic as she did after her earlier pregnancies. She also found that her little boy seemed much happier, more content, and calmer than her other two children did at the same age.

CORNELIA DALY, M.D.

Cornelia is a mother of four. She is the OB/GYN partner of Sheryl Ross, M.D., my very devoted medical consultant on this book. At age forty-three, Cornelia has been exercising religiously for more than twenty years. Her usual daily workout consists of thirty minutes of running, stair climbing, or swimming.

She continued exercising all the way through her four pregnancies. Each time, she modified her program by toning down the intensity, not the duration, of each activity. Also, she discontinued running after the twentieth week of her pregnancy. She is convinced that exercise is the reason she felt so good throughout all of her pregnancies.

Her age made her last pregnancy "high-risk." However, the only discomfort she felt was fatigue, which she believes would have been nonexistent if she did not have to work and care for three toddlers at the same time. This very petite woman delivered her fourth healthy baby—a seven-pound, five-ounce boy—at term.

Cornelia resumed a modified exercise routine two weeks after delivery, and was back up to her regular intensity after three months. She regained her normal weight and shape after eight months.

SUZANNE NOTTINGHAM

Suzanne is a mother of two. She teaches skiing, in-line skating, and step aerobics. She is a contributing editor to *Skiing* magazine and a fitness presenter for fitness organizations. She has been featured in advertisements for Power Bar, and is sponsored by the Roller Blade company. Needless to say, she is incredibly fit. Her workout, depending on the season, can consist of in-line skating, roller hockey, downhill skiing, walking, strength training, step aerobics, mountain biking, hiking, or snow shoeing.

Suzanne's second pregnancy was very healthy despite the fact that she is older than thirty-five and lives at the high altitude of 9,000 feet. She modified her exercise by discontinuing hockey and what she calls "hard-core" exercise. She decreased the intensity of her other activities, but increased their duration. Suzanne is such a pro on skates that she feels as comfortable skating as she does walking. She kept up a modified skating routine for seven and a half months of her pregnancy—literally skating her way through pregnancy! This is not recommended for anyone not as well trained as Suzanne.

Suzanne's labor was a very easy three hours, despite the fact that her baby was in the breech position and three weeks early (very common at high altitudes). She did not require an epidural. She felt fine after only three days postpartum, which is way beyond the norm, and resumed her regular exercise program after only a week. Suzanne attributes her easy labor and ultra-quick recovery in part to her workout program and in part to the luck of her genes.

SUSAN DODSON

Susan, a colleague of mine, is a mother of four (three biological, one adopted), who is very much in tune with her body. She exercised through her first pregnancy, and found that her son is much calmer and more relaxed compared to his friends whose mothers did not exercise during pregnancy. At age thirty-eight, pregnant with twins, she was able to continue her work as an aerobics instructor. She did, of course, modify her workouts. She taught two, rather than her usual five low-impact step classes a week, worked out with weights, and walked several times a week.

Unfortunately, like many fitness instructors, Susan thought she was indestructible. Twenty-one weeks into her pregnancy, she attended a fitness convention and participated in a slide aerobics class she had never taken before. After fifteen minutes she noticed some pubic pressure and quit. Three days later, she went into premature labor and was hospitalized for a week. She spent the rest of her pregnancy home on bed-rest.

Knowing how fast muscles atrophy when inactive, she was determined to keep her muscles toned even while stuck in bed. In addition to Kegels, she did various upper body and leg exercises using small hand weights, ankle weights, and rubber bands. She also did isometric contractions while lying or seated in bed, similar to the exercises for high-risk pregnancies described in this book.

Her labor took eighteen hours, but was fairly easy. She delivered two healthy baby girls. She lost twenty-five of her thirty-five pregnancy pounds in three days, and was back to normal weight within three weeks. However, she still waited six weeks before resuming regular workouts and eight weeks before going back to teaching. Over a year, she gradually built back up to teaching eight classes a week.

She attributes her ability to care for (and keep up with) her new twin girls to the modified workout she did while on bed-rest. Without it, she does not believe that she would have had the strength or energy to keep up after being bedridden for four months. Of course, the point of this story is that even someone as fit as an aerobics instructor should not attempt a new activity during pregnancy.

DIANE TERESI-WENSON

At thirty-six years of age, Diane was a borderline high-risk pregnancy. However, she was well prepared for any complications her body might throw her way. Diane was the 1993 and 1994 National Aerobics Pairs Champion. She became pregnant while she and her husband were at the end of a grueling national tour showing aerobic routines.

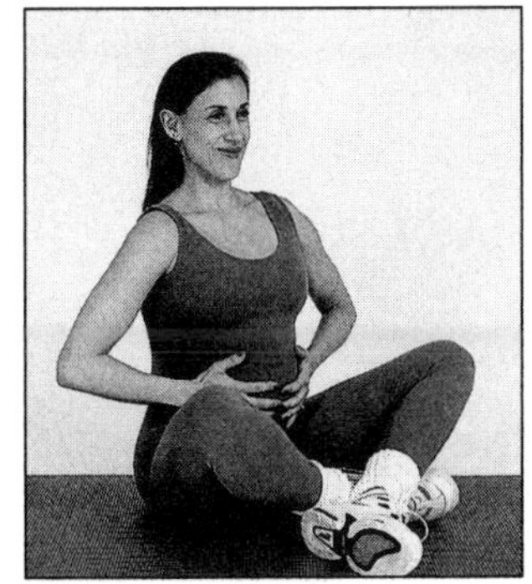

Diane Teresi-Wenson

When not touring, Diane teaches fitness classes. Her regular weekly schedule includes three hours of weight training and six step and slide classes. Throughout her pregnancy she continued her regular routine, but modified her workouts by lowering her step height. During her classes, when she felt the need to slow down, she would walk around the slide and describe the exercises to her class rather than demonstrate them. Otherwise, Diane taught and worked out until the day of her delivery.

I couldn't have designed a better fitness program for Terri than she did for herself. And she designed it by listening to her own body.

Her pregnancy was one we all wish to have. She felt very comfortable and fit throughout the entire nine months, without experiencing a single discomfort—no pain, cramps, backaches, fluid retention . . . nothing. She did miss being able to do full splits with her head touching the floor because her belly was in the way. Her labor was at term, but quite long and painful because her baby wanted to come out sideways. Little Frankie Lee eventually straightened out and is now a very alert and busy little girl.

Diane gradually got back into her routine two weeks later. After only four to six months postpartum, she felt better than ever. By then, her weight was seven pounds less than before her pregnancy, and her body fat was also lower. This is not something that most women should strive for, but it shows what our bodies can do.

TERRI BURSTEN

Terri is a mother of three boys. Her last pregnancy was at age thirty-three, during a very fit stage in her life. She deliberately prepared herself for this pregnancy by exercising four to five days a week prior to conceiving. Her workout consisted of high-impact aerobics classes, running, and weight training—all twice a week.

Terri reduced the speed and intensity of her exercises over the course of her pregnancy. She also lowered all the weights in her workout, especially those of the inner and outer thigh machine and the lat pulldown. Though she was accustomed to using these machines, they put too much strain on her joints. She quit all abdominal work halfway through her pregnancy, but did pelvic tilts on all fours instead because "it felt natural." She was quite surprised when she found out that pelvic tilts work the abdominals.

Except for the brief incidence of a small vessel blot clot, Terri went through pregnancy fairly easily. She had a much easier labor than with her two previous "less fit" pregnancies. Her little boy was perfectly healthy and weighed in at seven pounds.

Terri resumed her workout schedule with the bike and stair machine two weeks after delivery. At six weeks postpartum, she started to run and work out with weights again. She felt normal within six months. I couldn't have designed a better fitness program for Terri than she did for herself. And she designed it by listening to her own body.

JANE SEYMOUR

Jane Seymour does not really need an introduction. An actress, artist, wife, and mother of four children and two stepchildren, she is busy beyond belief. With ten- to fourteen-hour working days on the set of *Dr. Quinn, Medicine Woman*, being pregnant with twins at age forty-four was not an easy task. These factors also placed Jane in a high-risk category. Exercise became a necessity for Jane, who wanted to stay strong, energetic, healthy, and happy.

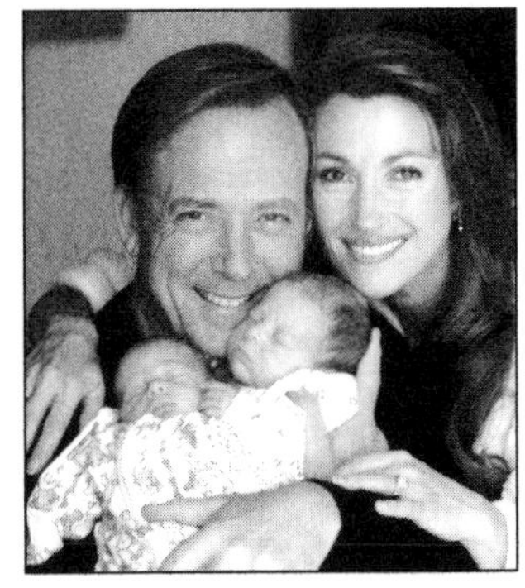

Jane Seymour, her husband, and their twins

Her pre- and postnatal workout program, which was medically supervised, consisted of daily walks on the set in between takes, seated abdominal contractions, and pelvic tilts. She also did Kegels while rehearsing her lines. She worked out three days a week, alternating between the gym and the pool.

Jane's major concern was her posture and gait. She also wanted to make sure that she would eventually get her slim waistline back. To prevent the late pregnancy waddle, I had her do a lot of abductor (outer thigh) exercises. To keep the abdominals elastic and prevent diastasis recti, she also did a lot of abdominal exercises.

Carrying twins meant that there was even more weight pulling Jane's shoulders forward. We counteracted this with upper back strengthening and lower back stretching. In the pool, we did water aerobics to music, and used all kinds of pool toys, such as webbed gloves and floaties, to add resistance. This helped to simulate those exercises that she did in the gym.

Throughout Jane's pregnancy, her workout had to be modified to suit her changing body and condition. This was true especially toward the end, when she was placed on partial bed-rest due to her high-risk factors. Her entire workout had to be performed in bed. I designed a special program for her, including resistance exercises using Dyna-Bands and ankle weights. She worked out until the day before her delivery. Jane had two bouncing baby boys, John and Kristopher, six weeks early through a C-section.

Three days after her delivery, she started doing Kegels, abdominal contractions, and pelvic tilts again. Her first real workout, two weeks postpartum, was easy for Jane. With a Golden Globe Award nomination (for *Dr. Quinn*), she wanted to look her best for the awards show—which was only five weeks away.

We concentrated mainly on abs, abs, and more abs, with some glutes and upper body exercises thrown in as well. We knew what dress Jane was going to wear, and we made sure that she would look fabulous in it. The hard work paid off when she won the award. People couldn't stop talking about how quickly she had regained her incredible figure.

After the awards, her goal shifted to getting strong again and being able to keep her energy level up. Postpartum, her upper back was very tired and sore from nursing, and needed quite a bit of work. (I am very pleased that Jane decided to nurse, which she continued for six months despite a grueling work schedule and very little privacy.)

Between nursing twins, rearing four other children, and becoming the toast of the town—doing interviews, commercials, promos, photo shoots, and more—exercise became the only time she had to herself. Hopefully, most of you can take things at a slower pace.

Jane is currently writing a book about twin pregnancy.

fit, trim, and healthy—for the rest of your life

As you see, it can take up to a year to feel normal again after a pregnancy. When you do get your old body back, do not change the wonderfully healthy lifestyle that you created for yourself during pregnancy. Contrary to what most people say, exercising and eating healthy has nothing to do with discipline and everything to do with priorities.

The tips described in this book can be followed for the rest of your life. A commitment to exercise and a well-balanced nutritional intake as a lifestyle, rather than as a temporary program, will reward you in the long term—by reducing your risk of heart disease, cancer, and other illnesses. It will add years to your life and life to your years.

You will also be providing a wonderful example for your children. They will learn to participate in an active, healthy lifestyle, gaining untold benefits to the quality of their lives and longevity. Now that you have the tools, it is up to you. Just do not forget those valuable Kegels. For the rest of your life—squeeze, squeeze, and squeeze. . . .

glossary

aerobic Exercise, such as walking, performed "with oxygen."

air embolism Abnormal presence of an air bubble in the bloodstream, obstructing bloodflow.

alignment Proper postural positioning.

amenorrhea Unusual absence of a period.

amino acid Organic compounds containing the building blocks of protein.

anaerobic Exercise, such as sprinting or weight lifting, that does not require the body to transport oxygen to the cells.

anemia Insufficient iron level—results in paleness, weakness, and other symptoms.

anorexia nervosa Eating disorder characterized by an obsession with weight loss, distorted body image, fear of obesity, and excessive exercise.

antagonist Muscle working in opposition to another.

Apgar score Measurements of activity, pulse, grimace, appearance, and respiration taken at one and five minutes after birth to assess a newborn's well-being.

artery Blood vessels supplying the body with blood from the heart.

biomechanics The mechanics of muscular function.

blood pressure The force with which the heart pumps blood through the body.

bradycardia Abnormally slow heart rate.

Braxton Hicks contraction Irregular tightening of the uterus during pregnancy. Also called "false labor."

breech position Presentation of the baby's buttocks or feet first at delivery.

cardiovascular Relating to the heart and blood vessels.

diastasis recti A separation of the abdominal muscles along the midline.

dynamic stretches Long, smooth stretching movements, gradually increasing in reach.

edema Swelling caused by water retention.

endorphin Hormone that stimulates alertness and reduces perception (feeling) of pain, including pregnancy discomforts and labor pain.

episiotomy An incision made to enlarge the vaginal opening during delivery.

estrogen A female hormone that stimulates growth and lining of the uterus.

fetal alcohol syndrome A disorder resulting from alcohol consumption by the mother during pregnancy. Complications can include brain damage, physical abnormalities, mental retardation, and miscarriage.

gestational diabetes Pregnancy-induced condition that occurs in about 3 percent of women. Onset is most likely after the twenty-fourth week of pregnancy.

hCG Human Chorionic Gonadotropin is a hormone produced by the placenta that stimulates the ovaries to produce estrogen and progesterone.

hyperglycemia High blood sugar level (diabetes).

hypertension High blood pressure.

hypoglycemia Low blood sugar level.

hypotension Inadequate (low) blood pressure, possibly from diminished blood supply.

incompetent cervix A weakened cervix that may be incapable of holding the fetus within the uterus for the full nine months.

incontinence Inability to control urination or defecation.

interval training Exercising with alternate periods of high and low intensity.

inverted position Positions in which the body is upside down or the head is below the level of the heart.

isometric contraction Holding a muscle contraction in a fixed position for a period of time.

Kegel exercise Contraction and release of the pelvic floor muscles.

levator ani The pelvic floor muscles. (Literally, "elevate the anus.")

linea alba The midline of the abdominal muscles.

linea negra The discoloration of the linea alba (dark brown) during pregnancy.

macrosomia An abnormally large fetus.

neurological Relating to the nervous system.

osteoporosis A disorder characterized by bone deterioration; found mostly in menopausal women.

pelvic organ prolapse Condition in which an organ, such as the uterus, slips from its usual position and protrudes through the vagina.

perineum The area between the vagina and anus.

placenta abruption Condition in which the placenta has broken away from the inner wall of the uterus.

placenta previa Condition in which the placenta covers the cervix.

plyometrics Movements that require both feet to be lifted off the ground simultaneously.

preeclampsia A condition in pregnancy characterized by abnormally high blood pressure, edema, and abnormal kidney function.

pregnancy-induced A condition, such as diabetes, brought about by a pregnancy.

progesterone A female hormone that maintains the pregnancy.

prone position Lying on the stomach.

pulmonary Relating to the lungs.

relaxin A hormone produced during pregnancy that softens the joints and ligaments.

retraction Contraction of back muscles.

sciatic nerve The primary nerve of the leg, the sciatic nerve originates in the lower back and extends down the muscles of the buttocks, thighs, legs, and feet.

static stretches Stretches that are held in a fixed position. Compare to dynamic stretches.

supine position Lying on the back.

tachycardia Abnormally rapid heart beat.

vena cava The major vein that returns blood to the heart from the lower body.

weight-bearing activity Activity in which the exerciser supports her own body weight (as in jogging) or adds weight to increase resistance. Swimming is an example of nonweight-bearing exercise.

bibliography

BOOKS

Artal, Raul, and Genell J. Subak-Sharpe. *Pregnancy & Exercise.* New York: Bantam Doubleday Dell, 1992.

Artal-Mittelmark, Raul, R. Wiswell, and B. Drinkwater. *Exercise in Pregnancy.* Baltimore: Williams & Wilkins, 1991.

Clapp III, James F. *Exercising Through Your Pregnancy.* Champaign, IL: Human Kinetics, 1998.

Creasy, Robert K. and Robert Resnik. *Maternal-Fetal Medicine: Principles and Practice.* 3rd edition. Philadelphia: W. B. Saunders Co., 1989.

Dale, Barbara, and Johanna Roeber. *The Pregnancy Exercise Book.* New York: Pantheon Books, 1993.

Dowling, A. *Basic Manual for Perinatal Health and Fitness Instructors.* Stony Creek, CT: Dancing Thru Pregnancy, Inc., 1994.

Dunne, L. J. *Nutrition Almanac.* 3rd edition. New York: McGraw-Hill, 1990.

Eisenberg, Arlene, Heidi E. Murkoff, and Sandee E. Hathaway. *What to Expect When You're Expecting.* 2nd edition. New York: Workman Publishing, 1991.

———. *What to Eat When You're Expecting.* New York: Workman Publishing, 1986.

Gabbe, Steven G., Jennifer R. Niebyl, and Joe Leigh Simpson. *Obstetrics: Normal & Problem Pregnancies.* Philadelphia: Churchill Livingstone, 1986.

Geelhoed, Glenn W., Robert D. Willix, and J. Barilla. *Natural Health Secrets from Around the World.* Boca Raton, FL: Shot Tower Books, 1994.

Hanlon, Thomas W., ed. *Fit for Two: The Official YMCA Prenatal Exercise Guide.* Champaign, IL: Human Kinetics, 1995.

Herbst, Arthur L., Daniel R. Mishell, Morton A. Stenchever, William Droegemuller. *Comprehensive Gynecology.* 2nd edition. St. Louis: Mosby-Year Book, 1992.

Holstein, Barbara B. *Shaping Up for a Healthy Pregnancy: Instructor Guide.* Champaign, IL: Human Kinetics, 1988.

Marshall, Connie. *From Here to Maternity.* Scottsdale, AZ: Conmar Publishing, 1994.

Noble, Elizabeth. *Essential Exercises for the Childbearing Year.* 3rd edition. Boston: Houghton Mifflin, 1988.

Powter, Susan. *Food.* New York: Simon & Schuster, 1995.

Stewart, Deborah D. *Baby & Me: The Essential Guide to Pregnancy.* Lake Forest Park, WA: The Willapa Bay Company, 1993.

Whitney, Hamilton. *Understanding Nutrition.* 4th edition. St. Paul: West Publishing, 1987.

MEDICAL STUDIES AND JOURNALS

American College of Obstetricians and Gynecologists (ACOG). "Early Pregnancy Loss." *ACOG Technical Bulletin* 212, September 1995.

———. "Exercise During Pregnancy and the Postpartum Period." *ACOG Technical Bulletin* 189, February 1994.

———. "Pelvic Organ Prolapse." *ACOG Technical Bulletin* 214, October 1995.

———. "Preconceptional Care." *ACOG Technical Bulletin* 205, May 1995.

———. "Preterm Labor." *ACOG Technical Bulletin* 206, June 1995.

———. "Substance Abuse." *ACOG Technical Bulletin* 194, July 1994.

———. "Substance Abuse in Pregnancy." *ACOG Technical Bulletin* 195, July 1994.

———. "Urinary Incontinence." *ACOG Technical Bulletin* 213, October 1995.

———. "Women and Exercise." *ACOG Technical Bulletin* 173, October 1992.

Artal, R. "Exercise and Pregnancy." *Clinics in Sports Medicine,* vol. 11 (1992): 363–76.

Artal, R., and P. J. Buckenmeyer. "Exercise During Pregnancy and Postpartum." *Contemporary OB/GYN,* vol. 40 (1995): 62–90.

Artal, R., N. Khodiguian, and R. H. Paul. "Intrapartum Fetal Heart Rate Responses to Maternal Exercise," vol. 22 (1993): 499–502.

Artal, R., V. Fortuanto, and A. Welton. "A Comparison of Cardiopulmonary Adaptations to Exercise in Pregnancy at Sea Level and Altitude." *American Journal of Obstetrics and Gynecology,* vol. 172 (April 1995): 1170–78.

Bonen, A., and P. D. Campagna. "Substrate and Hormonal Responses during Exercise Classes at Selected Stages of Pregnancy." *Canadian Journal of Applied Physiology,* vol. 20 (1995): 440–51.

Clapp III, J. F. "A Clinical Approach to Exercise During Pregnancy." *Clinics in Sports Medicine,* vol. 13 (1994): 443–57.

———. "Exercise and Fetal Health." *Journal of Developmental Physiology,* vol. 15 (1991): 9–14.

———. "Exercise in Pregnancy: Good, Bad, or Indifferent?" *Current Obstetric Medicine,* vol. 2 (1993): 25–49.

———. "The Changing Thermal Response to Endurance Exercise During Pregnancy." *American Journal of Obstetrics and Gynecology*, vol. 165 (1991): 1684–89.

Clapp III, J. F. and E. Capeless. "Neonatal Morphometrics After Endurance Exercise During Pregnancy." *American Journal of Obstetrics and Gynecology*, vol. 163 (1990): 1805–11.

———. "The VO2 Max of Recreational Athletes Before and After Pregnancy." *Medicine and Science in Sports and Exercise*, vol. 23 (1991): 1128–33.

Clapp III, J. F., and K. D. Little. "Effect of Recreational Exercise on Pregnancy Weight Gain and Subcutaneous Fat Deposition." *Medicine and Science in Sports and Exercise*, 1995: 170–177.

———. "Effect of Recreational Exercise on Pregnancy Weight Gain and Subcutaneous Fat Deposition." *Medicine and Science in Sports and Exercise*, vol. 27 (Feburary 1995): 170–77.

———. "The Effect of Regular Maternal Exercise on Erythropoietin in Cord Blood and Amniotic Fluid." *American Journal of Obstetrics and Gynecology*, vol. 172 (May 1995): 1445–51.

———. "The Physiological Response of Instructors and Participants to Three Aerobics Regimens." *Medicine and Science in Sports and Exercise*, 1994: 1041–46.

Clapp III, J. F., and K. H. Rizk. "Effect of Recreational Exercise on Midtrimester Placental Growth." *American Journal of Obstetrics and Gynecology*, vol. 167 (1992): 1518–22.

Clapp III, J. F. "Morphometric and Neurodevelopmental Outcome at Age Five Years of the Offspring of Women Who Continued to Exercise Regularly Throughout Pregnancy." *Mosby-Year Book*, 1996: 856–63.

Clapp III, J. F., K. D. Little, and E. Capeless. "Fetal Heart Rate Response to Sustained Recreational Exercise." *American Journal of Obstetrics and Gynecology*, vol. 168 (1993): 198–206.

Clapp, J. F., K. D. Little, S. K. Appleby-Wineberg, and J. A. Widness. "The Effect of Regular Maternal Exercise on Erythopoietin in Cord Blood and Amniotic Fluid." *American Journal of Obstetrics and Gynecology*, vol. 172 (1995): 1445–51.

Clark, A. M., W. Ledger, and C. Galletly. "Weight Loss Results in Significant Improvement in Pregnancy and Ovulation Rates in Anovulatory Obese Women." *Human Reproduction* (England), vol. 10 (October 1995): 2705–12.

"Folic Acid for Prevention of Neural Tube Defects." *The Contraception Report*, vol. 4 (1993): 11–13.

Gibson, R. A., M. Makrides, M. A. Neumann, and K. Simmer, et al. "Ratios of Linoleic Acid to A-Linolenic Acid in Formulas for Term Infants." *Department of Pediatrics and Child Health, Flinders Medical Center* (Adelaide, Australia), 1994: 3472–76.

Hall, B. "Changing Composition of Human Milk and Early Development of and Appetite Control." *The Lancet*, April 5, 1975, 779–81.

Hall, D. C., and D. A. Kaufmann. "Effects of Aerobic and Strength Conditioning on Pregnancy Outcomes." *American Journal of Obstetrics and Gynecology*, vol. 157 (1987): 1199–1203.

James, M. J., R. A. Gibson, and M. A. Neumann, et al. "Inhibition of Human Neutrophil Leukotriene B4 Synthesis in Essential Fatty Acid Deficiency: Role of Leukotriene A Hydrolase." *Lipids*, vol. 299 (1994): 151–55.

Levine, J. J., and N. T. Ilowite. "Sclerodermalike Esophageal Disease in Children Breast-Fed by Mothers with Silicone Breast Implants." *Journal of the American Medical Association*, vol. 271 (1994): 213–16.

Makrides, M., K. Simmer, M. Goggin, R.A. Gibson. "Erythrocyte Docosahexaenoic Acid Correlates with the Visual Response of Healthy, Term Infants." *Pediatric Research*, vol. 33 (1993): 425–27.

Makrides, M., M. Neumann, K. Simmer, et al. "Long Chain Polyunsaturated Fatty Acids: Essential Nutrients in Infancy." *Department of Pediatrics and Child Health and Department of Ophthalmology, Flinders Medical Center* (Adelaide, Australia), 1994.

Makrides, M., M. Neumann, R. W. Byard, et al. "Fatty Acids Composition of Brain, Retina, and Erythrocytes in Breast- and Formula Fed Infants." *American Journal of Clinical Nutrition*, vol. 60 (1994): 189–94.

Mayberry, L. J., M. Smith, and P. Gill. "Effect of Exercise on Uterine Activity in the Patient in Preterm Labor." *Journal of Perinatology*, vol. 12 (1993): 354–58.

McMurray, R.G., V. L. Katz, and W. E. Meyer-Goodwin. "Thermo-Regulation of Pregnant Women During Aerobic Exercise on Land and in the Water." *American Journal of Perinatology*, vol. 10 (1993): 178–82.

O'Neill, M. E., K. A. Cooper, C. M. Mills, et al. "Accuracy of Borg's Ratings of Perceived Exertion in the Prediction of Heart Rates During Pregnancy." *British Journal of Sports Medicine*, vol. 26 (1992): 121–24.

O'Neill, M., K. A. Cooper, S. N. Hunyor, and S. Boyce. "Cardiorespiratory Response to Walking in Trained and Sedentary Pregnant Women." *The Journal of Sports Medicine and Physical Fitness*, vol. 33 (1993): 40–43.

Ohlin, A., and S. Rossner. "Trends in Eating Patterns, Physical Activity, and Sociodemographic Factors in Relation to Postpartum Body Weight Development." *British Journal of Nutrition*, vol. 71 (1994): 457–70.

Orange, L. M. "Guidelines on Exercise in Pregnancy Updated." *OB/GYN News*, May 1, 1994, 3.

Ostgaard, H. C., G. Zetherstrom, E. Roos-Hanson, and B. Svanberg. "Reduction in Back and Posterior Pelvic Pain in Pregnancy." *Spine*, vol. 19 (1994): 894–900.

Ramin, S. M., and F. G. Cunningham. "Obesity in Pregnancy." *Williams Obstetrics Supplement*, vol. 13 (1995): 1–14.

Rauramo, I., S. Ilmonen, and L. Viinikka. "Prostacyclin and Thromboxane in Pregnant and Non-Pregnant Women in Response to Exercise." *American Journal of Obstetrics and Gynecology*, vol. 85 (June 1995): 1027–30.

Schramm, H.F., J. W. Stockbauer, and H. J. Hoffman. "Exercise, Employment, Other Daily Activities, and Adverse Pregnancy Outcomes." *American Journal of Epidemiology*, vol. 143 (February 1996): 211–18.

Spinnewijn, W. E., and F. K. Lotgering. "Fetal Heart Rate and Uterine Conractility During Maternal Exercise at Term." *American Journal of Obstetrics and Gynecology*, vol. 174 (January 1996): 43–48.

Sternfeld, B. "Exercise and Pregnancy Outcome." *IDEA Today*, October 1995: 34–35.

Sternfeld, B., C.P. Duesenberry Jr., and B. Eskenazi. "Exercise During Pregnancy and Pregnancy Outcome." *Medicine and Science in Sports and Exercise*, vol. 27 (May 1995): 634–40.

Turner, T. "Muscle Control." *Nursing Times*, vol. 90 (1994): 64–69.

Zurawski, G. F. and S. M. Shnider. "How Anesthetic Drugs Affect Neonatal Neurobehavior." *Contemporary OB/GYN*, vol. 17 (1981): 179–87.

MAGAZINE, NEWSPAPER, AND NEWSLETTER ARTICLES

Blasutta, M. L. "Behind Closed Doors: Your Sex Clock." *Fitness*, September 1994, 38.

Brundage, M. A. "Good News About Exercise and Pregnancy." *PHFN News*, Winter/Spring 1993, 3–4.

Cardozo, C. "Pregnancy Report: Your Baby, Your Skin." *Self*, January 1995, 43.

Cohen, S. "Toxic Legacy?" *Shape*, May 1996, 50–54.

Cole, M. "Aquatic Exercise: Come On In—The Water's Fine." *NASM News*, vol. 1 (1994): 1–2.

Condon, G. "Expecting & Exercising." *The Hartford Courant*, November 25, 1993, E1, E3.

Depken, D., and C. Zelasko. "Exercise During Pregnancy: Concerns for Fitness Professionals." *Strength and Conditioning*, October 1996, 43–50.

Doheny, K. "Pre-Conception Health Is Vital Too." *Los Angeles Times*, 1995.

Edward-Bullen, S., and C. Graham. "Step Moms." *IDEA Today*, April 1992, 19–20.

Gordon, M. "Baby Fat?" *Harper's Bazaar*, November 1995, 76–80.

Graham, J. "Walking Mother." *Walking*, January 1993, 43–48.

Greider, K. "How Dangerous Is It to Drink When You're Pregnant?" *Self*, June 1994, 106–11.

Johnson, T. and B. Apgar. "Exercise During Pregnancy." *The Female Patient*, vol. 21, August 1996, 61–76.

Knowlton, L. "Body Watch: The ABC's of Good Nutrition." *Los Angeles Times*, August 16, 1994, E3.

Maugh, Thomas H. "Study Finds Slight Vitamin A Excess Hikes Birth Defect Risk." *Los Angeles Times*, October 7, 1995, A1, A19.

McCarthy, L. F. "The New Stretch Mark Removers." *Fitness*, July 1995, 30.

Myers, C. "Labor Intensive." *Mirabella*, November 1994, 98.

———. "New Solutions for Morning Sickness." *Tufts University Diet & Nutrition Letter*, vol. 11 (1994): 6–7.

Occhipinti, Mark. "Does Milk Really Do the Body Good?" *Women's Fitness*, date unknown, 76–78.

Rodriguez, N. "Food or Fiction?" *IDEA Personal Trainer*, September 1995, 26–33.

Schlosberg, S. "Body Language." *Los Angeles Times*, October 3, 1995, E1–5.

Smith, L. "Breastfeeding." *Los Angeles Times*, April 12, 1995, E3.

Sower, E. "Most-Wanted Mineral: Calcium." *Fit Pregnancy*, Winter 1995, 42–43.

Stolberg, S. "Fetus Found Affected by Secondhand Smoke." *Los Angeles Times*, February 23, 1994, A1, A19.

Turner, Lisa. "Bone Up on Osteoporosis." *Let's Live*, March 1999, 42–47.

Williams, S. "Fewer C-Sections, But Still Too Many." *Self*, September 1994, 64.

NEWSLETTERS AND FACT SHEETS

Stress and Pregnancy. March of Dimes, 1989.

Eating for Two: Nutrition During Pregnancy. March of Dimes, 1992.

Exercise and Fitness: A Guide for Women. ACOG, 1992.

Fitness for Two. March of Dimes, 1992.

Folic Acid: Good News for Women and Babies. March of Dimes, 1992.

How Your Baby Grows. March of Dimes, 1992.

Smoking and Pregnancy. American Lung Association, 1992.

INTERVIEWS

Crane, Paul, M.D., Beverly Hills, CA.

Kerin, John F., M.D., Professor, SA. Australia.

Kooperman, Sara, J. D., Sara's City Work Out, Inc., Chicago, IL.

Notes

Notes

Notes

Notes

Notes

Notes